# Uveal Melanoma: A Model for Exploring Fundamental Cancer Biology

# Uveal Melanoma: A Model for Exploring Fundamental Cancer Biology

EDITORS

M.J. Jager

*Department of Ophthalmology*
*Leiden University Medical Center*
*Leiden, The Netherlands*

J.Y. Niederkorn

*Department of Ophthalmology*
*University of Texas Southwestern Medical Center*
*Dallas, Texas, USA*

B.R. Ksander

*Schepens Eye Research Institute*
*Harvard Medical School*
*Boston, USA*

Taylor & Francis
Taylor & Francis Group
LONDON AND NEW YORK

*Library of Congress Cataloging-in-Publication Data*

Uveal melanoma : a model for exploring fundamental cancer biology / editors, M.J. Jager, J.Y. Niederkorn, B.R. Ksander.
p. ; cm.
Includes bibliographical references and index.
ISBN 90-265-1962-1
1. Uvea--Cancer--Molecular aspects 2. Melanoma--Molecular aspects I. Jager, Martine. II. Niederkorn, J.Y. (Jerry Y.), 1946- III. Ksander, Bruce R.
[DNLM: 1. Melanoma. 2. Uveal Neoplasms. WW 240 U 937 2003]
RC280.E9U95 2003
616.99'484--dc22

2003067392

Typesetting: Charon Tec Pvt. Ltd, Chennai, India



Published by: Taylor & Francis The Netherlands, Lisse
http://www.tandf.co.uk/books

ISBN 90 265 1962 1

# Contents

# Preface

Uveal melanoma is the most common intraocular malignancy in adults and presents with an unusual clinical pattern that is completely unique and distinct from cutaneous melanoma. Primary uveal melanomas grow rather slowly and metastases may not appear for many years. However, when metastases finally develop, they occur almost exclusively in the liver, are highly aggressive, and fail to respond to current treatments. Unfortunately, there are few treatment options available to patients with metastatic uveal melanoma. The development of successful therapies will certainly require a better understanding of the pathobiology of this unusual disease.

There are many features of these tumours that make them an ideal target for further research. As compared with other tumours, uveal melanomas are easily visualised and since larger tumours are still being treated by enucleation, primary tumour tissue is available for research studies. The relative homogeneity of these tumours allows different parts to be used for histologic, genetic, and immunological studies. In addition, cell lines have been made from primary tumour specimens and have fostered many *in vitro* and *in vivo* studies.

Excellent patient registries have made it possible to correlate tumour parameters with patients survival. This will certainly aid in making similar correlations between the molecular genetics of these tumours and the clinical pattern of tumour progression. Due to the presence of good registries and the exchange of cell lines, the use of uveal melanoma as a model for basic cancer research has greatly increased over the last ten years. Following a successful basic research meeting at the Leiden University Medical Center in Leiden, the Netherlands, in 2001, a large number of scientists with an interest in uveal melanoma collaborated to synthesize their perceptions regarding the genetics, immunology and angiogenesis of uveal melanoma. As editors, we think this collection of manuscripts is a good representation of the current research in this field. As these research projects mature, we predict it will spawn novel therapies that will benefit not only uveal melanoma patients, but patients with other types of tumours as well.

*Martine J. Jager*
*Jerry Y. Niederkorn*
*Bruce R. Ksander*

# Authors' Addresses

G. Anastassiou, MD—Augenklinik, Universitätsklinikum Essen 45122, Hufeland strasse 55, Essen 0-45122, Germany. E-mail: anastassiou@uni-essen.de

D.-U. Bartsch, PhD—University of California San Diego, La Jolla, CA, USA.

M.A. Blasi, MD—Department of Ophthalmology, Universita degli Studi di L'Aquila, Via Vetoio Pal 11/a, L'Aquila 67100, Italia.

S.R. Boyd, MD—St. Michael's Hospital, University of Toronto, Toronto, Ontario, Canada. E-mail: boyds@smh.toronto.on.ca

R. Clarijs, MD—Department of Pathology, University Medical Center St Radboud, PO Box 9101, 6500 HB Nijmegen, The Netherlands. E-mail: r.clarijs@pathol.umcn.nl.

I.A. Cree, MD—Department of Pathology, Institute of Ophthalmology, Bath Street, London EC1V 9EL, England and Translational Oncology Research Centre, Department of Histopathology, Michael Darmady Laboratory, Queen Alexandra Hospital, Cosham, Portsmouth, United Kingdom. E-mail: ian.cree@port.ac.uk

M. Deckers, PhD—Department of Endocrinology and Metabolic Diseases, Leiden University Medical Center, PO Box 9600, 2300 RC Leiden, The Netherlands.

F. Di Nicolantonio, BSc—Translational Oncology Research Centre, Department of Histopathology, Michael Darmady Laboratory, Queen Alexandra Hospital, Cosham, Portsmouth, United Kingdom.

A.E. Director-Myska, PhD—Department of Cellular Pathology and Genetics, Armed Forces Institute of Pathology, 1413 Research Bvd., Bldg. 102, Rockville, MD 20850, USA.

R. Folberg, MD—Department of Pathology, University of Illinois at Chicago, Chicago, IL 60612–7335, USA. E-mail: rfolberg@uic.edu

W.R. Freeman, MD—University of California San Diego, La Jolla, CA, USA.

P. Grammatico, PhD—Department of Medical Genetics, University 'La Sapienza', Rome, Italy.

N.A. Gruis, PhD—Departments of Dermatology and Human and Clinical Genetics, Leiden University Medical Center, Wassenaarseweg 72, 2333 AL Leiden, The Netherlands. E-mail: n.a.gruis@lumc.nl

J.W. Harbour, MD—Ocular Oncology Service, Washington University School of Medicine, Box 8096, 660 South Euclid Avenue, St Louis, MO 63110, USA. E-mail: harbour@vision.wustl.edu

H.M.H. Hurks, PhD—Department of Ophthalmology, Leiden University Medical Center, PO Box 9600, 2300 RC Leiden, The Netherlands.

M.J. Jager, MD, PhD—Department of Ophthalmology, Leiden University Medical Center, PO Box 9600, 2300 RC Leiden, The Netherlands. E-mail: m.j.jager@lumc.nl

A. Kampik, MD, PhD—Augenklinik der Universität, München, Germany.

T. Kivelä, MD, PhD—Ocular Oncology Service and Ophthalmic Pathology Laboratory, Department of Ophthalmology, Helsinki Univeristy Central Hospital, Haartmaninkatu 4 C, PL 220, FIN-00029 HUS, Helsinki, Finland. E-mail: tero.kivela@helsinki.fi

C. Löwik, PhD—Department of Endocrinology and Metabolic Diseases, Leiden University Medical Center, PO Box 9600, 2300 RC Leiden, The Netherlands.

T. Mäkitie, MD, PhD—Ocular Oncology Service and Ophthalmic Pathology Laboratory, Department of Ophthalmology, Helsinki University Central Hospital, Helsinki, Finland.

A.J. Maniotis, PhD—Department of Pathology, University of Illinois at Chicago, Chicago, IL, USA.

I.W. McLean, MD—Department of Ophthalmic Pathology, Armed Forces Institute of Pathology, 6825 14th Street NW, Washington, DC 20306-6000, USA. E-mail: mclean@afip.osd.mil

J.A.W. Metzelaar-Blok, MD—Department of Ophthalmology, Leiden University Medical Center, Leiden, The Netherlands.

A.J. Mueller, MD—Augenklinik der Universität, Mathildenstr. 8, 80335 München, Germany. E-mail: amueller@ak-i.med.uni-muenchen.de

N. Naus, MD, PhD—Department of Ophthalmology, University Hospital Rotterdam, The Netherlands.

M.H. Neale, PhD—Translational Oncology Research Centre, Department of Histopathology, Michael Darmady Laboratory, Queen Alexandra Hospital, Cosham, Portsmouth, United Kingdom.

J.Y. Niederkorn, PhD—University of Texas Southwestern Medical Center, 5323 Harry Hines Blvd., Dallas, TX 75235-9057, USA. E-mail: Jerry.Niederkorn@UTSouthwestern.edu

R. Parys-Van Ginderdeuren, MD—Dienst Oogziekten, Kapucijnenvoer 35, UZ Leuven, B3000 Leuven, Belgium. E-mail: Rita.Vanginderdeuren@uz.kuleuven.ac.be

J. Pe'er, MD—Department of Ophthalmology, Hadassah University Hospital, PO Box 12000, Jerusalem 91120, Israel. E-mail: peer@md.huji.ac.il

G. van der Pluijm, PhD—Department of Endocrinology and Metabolic Diseases C4-R, Leiden University Medical Center, Albinusdreef 2, 2333 ZA Leiden, PO Box 9600, 2300 RC Leiden, The Netherlands. E-mail: G.van_der_Pluijm@lumc.nl

D.J. Ruiter, MD, PhD—Department of Pathology, University Medical Center St Radboud, PO Box 9101, 6500 HB Nijmegen, The Netherlands. E-mail: d.ruiter@pathol.umcn.nl

U. Schaller, MD—Augenklinik der Universität, München, Germany.

A.D. Singh, MD—Department of Ophthalmic Oncology, Cole Eye Institute, Cleveland Clinic, Cleveland, Ohio, USA. E-mail: arunsingh@eyetumors.com

K. Sisley, PhD—Academic Unit of Ophthalmology and Orthoptics, University of Sheffield, United Kingdom. E-mail:k.sisley@sheffield.ac.uk

P. Toivonen, MD—Ocular Oncology Service and Ophthalmic Pathology Laboratory, Department of Ophthalmology, Helsinki University Central Hospital, Helsinki, Finland.

R.M.W. de Waal, PhD—Department of Pathology, University Medical Center St Radboud, PO Box 9101, 6500 HB Nijmegen, The Netherlands. E-mail: R.dewaal @pathol.umcn.nl

J.S. White—Department of Cellular Pathology and Genetics, Department of Cellular Pathology and Genetics, Armed Forces Institute of Pathology, 1413 Research Bvd., Bldg. 102, Rockville, MD 20850, USA.

TEEMU MÄKITIE, MARTINE J. JAGER AND TERO KIVELÄ

# 1. Prognostic Indicators in Choroidal and Ciliary Body Melanoma

## INTRODUCTION

Cancer and blindness are among the most feared diseases,[1,2] and these two features are combined in intraocular tumours. The most common intraocular tumours are benign melanocytic uveal nevi and metastases derived from malignancies elsewhere in the body.[3] Malignant melanoma of the uvea is, however, the most common primary malignant intraocular tumour in adults, and often deadly.[4,5]

Uveal melanoma is related to cutaneous melanoma, but differs from it in many aspects, although both originate from melanocytes.[3,6] Unlike the situation in cutaneous melanoma, UV light and a hereditary predisposition have little or no effect on the development of a uveal melanoma.[4,7,8] While cutaneous and conjunctival melanoma initially spread locally via the lymphatic vessels, uveal melanoma disseminates hematogeneously, because the inside of the eye lacks lymphatics. Because of this, uveal melanoma has a great propensity to develop distant metastases, particularly in the liver, whereas cutaneous and conjunctival melanoma tend to disseminate in regional lymph nodes.[9–12]

Recent studies have revealed substantial cytogenetic, immunologic and molecular differences between these tumours, which probably explain their divergent biological behaviour.[13–16] As regards uveal melanoma, histopathologic examinations are performed according to internationally set standards, and many countries provide excellent survival data on the patients (Fig. 1.1). Because of this, many basic studies regarding the pathobiology take place, and much information is available on the relevance to patient survival of biological pathways. All of this makes this tumour an excellent model for the study of cancer biology in general.

## HISTOLOGY

Neuroectodermally derived melanocytes of the choroid, ciliary body and iris give rise to uveal melanoma.[3] The highly vascularised choroid is the largest part of the uveal tract and the most common site for intraocular melanoma. Of uveal melanomas, 80% grow in the choroid, 15% involve both the choroid and the ciliary body, and 5% are confined to the ciliary body, iris, or both.[17]

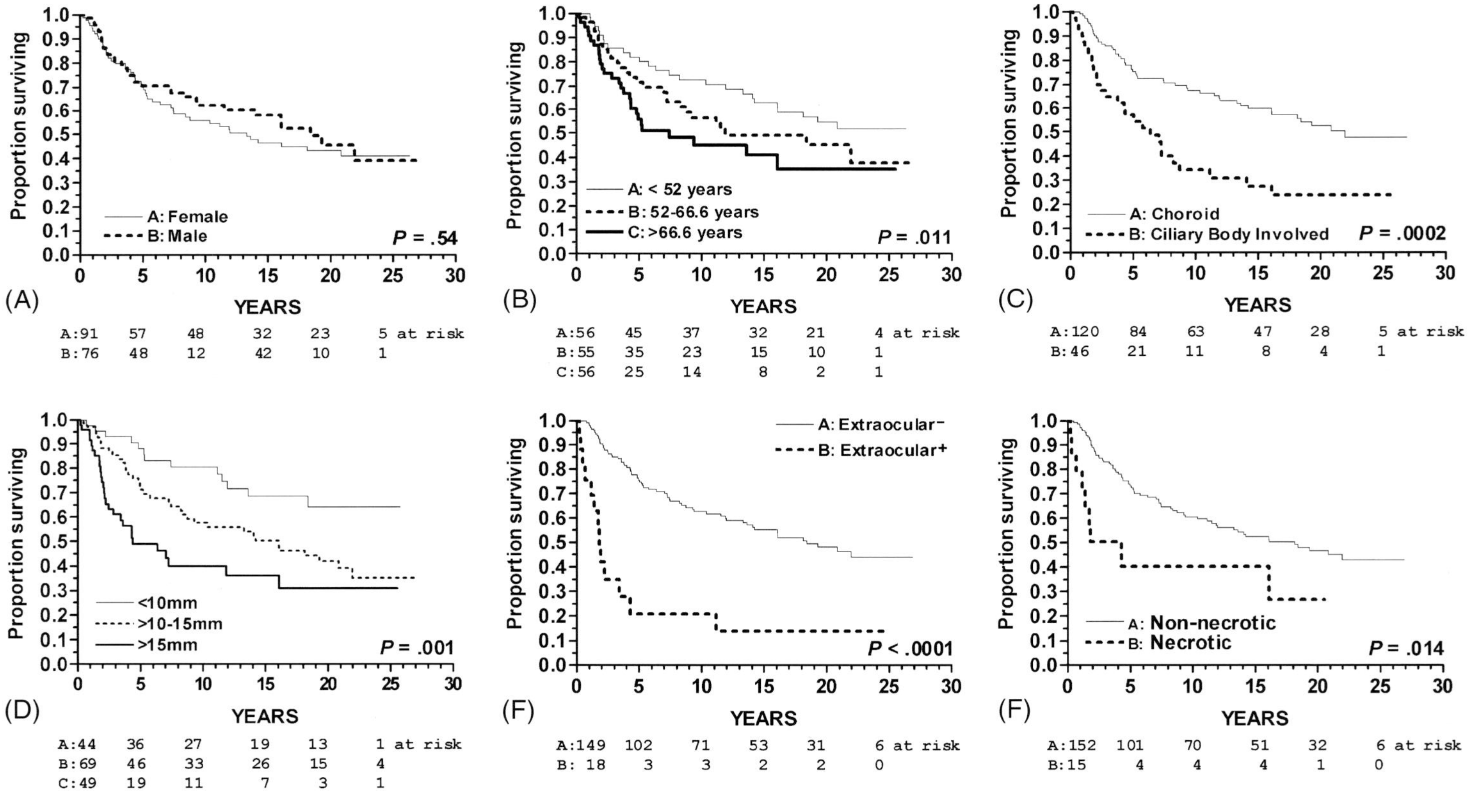


Fig. 1.1 Melanoma-specific survival in an unselected cohort of 167 consecutive uveal melanoma patients (Kaplan–Meier plots) according to (A) gender, (B) age, (C) ciliary body involvement, (D) largest basal tumour diameter, (E) extraocular extension, (F) presence of necrosis.

Uveal melanoma can break out into two different directions: towards the centre of the eye, i.e. through the overlying Bruch's membrane and outwards, through the underlying sclera. Having broken through Bruch's membrane, choroidal melanoma has access to the subretinal space, immediately achieving a shape of a 'collar button' or 'mushroom', which is highly characteristic, even pathognomonic, of choroidal melanoma (Fig. 1.2). It may then also erode the overlying retina and extend into the vitreous cavity. The outermost layer of the eye, the sclera, can resist local invasion into the orbit for years, except close to the optic disc and around the corneoscleral limbus. Often, growth occurs along the intrascleral vessels.

Diffuse uveal melanoma has an uncommon growth pattern, representing approximately 5% of posterior uveal melanomas. It is named for its flat shape and small height and it may affect large areas of the choroid.[18] Variants of diffuse uveal melanoma are a ring melanoma that grows circumferentially in the ciliary body and a retinoinvasive melanoma that invades within the retina and extends into the optic nerve.[19,20]

The earliest prognostic factors identified, in addition to anatomical extent of the tumour, was its cell type. Initially divided into several categories by Callender (1931), two main types are currently recognised (Fig. 1.3). The spindle cell is thought to be slowly growing and to be associated with a more favourable prognosis, whereas the more noncoherently growing epithelioid cell is associated with brisk growth and a worse prognosis. In many uveal melanomas, both cell types occur in varying proportions. Such melanomas are described as having a 'mixed' cell type.

Rarely, cutaneous melanoma can metastasize intraocularly.[21] These metastatic melanomas often grow in the retina and vitreous body, both of which are rarely invaded by uveal melanomas.

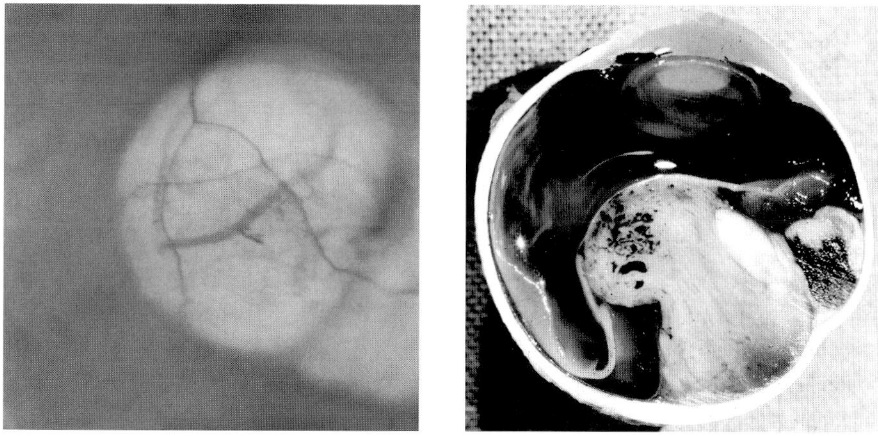

(A) (B)

Fig. 1.2 (A) Clinical picture of a mushroom-shaped intraocular uveal melanoma. (B) Macroscopic histological picture. 'Collar button' or 'mushroom' shape of an intraocular uveal melanoma. The cornea and lens are seen in the top area of the figure.

(A)

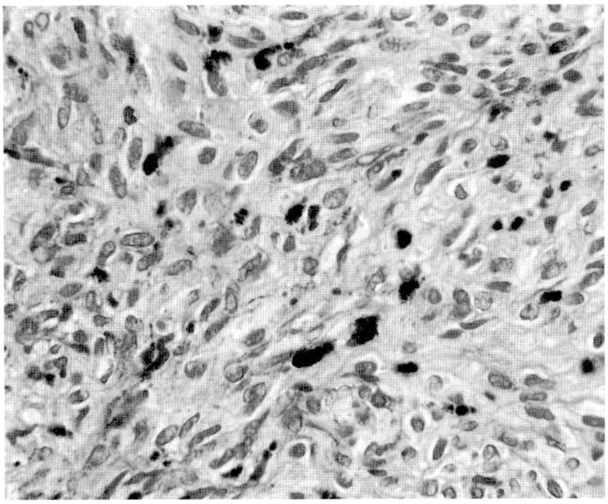

(B)

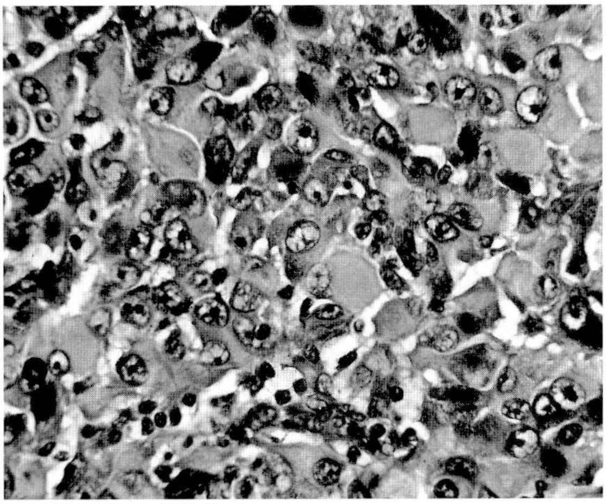

Fig. 1.3 (A) Example of uveal melanoma spindle cells. (B) Example of uveal melanoma epithelioid cells.

## MALIGNANT UVEAL MELANOMA: EPIDEMIOLOGY

The uvea consists of three elements: the iris, the ciliary body and the choroid, all three of which contain melanocytes. Melanomas that arise from the iris differ markedly from those of the choroid and ciliary body. Due to their anatomic location that favours early diagnosis and, perhaps, their relatively benign cellular composition, death from iris melanoma is markedly less common than death from choroidal and ciliary body melanoma.[3,22–24] Consequently, iris melanomas are not included in this book, and uveal melanoma refers to choroidal and ciliary body melanomas.

Uveal melanoma is the most common malignant primary tumour of the eye in Caucasian adults.[4] The annual incidence of malignant uveal melanoma ranges from six to ten new cases per million Caucasians, being particularly common in

Scandinavia[25] where people are fair-haired and blue-eyed. Its incidence is 15 to 50 times lower in Africans and Orientals. Retinoblastoma exceeds uveal melanoma in frequency among non-Caucasians.[26] In contrast to the strikingly increasing incidence of cutaneous melanoma, the frequency of uveal melanoma has not changed during the last two decades according to several studies.[4,27] In systematic reviews of databases in the United States, an incidence of 4.3 per million was found,[27] with no changes between 1973 and 1997. In Sweden, the age-standardised incidence of uveal melanoma even declined significantly in the male population, from 11.7 cases/million to 8.4 cases/million from 1960 to 1998.[25]

The incidence of uveal melanoma depends on age: uveal melanoma is very rare in childhood, but its incidence increases in older age groups achieving a peak in late middle age (50–60 year old). Persons with lightly pigmented skin, hair, and irises, are at a slightly increased risk of developing uveal melanoma.[28–30] In a study in the USA, 98% of cases occurred in Caucasians.[25] A slight predominance of male gender is evident from large series of uveal melanoma, but the reason for the male predominance is unknown.[4,27]

## AETIOLOGY AND PREDISPOSITION

In addition to age and race, one of the best-documented predisposing lesions is the relatively common choroidal nevus; 3–20% of the population has at least one choroidal nevus.[3] However, only a small minority of nevi (1 in 15000 per year) transforms to malignant melanoma. In contrast to cutaneous melanoma, exposure to ultraviolet light is not related to uveal melanoma, but contradictory reports also exist.[4,29] Conditions with congenitally increased numbers of melanocytes, known as congenital ocular melanocytosis and congenital oculodermal melanocytosis (nevus of Ota) are more common among patients with uveal melanoma than in the general population.[4] The lifetime risk for developing uveal melanoma is 1:400 for a patient with ocular melanocytosis.[31] The dysplastic nevus syndrome or FAMMM syndrome is also associated with an increased risk of uveal melanoma.[32,33] Hormonal factors, like childbearing history and hormonal therapy have been studied as etiological factors, but no convincing relationship has been established.[34,35]

Even though knowledge of cancer genetics has markedly increased, the specific genes involved in the development and progression of uveal melanoma are not yet known. Some frequent chromosomal changes, such as monosomy of chromosome 3 and structural alterations of chromosomes 6 and 8 are distinctly connected with uveal melanoma.[36–39] Many research groups are focussing on the genes that are missing in case of monosomy 3, as such genes might be cancer suppressor genes. While two areas with potential cancer suppressor genes have been identified, no genes have as yet been identified.[40,41] In spite of occasional uveal melanomas in first-degree relatives, no convincing evidence for familial inheritance exists.[7,42]

## DIAGNOSIS

Most patients with uveal melanoma have symptoms of blurred vision, visual field loss, photopsia, floaters, and rarely, pain before diagnosis; 10–30% of uveal melanomas are diagnosed during routine ophthalmologic examination in the absence of any preceding symptoms.[43–45] Indirect ophthalmoscopy is widely used in making the diagnosis of choroidal melanoma.[19] Of medium-sized and large uveal melanoma, up to 99% are diagnosed correctly by clinical methods.[46] It may, however, be difficult to differentiate between a small melanoma and a nevus.[19,47] Documented growth is often needed to confirm the diagnosis of small melanomas, but also nevi may slowly grow during follow-up. Exudative retinal detachment is frequently associated with choroidal melanoma, which may help in diagnosis of a small melanoma, but it may also obscure an underlying larger tumour and delay diagnosis.[48]

Transillumination of the eye helps to determine the anterior margins of the tumour in lightly pigmented individuals. Development of B-scan ultrasonography has greatly helped ophthalmologists in diagnosing choroidal tumours. High frequency ultrasonography also helps in the diagnosis of ciliary body tumours.[49] Computed tomography and magnetic resonance imaging are further options.[47] The cellular composition of the intraocular tumour can be assessed by fine-needle aspiration biopsy performed either via a transscleral or a transvitreal route, but this method has so far been limited to patients whose clinical diagnosis is in doubt and to experimental applications.[50–52] 'Double circulation' consisting of choroidal and tumour vessels that are leaky in late phases of a fluorescein fundus angiography is characteristic of uveal melanoma, but angiography does not reliably differentiate a malignant lesion from a benign one.

The diagnosis of metastatic disease has been based on liver function tests and chest x-ray examination.[53–55] However, recently, abdominal ultrasonography and computed tomography were found to be more sensitive as methods for screening for metastases of uveal melanoma.[11,56–58] Liver function tests, nevertheless, provide confirmatory evidence.[11]

## LOCAL TREATMENT

Enucleation was the standard and only treatment of uveal melanoma for decades until eye-conserving methods, developed in the 1950s, came to clinical use in the late 1960s.[59] Enucleation is still an effective and acceptable treatment modality, especially for large melanomas and under circumstances in which the availability of conservative methods is limited, like in developing countries.[19] Enucleation results in excellent local tumour control, approaching 100% success if no extraocular extension is present at the time of surgery.[60]

The American Collaborative Ocular Melanoma Study (COMS) was initiated in 1986 to resolve whether or not any difference in survival exists between enucleation and radiotherapy.[61] A large number of patients with medium-sized melanoma was randomised either to enucleation or to iodine plaque radiotherapy, and preliminary results indicate no difference in survival.[62] Retrospective studies on effectiveness and safety of radiotherapy as compared to enucleation likewise have shown that a significant difference between these two treatment methods is unlikely, which has led to a decline in enucleation rates in European and American ophthalmic centres.[19,63–69]

Radiotherapy given either with episcleral radioactive plaques (cobalt-60, iodine-125, ruthenium-106, iridium-192 or palladium-103) or with accelerated protons or helium ions often saves some functional vision in the eye with uveal melanoma particularly when the tumour is small.[70–73] Uveal melanoma is, however, resistant to higher doses of irradiation than the retina and the optic nerve, which increases the risk for visual impairment due to radiation retinopathy and optic neuropathy.[71,72,74] Local recurrences of uveal melanoma after radiotherapy range from 5% to 10% within five years and local recurrences may indicate even a five-fold risk for metastatic disease.[75,76] Another possibility is that tumours which recur are initially more malignant. Low-dose (4–8 Gy) irradiation before enucleation had no effect on survival.[77,78]

Thermotherapy given through a dilated pupil (transpupillary thermotherapy) has been shown to be an effective treatment for selected small choroidal melanomas and in combination with brachytherapy also for larger ones.[79–82] Tumour resection under arterial hypotension in otherwise healthy patients is another type of eye-conserving treatment of uveal melanoma.[83–87] More recently, studies on gamma-knife techniques and photodynamic therapy have been published.[88,89] Due to small sample sizes and short follow-up times their eventual place in clinical ophthalmic oncology is not yet established.

## TREATMENT OF METASTATIC DISEASE

Even though new local treatment options have shown their safety as compared to traditional enucleation, no significant improvement has taken place with regard to survival of patients with uveal melanoma.[64,65,90] Obviously, in most cases, intraocular melanoma has already disseminated at the time when treatment of the primary tumour takes place.[91] The choice between radical and conservative therapy does not seem to influence survival.

Manifest disseminated uveal melanoma is still an unbeatable challenge for oncologists; the median survival after metastatic disease is only from a few months to one year.[53,92,93] Recently, a clinical staging system was proposed to enable the clinician to better estimate the survival time after diagnosis of metastases.[58]

Chemotherapy and chemoembolization to the hepatic artery with or without interferon have lengthened the mean survival time to 12 months and up to 20% of metastases have regressed at least partially during treatment, but the disease later always has progressed and killed the patient.[93] Only a few patients treated with surgery for a solitary, slowly growing metastasis, have survived long term.[94–96]

A combination of BOLD therapy and recombinant interferon alpha-2b did not achieve any objective responses in a multicentre setting, but the survival time was comparable to that achieved with intra-arterial therapies.[97] Liver perfusion with fotemustine for liver metastases only is another option that is investigated at the moment, together with interferon alpha and interleukin 2.[57,95,98] One of the reasons that the different chemotherapy regimens do not have a significant influence on survival may be that uveal melanoma cells carry many different multidrug resistance molecules, which are able to remove the drugs from tumour cells.[99] In a recent study, the feasibility of a combination of treosulfan and gemcitabine as treatment for uveal melanoma metastases was determined.[100] The basis of this approach is discussed by Cree later in this book, and multicentre studies seem to be warranted.

## NATURAL COURSE OF THE DISEASE

Because uveal melanomas are treated promptly after diagnosis, its natural course is a matter of dispute. In several series of treated patients, the 10-year cumulative melanoma-specific survival has been close to 60%, and it has thereafter decreased by about 1% per year.[101–103] but these estimates are biased high because of competing-risk events. Analyses which take competing risks into account estimate that mortality will eventually be around 50%.[104] Deaths from metastatic uveal melanoma have been reported even decades after enucleation.[104–106]

Uveal melanoma has a remarkably strong tendency to produce liver metastases.[9,11,107] In over 50% of the patients, the liver is involved as the only metastatic site, and only 5% of patients who have disseminated uveal melanoma do not eventually have liver metastases. Other preferred sites for metastases are skin, lung, and bone. The median expected lifetime after diagnosing metastatic uveal melanoma is in most cases less than a year, but single patients with few, slowly growing metastases are known to have survived even for three to four years.[92,96]

As documented in many series, the melanoma-specific mortality is highest within the first two to three years after enucleation, which led Lorenz E. Zimmerman to suggest that removal of the tumour-containing eye might cause tumour dissemination and increase melanoma-specific mortality.[108,109] The natural history of uveal melanoma is traditionally inferred based on tumour size and how long it takes for a tumour to grow from a medium-sized to a large one, because large series of untreated patients have not been published.[109,110] The average survival time of patients who have refused all treatments for intraocular melanoma was five years and some patients have survived even 15 years.[111] McLean and collaborators have estimated that it takes seven years of a small tumour (LBD <10 mm) to grow into a large one (LBD >15 mm). Manschot,[112–114] on the other hand, has strongly supported radical therapy (enucleation) even for small tumours (<7 mm), because he believes that they might then be treated before dissemination has occurred.

Empirical data based on tumour doubling times of metastases suggest that clinically undetectable micrometastases probably initiate on average two to three years prior to the detection of the primary tumour.[91] To improve survival of patients with uveal melanoma, it seems prudent to minimise delays in the treatment of the primary tumour as much as possible and to screen high-risk patients for metastatic disease, hoping that one day an effective adjuvant therapy may become available, which would be more efficient than the current chemotherapy regimens for distant metastasis.[11,43,91] The course of the disease is, however, also modulated by tumour and host characteristics. A specific patient with a large tumour may survive much longer than another patient with a small tumour, and this applies to other prognostic factors as well.

## PROGNOSTIC INDICATORS OF UVEAL MELANOMA
## PATIENT-RELATED FACTORS

### AGE AND SEX

Increasing age is associated with poorer melanoma-specific survival, which may result from a decreased effectiveness of the immune system associated with old age.[115,116] The short term prognosis (five-year) of young patients (<20 years) is better than that of adults, but the long-term prognosis (15-year) is similar.[117,118] Whether women have a better survival than men, as some studies suggest,[119,120] has remained controversial since other studies have not found such a relationship.[121–124]

## REPRODUCTIVE FACTORS

Some uveal melanomas have progressed during pregnancy, possibly coincidentally, because the childbearing history and the use of oral contraceptives do not increase the risk for metastatic disease.[34,35,125] In fact, a recent paper suggested that childbearing may even improve the prognosis of uveal melanoma patients.[120] The protective influence of parity was highest in the period directly following treatment, and it increased with the number of live births. In a Cox regression analysis, however, men and nulliparous women had only a borderline higher risk for metastatic death than women who had given birth.

## IMMUNOLOGICAL FACTORS

The onset of clinical metastatic disease many years after enucleation and the rare spontaneous regression of uveal melanoma has been cited as indirect evidence for a role of the immune system in progression of this tumour.[126] Immune responses may play a role here. Such responses could be mediated by tumour-infiltrating and circulating immune cells. Of lymphocytes infiltrating uveal melanoma, the majority are CD4+ and CD8+ T-cells that may modulate the immune response and may have direct cytotoxic effects on tumour cells.[127–129] A dense infiltration of lymphocytes has been associated with shorter survival time by univariate analysis.[119,130]

Tumour-infiltrating macrophages have not been studied to the same extent as lymphocytes, but some reports have mentioned sparse to marked infiltration by CD68+ macrophages in uveal melanoma.[129,131–133] The possible functions of macrophages in malignant tumours are thought to be variable and even contradictory: on the one hand they might be directed against the tumour, on the other hand they might promote tumour growth.[134,135] Other leukocytes, such as granulocytes, B-lymphocytes, and natural killer cells seem to be present to a smaller extent than T-lymphocytes and macrophages in these tumours and their role is even more uncertain.[127] An increased density of T cells and macrophages has been found to be associated with an increased expression of HLA Class I antigens.[127]

Human leukocyte-associated (HLA) antigens are essential for immune cells to recognise neoplastic cells.[136] Regarding the HLA Class I antigens, low expression of HLA-A and HLA-B antigens in uveal melanoma has been associated with an improved survival.[13,137,138] This inverse correlation was explained by dual functions of HLA antigens. Whereas lymphocytes need HLA antigens to recognise tumour cells, the presence of HLA Class I antigens may block natural killer cell mediated lysis of tumour cells.[139] A high expression of HLA-B was associated with the epithelioid cell type and inversely correlated with expression of the *c-Myc* oncogene.[140] The type of HLA antigen was not related to the development of a uveal melanoma, but it might play a role in the development of metastases.[141]

## MISCELLANEOUS FACTORS

The presence of cutaneous dysplastic nevi not only increases the risk for developing primary uveal melanoma, but it may also be associated with the epithelioid cell type, a traditionally poor prognostic indicator of uveal melanoma.[33,142] Patients with cutaneous melanoma did not show an increased incidence of uveal melanoma, although patients with a uveal melanoma clearly were at higher risk to develop cutaneous melanoma.[42,143] In a large series of proton beam irradiated uveal melanomas, patients with blue and grey irises were at 1.9 times higher risk of dying of metastatic uveal melanoma than patients with brown irises.[30] No relationship was observed between smoking and risk of metastatic death.[144]

# TUMOUR-RELATED FACTORS

## TUMOUR LOCATION

Anterior tumour location within the ciliary body or with ciliary body involvement has often been linked to an increased melanoma-specific mortality.[101,102,119,145,146] According to Li et al.[146] a melanoma of presumed ciliary body origin (>50% tumour base anterior to the ora serrata) had a 1.6 to 2.3 times higher chance to metastasise than a choroidal tumour (<50% tumour base anterior to the ora serrata). Choroidal tumours extending into the ciliary body tend to be larger than posteriorly located ones, but tumour size alone does not explain such an association. Ciliary body involvement has been an independent predictor of survival in many multivariate models in addition to LBD.[102,115,147,148] A high frequency of microvascular networks and chromosomal changes, especially monosomy of chromosome 3 and gain of chromosome 8, have in some data sets been put forward as factors underlying the more aggressive nature of ciliary body melanomas.[36,147,149] It is clear from iris melanoma that the determining factor must be different from location. Iris melanomas metastasise very rarely and the reported 10-year mortality is only 5%.[23]

When a ciliochoroidal or iris melanoma that invades the ciliary body is diagnosed, the original uveal compartment where the tumour initiated may be difficult to recognise. Such tumours are therefore often acknowledged as being of choroidal-ciliary body origin. Of posterior tumours, those located adjacent to the optic disc may have a worse prognosis because of more frequent extrascleral extension.

## EXTRAOCULAR EXTENSION

The fibrous outer layer of the eye, the sclera, resists the growth of intraocular melanoma effectively, but sometimes intraocular melanoma invades the orbit along emissaries such as posterior ciliary arteries and vortex veins.[3] Juxtapapillary choroidal melanoma may invade the orbit adjacent to the optic disc and, rarely, through the optic nerve.[20] Choroidal and ciliary body melanomas that infiltrate the chamber angle may grow into subconjunctival tissue to cause local lymph node metastases, which otherwise do not develop from uveal melanoma.[150] Intraocular melanoma disseminates mostly hematogenously.

Extraocular extension is an unfavourable prognostic sign. Conservative treatment is traditionally not recommended and radical surgery combined with irradiation therapy is suggested instead.[151,152] However, if extraocular extension is small (<3 mm), plaque or charged particle irradiation may still be effective.[153]

## TUMOUR SIZE

One of the most consistent prognostic indicators for high risk of metastasis from uveal melanoma is tumour size.[101,103,119,121,122,145,154,155] Of the various ways to classify tumour size (Table 1.1), largest basal tumour diameter (LBD) and tumour height are used most commonly. With regard to LBD, melanomas are now divided into small (<10 mm), medium-sized (10–16 mm), and large (>16 mm) tumours (Table 1.1). Evaluation of tumour volume and recently presented computer-assisted quantification of cross-sectional tumour area are other ways of measuring tumour size.[156,157] So far, results have been most consistent for LBD and, from a clinical point of view, it can be conveniently measured by indirect ophthalmoscopy and B-scan ultrasonography. LBD is also related to the success of local resection. Tumour height largely determines the dose in plaque brachytherapy.

Formal classifications, such as the TNM system and COMS classifications also take into account tumour height (Table 1.1). The 10-year melanoma-specific mortality is as high as 60% among patients with large tumours, whereas it is only 10–15% in cases with a small melanoma.[62,78,101,102,121,158]

## CELL TYPE

G.R. Callender comprehensively described the cytological features of uveal melanoma cells in 1931. The classification that still carries his name is based on the shape

Table 1.1 Classifications of tumour size in choroidal and ciliary body melanomas.

| | Category | | |
|---|---|---|---|
| Classification | Small | Medium-sized | Large |
| TNM (5th ed.)[159] | LBD ≤ 10 mm and Hght ≤ 3 mm (T1) | LBD > 10–15 mm and Hght > 3–10 mm (T2) | LBD > 15 mm and Hght > 5 mm (T3) |
| TNM (6th ed.)[160] | LBD ≤ 10 mm and Hght ≤ 2½ mm (T1) | LBD > 10–16 mm and Hght > 2½–10 mm (T2) | LBD > 16 mm and Hght > 10 mm (T3) |
| Collaborative ocular melanoma study | LBD ≤ 16 mm and Height < 2.5 mm | LBD ≤ 16 mm and Height ≥ 2.5 but ≤ 10 mm | LBD > 16 mm and Height ≥ 2 mm or Height > 10 mm |
| Common classification based on LBD[119] | LBD ≤ 10 mm | LBD > 10–15 mm | LBD > 15 mm |
| Tumour cross-sectional area[157] | <16 mm | ≥16 mm but <61.4 mm | ≥61.4 mm |

and other cytological features of melanoma cells, but it has since then been modified by ophthalmic pathologists of the Armed Forces Institute of Pathology (AFIP). Callender defined two main cell types: the spindle and the epithelioid cell.[3] Spindle cells typically grow in a compact cohesive fashion and they were originally subdivided into spindle-A and spindle-B type.[3] Patients with spindle-A type melanoma have a significantly more favourable clinical course than patients with spindle-B type melanoma.[155] In the modified AFIP classification, most spindle-A cell type tumours were reclassified as nevi rather than as a malignant melanoma, and the diagnosis of spindle cell type melanoma usually required spindle-B cells.[161] The malignant potential of the less cohesive epithelioid cells has been established in many independent studies.[102,119,145,154,156,162,163]

In addition, the original Callender classification included mixed, fascicular, and necrotic types of uveal melanoma cells. The presence of the necrotic cell type indicated a higher mortality than the presence of non-necrotic cell types only, but the association was non-significant after controlling for tumour size.[164] A matter of controversy has been which amount of epithelioid cells is to be considered a sign of poor prognosis.[165–167] In recent studies, the mixed and epithelioid cell types have often been combined in the same category, and the presence of even a single well-defined epithelioid cell in a section may lead to classifying the tumour as nonspindle instead of spindle.[119,168,169] This two-category classification is also convenient for use in multivariate analysis.[119]

Interestingly, using modern techniques such as the microarray test, tumours with a similar cell type express similar sets of specific mRNAs, indicating that the cell types identify specific biological types of tumours[41] (N.A. Gruis, J.W. Harbour, personal communications). This means that there is an association between cell type and the expression patterns of certain protein families and, once we can better identify the relevant proteins, we may develop a better insight into the molecular basis of the association between cell type and the development of metastases.

## TUMOUR PIGMENTATION

Heavy tumour pigmentation has been associated with decreased survival in several univariate studies, but different classifications of the amount of pigmentation make comparisons between cohorts difficult.[101,132,155,156] The relationship between heavy tumour pigmentation and two other prognostic indicators, i.e. epithelioid cell type and large LBD, suggests that prognostic significance of tumour pigmentation may be secondary to other tumour characteristics.[131] Cutaneous melanomas with a high melanin content are more resistant to irradiation than lightly pigmented ones, but the significance of this observation with regard to uveal melanoma is unknown.[170]

## MICROVASCULAR PATTERNS

Studies on tumour blood vessel morphology in uveal melanoma were introduced by Robert Folberg and colleagues in 1992 when they presented nine morphological types of microvessel architecture which they designated microvascular patterns.[171]

The patterns were identified by fluorescein-conjugated *Ulex europaeus* I using laser scanning confocal microscopy and by periodic acid-Schiff stain (PAS) that stains basement membranes and collagen.[172] Specific patterns were shown to have an association with survival (see Chapters 11, 14). In a matched case-control study of 40 patients, patients who survived over 15 years had more frequently the normal and silent pattern than patients who died of metastatic uveal melanoma. Furthermore, melanocytic nevi did not contain any parallel with cross-linking, arcs, arcs with branching, loops, or networks, consistent with the finding that these latter patterns would be associated with melanoma deaths.[173]

In uveal, cutaneous and conjunctival melanoma, parallel vessels with cross-linking or networks gained independent prognostic significance in multivariate analysis, adjusting for the important conventional prognostic indicator, tumour thickness.[119,174,175] All nine microvascular patterns were found in these tumours proving that their formation is not restricted to intraocular melanoma. Many different hypotheses regarding the biological nature of the patterns have been put forward, and will be discussed in further chapters.

Preliminary investigations have revealed differences in gene expression between melanomas that form microvascular networks and melanomas that are incapable of doing that.[15] For example, a specific profile of protein tyrosine kinases was associated with the ability of uveal melanoma cells for vasculogenic mimicry.[176]

## MICROVASCULAR DENSITY

The concept of microvascular density (MVD) and methods for measuring it were explored in the 1990s.[177,178] High numbers of immunolabeled microvessels counted in the area of densest vascularization, designated a 'hot spot', were associated with an increased risk of metastatic death, and this was taken as evidence of active angiogenesis in many types of cancer.[178,179] The majority of studies have shown that a high MVD is associated with a worse survival, but contradictory reports are not uncommon.[179] In particular, reports of cutaneous melanoma have been controversial.[180,181] Initial studies suggested that high vascularization had a significant influence on survival, but no consensus has been reached. This may be due to the fact that cutaneous melanoma cells can also use lymphatic vessels in their dissemination, which likely blurs an association with the density of microvessels.[182] The theoretical background of MVD has been criticized for lack of a well-proved link with angiogenesis, poor reproducibility, and the questionable specificity of some of the antibodies used in highlighting microvessels.[181,183,184]

Foss and colleagues[122] reported that high MVD was associated with a shorter survival in patients with uveal melanoma. They also looked at the PAS patterns, but did not find any relationship between microvascular patterns and survival in their data set after adjusting for MVD. MVD was higher in tumours with microvascular loops and networks, suggesting that the effect on prognosis of microvascular patterns might be secondary to high MVD.[185] Two other groups have presented opposite results on the prognostic significance of MVD in uveal melanoma.[186,187] More recently, the findings of Foss have been independently confirmed,[163,188] and Al Jamal et al.[189] have reported that microvascular density is a significant prognostic indicator even when controlling for the mean of the ten largest nucleoli.

## CELL–MATRIX INTERACTION

Interactions between tumour cells and surrounding stroma are considered essential for tumour progression and dissemination. Recent studies using microarrays have helped to determine pathways that play a role in tumour cell dissemination. Microarrays can help to identify multiple molecules that differentiate between an aggressive and non-aggressive phenotype.[190] Many differences have also been identified by applying immunohistochemistry and survival analyses.

A decade ago it was documented that some uveal melanomas co-express vimentin (typical of melanocytes) and cytokeratin 8 and 18 (typical of carcinomas) intermediate filaments.[168] Recently, *in vitro* studies showed that uveal melanoma cells that express both types of intermediate filaments had a six-fold increased capacity of invasion as compared to melanoma cells that expressed vimentin only.[191,192] Cells that expressed both intermediate filaments were named 'interconverted cells'.[191,192] Clinical evidence for an association between the interconverted phenotype and prognosis is still missing, perhaps due to the small number of tumours studied so far.[168]

Of the cell adhesion molecules, neural cell adhesion molecule (NCAM) is expressed especially on rapidly metastasising uveal melanomas.[193] The HNK-1 epitope, which is part of the NCAMs, was more frequently expressed on larger tumours, but seldom in liver metastases. Another report, however, failed to document any relationship between NCAM expression and survival, but instead reported that expression of the intercellular cell adhesion molecule-1 (ICAM-1) was linked with the development of metastases.[124]

Expression of VLA-2 integrin receptor was associated with the presence of microvascular networks, but none of the integrin receptors studied [VLA-2, VLA-3, and alpha (v)] seemed to have prognostic significance.[124]

Both primary and metastatic uveal melanomas lack estrogen and progesterone receptors, and potential effects of anti-estrogens on uveal melanoma cannot be mediated by conventional mechanisms.[194,195] Positive cytoplasmic immunostaining with an antibody to estrogen receptors was shown to result from cross-reacting CD68-positive macrophages.[195]

Expression of epidermal growth factor receptor (EGFR) in uveal melanoma cell lines correlated with metastatic potential and liver-targeted metastasis in mice.[196] Moreover, EGFR expression correlated with metastatic death in a small clinical series of uveal melanomas.[197] However, EGFR expression in uveal melanoma also may be confined to tumour-infiltrating macrophages.[198]

Expression of matrix metalloproteinase-2 (MMP-2) was recently linked with decreased uveal melanoma-specific survival, but the sample size was not large enough to test the independent prognostic significance of MMP-2 in multivariate analysis.[199] On the other hand, the presence of TIMP-3 (an inhibitor of MMP expression) was markedly decreased on metastatic uveal melanoma cell lines,[200] and this suggests that regulation of expression of MMPs may play a role in the formation of metastases.

## MARKERS OF CELL PROLIFERATION

The development of antibodies to proteins, such as PC-10 and Ki-67, which identify cells in the proliferative phase of the cell cycle, prompted studies to resolve the prognostic significance of the presence of proliferating tumour cells in uveal melanoma and in other cancers.[201–203] A high fraction of PC-10 and Ki-67 immunopositive uveal melanoma cells has been associated with decreased melanoma-specific survival in many cohorts of uveal melanoma. In one particular study, a high fraction of PC-10 immunopositive tumour cells was associated with a 40% increase in 10-year melanoma-specific mortality.[203] A high PC-10 count was an independent prognostic factor by multivariate analysis adjusted for LBD, presence of microvascular networks, and the mean diameter of the largest nucleoli.[123] Similarly, a high expression of cyclin D1, a protein involved in the cell cycle, indicated an unfavourable outcome in uveal melanoma.[204] Moreover, cyclin D1 positivity was associated with the epithelioid cell type and a high index of Ki-67 positive tumour cells.[205,206]

## NUCLEAR MORPHOMETRY

A high number of mitoses has been associated with increased mortality in uveal melanoma.[102,156,201] Several studies have indicated that higher than average indices of cytomorphometric parameters, such as nuclear and nucleolar area of randomly selected cells, are associated with higher than average melanoma-specific mortality.[103,207–210] In particular, the mean of the ten largest nucleoli and the standard deviation of nucleolar areas have retained independent prognostic value in multivariate analyses, and computer-assisted measurements have been reproducible between different laboratories. However, the methodology of nuclear morphometry assessment is still variable. Recently silver-stained sections were found superior to HE-stained sections.[164]

Regarding the relative importance of nuclear morphometry and other tumour characteristics, Pe'er and associates[211] reported that, in their data set, the network and the parallel vessels with cross-link microvascular patterns were more powerful prognostic indicators than the mean of the ten largest nucleoli. Other investigators have found that the mean of the ten largest nucleoli is an independent indicator of prognosis even when microvascular loops and networks and microvascular density are included in the multivariate model.[189]

# CYTOGENETICS

## DNA ANEUPLOIDY

A DNA content deviating from the normal amount (aneuploid instead of the normal diploid) reflects the genetic instability of tumour cells and impaired control of the cell cycle, which are characteristics of malignant cells. Aneuploid DNA and a high fraction of cells in the S-phase of the cell cycle have been associated with the epithelioid cell type and decreased survival in uveal melanoma.[212,213] Flow cytometry can be used to assess the DNA content and proliferative activity of tumour cells.[214]

## CHROMOSOMAL ABNORMALITIES

Specific chromosomal changes, in particular loss of one copy of chromosome 3 and gain of the long arm of chromosome 8 are emerging as particularly significant prognostic indicators in several independent studies of non-consecutive series of surgically treated uveal melanomas.[38,149,215,216] These chromosomal changes are more frequent in tumours with ciliary body involvement than in choroidal tumours, which may explain the worse prognosis of ciliary body melanomas as compared to choroidal melanomas. So far, studies of chromosomal changes concern predominantly large melanomas, because small and medium-sized melanomas are mostly treated by irradiation. Thus, the results can not be generalized to all uveal melanomas, but chromosomal changes certainly play an important role in tumour progression. A study based on a consecutive series of uveal melanomas that are studied regardless of tumour size is needed to establish the role and sequence of chromosomal changes among uveal melanomas of all sizes.

Recently, analysis of the partial deletion of the long and short arm of chromosome 3 suggested the presence of a tumour suppressor gene locus at 3q24–q26 and 3p25.[40] The long-term follow-up data were not yet available for patients whose tumour had a partial deletion. The growth restricting effect of TGF-beta may be lost in deletions involving chromosome 3p22 in which the gene for TGF-beta receptor is located.[217] An abnormality of the TGF-beta pathway was found in 61% of uveal melanomas, but the authors did not relate monosomy 3 to TGF-beta function.

# MOLECULAR PATHOLOGY

## ONCOGENE ACTIVATION

A potential role for the tumour-suppressor gene nm23 has been suggested in uveal melanomas that were small in size and showed no extraocular extension.[218,219] In an animal model, the expression of nm23 gene was associated with reduced metastatic potential and fewer liver metastases. No association was found between nm23 expression and conventional prognostic indicators, such as cell type and ciliary body involvement.

A high expression of the *c-Myc* oncogene is known to have an influence on survival in a number of cancers, including cutaneous melanoma. In case of uveal melanoma, the results have been opposite; a low expression of *c-Myc* is associated with higher mortality.[220,221] Nuclear *c-Myc* expression was found in every case of 71 studied uveal melanomas, but cytoplasmic *c-Myc* expression was much more prominent than nuclear expression in another study.[201,221] The presence of *c-Myc* positive cells was associated with decreased survival after adjusting for LBD and Ki-67 positive cells in a multivariate analysis.

## PROGRAMMED CELL DEATH

Expression of Bcl-2 protein, a proto-oncogene that blocks programmed cell death (apoptosis), has been documented convincingly in uveal melanoma, but its prognostic significance is lacking.[201,221–223] On the other hand, very few melanomas have been shown to express p53, a nuclear phoshoprotein that induces apoptosis and cell-cycle arrest.[224] The treatment effect of irradiation and transpupillary thermotherapy may be mediated by apoptosis.[221,224–226] Dendritic cells effectively stimulated lymphocyte proliferation and phagocytosed melanoma cells after uveal melanoma cells had undergone apoptosis due to irradiation. This finding suggests that dying intraocular melanoma can serve as an autologous stimulus for immune cells against tumour cells. Recently, overexpression of beta-catenin, a molecule involved in cell adhesion and signal transduction, induced apoptosis in uveal melanoma cells.[227]

## CONCLUSION

Metastatic uveal melanoma is among the few malignancies that are not yet susceptible to modern anti-cancer therapies. A few markers such as the presence of congenital ocular melanocytosis and the FAMMM syndrome are associated with an increased risk to develop a uveal melanoma, but no specific genes have as yet been found. A wide range of patient and tumour-characteristics are known to be prognostic factors in the development of metastases. Several of these are found to be associated with one another, such as a large diameter, large tumour height, chromosome 3 monosomy, involvement of the ciliary body, presence of epithelioid cells, heavy pigmentation, high numbers of infiltrating macrophages, microvascular loops and networks, and high microvascular density.

It is likely that biochemical analyses following microarray-RNA studies will show us the biochemical mechanisms that play a role in the development of metastases in uveal melanoma, and this will hopefully help us to find ways to treat the metastases of this deadly but intriguing malignancy.

## REFERENCES


1. Borland R, Donaghue N, Hill D. Illnesses that Australians most feared in 1986 and 1993. *Aust J Public Health.* 1994; 18: 366–369.
2. Folberg R. Tumor progression in ocular melanomas. *J Invest Dermatol.* 1993; 100: 326S–331S.
3. Zimmerman LE. Malignant melanoma. In: Spencer WH, ed. *Ophthalmic Pathology.* Philadelphia: W.B. Saunders Company, 1986; 2072–2139.
4. Egan KM, Seddon JM, Glynn RJ, Gragoudas ES, Albert DM. Epidemiologic aspects of uveal melanoma. *Surv Ophthalmol.* 1988; 32: 239–251.
5. Hungerford J. Uveal melanoma. *Eur J Cancer.* 1993; 29A: 1365–1368.
6. McKee PH. *Pathology of the skin.* Philadelphia: JB Lippincott, 1989.
7. Singh AD, Shields CL, De Potter P, Shields JA, Trock B, Cater J, Pastore D. Familial uveal melanoma. Clinical observations on 56 patients. *Arch Ophthalmol.* 1996; 114: 392–399.
8. Platz A, Ringborg U, Hansson J. Hereditary cutaneous melanoma. *Semin Cancer Biol.* 2000; 10: 319–326.
9. Einhorn LH, Burgess MA, Gottlieb JA. Metastatic patterns of choroidal melanoma. *Cancer.* 1974; 34: 1001–1004.
10. McLean IW. The biology of haematogenous metastasis in human uveal malignant melanoma. *Virchows Arch A.* 1993; 422: 433–437.
11. Eskelin S, Summanen P, Pyrhönen S, Tarkkanen A, Kivelä T. Screening for metastatic uveal melanoma revisited. *Cancer.* 1999; 85: 1151–1159.

12. Clarijs R, Schalkwijk L, Ruiter DJ, de Waal RM. Lack of lymphangiogenesis despite coexpression of VEGF-C and its receptor Flt-4 in uveal melanoma. *Invest Ophthalmol Vis Sci.* 2001; 42: 1422–1428.
13. Blom DJ, Luyten GP, Mooy C, Kerkvliet S, Zwinderman AH, Jager MJ. Human leukocyte antigen class I expression. Marker of poor prognosis in uveal melanoma. *Invest Ophthalmol Vis Sci.* 1997; 38: 1865–1872.
14. Naus NC, Zuidervaart W, Rayman N, Slater R, Van Drunen E, Ksander B, Luyten GP, Klein A. Mutation analysis of the PTEN gene in uveal melanoma cell lines. *Int J Cancer.* 2000; 87: 151–153.
15. Bittner M, Meltzer P, Chen Y, Jiang Y, Seftor E, Hendrix M, Radmacher M, Simon R, Yakhini Z, Ben Dor A, Sampas N, Dougherty E, Wang E, Marincola F, Gooden C, Lueders J, Glatfelter A, Pollock P, Carpten J, Gillanders E, Leja D, Dietrich K, Beaudry C, Berens M, Alberts D, Sondak V. Molecular classification of cutaneous malignant melanoma by gene expression profiling. *Nature.* 2000; 406: 536–540.
16. Cree IA. Cell cycle and melanoma — two different tumours from the same cell type. *J Pathol.* 2000; 191: 112–114.
17. Li W, Judge H, Gragoudas ES, Seddon JM, Egan KM. Patterns of tumor initiation in choroidal melanoma. *Cancer Res.* 2000; 60: 3757–3760.
18. Shields CL, Shields JA, De Potter P, Cater J, Tardio D, Barrett J. Diffuse choroidal melanoma. Clinical features predictive of metastasis. *Arch Ophthalmol.* 1996; 114: 956–963.
19. Shields JA, Shields CL, Donoso LA. Management of posterior uveal melanoma. *Surv Ophthalmol.* 1991; 36: 161–195.
20. Kivelä T, Summanen P. Retinoinvasive malignant melanoma of the uvea. *Br J Ophthalmol.* 1997; 81: 691–697.
21. Gunduz K, Shields JA, Shields CL, Eagle RC, Jr. Cutaneous melanoma metastatic to the vitreous cavity. *Ophthalmology.* 1998; 105: 600–605.
22. Jensen OA. Malignant melanoma of the iris. A 25-year analysis of Danish cases. *Eur J Ophthalmol.* 1993; 3: 181–188.
23. Shields CL, Shield JA, Materin M, Gershenbaum E, Singh AD, Smith, A. Iris melanoma. Risk factors for metastasis in 169 consecutive patients. *Ophthalmology.* 2001; 108: 172–178.
24. Chowers I, Folberg R, Livni N, Pe'er J. Comparison of microcirculation patterns and MIB-1 immunoreactivity in iris and posterior uveal melanoma. *Ophthalmology.* 2001; 108: 367–371.
25. Bergman L, Seregard S, Nilsson B, Ringborg U, Lundell G, Ragnarsson-Olding B. Incidence of uveal melanoma in Sweden from 1960 to 1998. *Invest Ophthalmol Vis Sci.* 2002; 43: 2579–2583.
26. Lee SB, Au Eong KG, Saw SM, Chan TK, Lee HP. Eye cancer incidence in Singapore. *Br J Ophthalmol.* 2000; 84: 767–770.
27. Singh AD, Topham A. Incidence of uveal melanoma in the United States: 1973–1997. *Ophthalmology.* 2003; 110: 956–961.
28. Jensen OA. Malignant melanomas of the uvea in Denmark 1943–1952. A clinical, histopathological, and prognostic study. *Acta Ophthalmol (Suppl).* 1963; 75: 1–220.
29. Holly EA, Aston DA, Char DH, Kristiansen JJ, Ahn DK. Uveal melanoma in relation to ultraviolet light exposure and host factors. *Cancer Res.* 1990; 50: 5773–5777.
30. Regan S, Judge HE, Gragoudas ES, Egan KM. Iris color as a prognostic factor in ocular melanoma. *Arch Ophthalmol.* 1999; 117: 811–814.
31. Singh AD, De Potter P, Fijal BA, Shields CL, Shields JA, Elston RC. Lifetime prevalence of uveal melanoma in white patients with oculo(dermal) melanocytosis. *Ophthalmology.* 1998; 105: 195–198.

32. Van Hees CL, De Boer A, Jager MJ, Bleeker JC, Kakebeeke HM, Crijns MB, Vandenbroucke JP, Bergman W. Are atypical nevi a risk factor for uveal melanoma? A case-control study. *J Invest Dermatol.* 1994; 103: 202–205.
33. Hammer H, Olah J, Toth-Molnar E. Dysplastic nevi are a risk factor for uveal melanoma. *Eur J Ophthalmol.* 1996; 6: 472–474.
34. Holly EA, Aston DA, Ahn DK, Kristiansen JJ, Char DH. Uveal melanoma, hormonal and reproductive factors in women. *Cancer Res.* 1991; 51: 1370–1372.
35. Egan KM, Walsh SM, Seddon JM, Gragoudas ES. An evaluation of the influence of reproductive factors on the risk of metastases from uveal melanoma. *Ophthalmology.* 1993; 100: 1160–1165.
36. Prescher G, Bornfeld N, Becher R. Nonrandom chromosomal abnormalities in primary uveal melanoma. *J Natl Cancer Inst.* 1990; 82: 1765–1769.
37. Sisley K, Cottam DW, Rennie IG, Parsons MA, Potter AM, Potter CW, Rees RC. Nonrandom abnormalities of chromosomes 3, 6, and 8 associated with posterior uveal melanoma. *Genes Chromosomes Cancer.* 1992; 5: 197–200.
38. Aalto Y, Eriksson L, Seregard S, Larsson O, Knuutila S. Concomitant loss of chromosome 3 and whole arm losses and gains of chromosome 1, 6, or 8 in metastasizing primary uveal melanoma. *Invest Ophthalmol Vis Sci.* 2001; 42: 313–317.
39. Scholes AG, Liloglou T, Maloney P, Hagan S, Nunn J, Hiscott P, Damato BE, Grierson I, Field JK. Loss of heterozygosity on chromosomes 3, 9, 13, and 17, including the retinoblastoma locus, in uveal melanoma. *Invest Ophthalmol Vis Sci.* 2001; 42: 2472–2477.
40. Tschentscher F, Prescher G, Horsman DE, White VA, Rieder H, Anastassiou G, Schilling H, Bornfeld N, Bartz-Schmidt KU, Horsthemke B, Lohmann DR, Zeschnigk M. Partial deletions of the long and short arm of chromosome 3 point to two tumor suppressor genes in uveal melanoma. *Cancer Res.* 2001; 61: 3439–3442.
41. Tschentscher F, Husing J, Holter T, Kruse E, Dresen IG, Jockel KH, Anastassiou G, Schilling H, Bornfeld N, Horsthemke B, Lohmann DR, Zeschnigk M. Tumor classification based on gene expression profiling shows that uveal melanomas with and without monosomy 3 represent two distinct entities. *Cancer Res.* 2003; 63: 2578–2584.
42. Van Hees CL, Jager MJ, Bleeker JC, Kemme H, Bergman W. Occurrence of cutaneous and uveal melanoma in patients with uveal melanoma and their first degree relatives. *Melanoma Res.* 1998; 8: 175–180.
43. Holden R, Damato B. Preventable delays in the treatment of intraocular melanoma in the UK. *Eye.* 1996; 10: 127–129.
44. Ah-Fat FG, Damato BE. Delays in the diagnosis of uveal melanoma and effect on treatment. *Eye.* 1998; 12: 781–782.
45. Eskelin S, Kivelä T. Mode of presentation and time to treatment of uveal melanoma in Finland. *Br J Ophthalmol.* 2002; 86: 333–338.
46. The Collaborative Ocular Melanoma Study Group. Accuracy of diagnosis of choroidal melanomas in the Collaborative Ocular Melanoma Study. COMS report no. 1. *Arch Ophthalmol.* 1990; 108: 1268–1273.
47. Shields JA, Shields CL, De Potter P, Singh AD. Diagnosis and treatment of uveal melanoma. *Semin Oncol.* 1996; 23: 763–767.
48. Shields CL, Shields JA, Kiratli H, De Potter P, Cater JR. Risk factors for growth and metastasis of small choroidal melanocytic lesions. *Ophthalmology.* 1995; 102: 1351–1361.
49. Maberly DA, Pavlin CJ, McGowan HD, Foster FS, Simpson ER. Ultrasound biomicroscopic imaging of the anterior aspect of peripheral choroidal melanomas. *Am J Ophthalmol.* 1997; 123: 506–514.
50. Folberg R, Augsburger JJ, Gamel JW, Shields JA, Lang WR. Fine-needle aspirates of uveal melanomas and prognosis. *Am J Ophthalmol.* 1985; 100: 654–657.

51. Char DH, Kroll SM, Stoloff A, Crawford JB, Miller TR, Howes EJ, Crawford P. Cytomorphometry of uveal melanomas: fine needle aspiration biopsy versus standard histology. *Trans Am Ophthalmol Soc.* 1989; 87: 197–210.
52. Jensen OA, Prause JU, Scherfig E. Transvitreal retino-choroidal biopsy of suspected malignant lesions of the choroid. Follow-up of cases over 7 years. *Acta Ophthalmol Scand.* 1997; 75: 409–411.
53. Gragoudas ES, Egan KM, Seddon JM, Glynn RJ, Walsh SM, Finn SM, Munzenrider JE, Spar MD. Survival of patients with metastases from uveal melanoma. *Ophthalmology.* 1991; 98: 383–389.
54. Albert DM, Niffenegger AS, Willson JKV. Treatment of metastatic uveal melanoma: review and recommendations. *Surv Ophthalmol.* 1992; 36: 438.
55. The Collaborative Ocular Melanoma Study Group. Assessment of metastatic disease status at death in 435 patients with large choroidal melanoma in the Collaborative Ocular Melanoma Study (COMS): COMS report no. 15. *Arch Ophthalmol.* 2001; 119: 670–676.
56. Lorigan JG, Wallace S, Mavligit GM. The prevalence and location of metastases from ocular melanoma: imaging study in 110 patients. *Am J Roentgenol.* 1991; 157: 1279–1281.
57. Leyvraz S, Spataro V, Bauer J, Pampallona S, Salmon R, Dorval T, Meuli R, Gillet M, Lejeune F, Zografos L. Treatment of ocular melanoma metastatic to the liver by hepatic arterial chemotherapy. *J Clin Oncol.* 1997; 15: 2589–2595.
58. Eskelin S, Pyrhönen S, Hahka-Kemppinen M, Tuomaala S, Kivelä T. A prognostic model and staging for metastatic uveal melanoma. *Cancer.* 2003; 97: 465–475.
59. Rennie IG. The Ashton Lecture. Uveal melanoma: the past, the present and the future. *Eye.* 1997; 11: 255–264.
60. The Collaborative Ocular Melanoma Study Group. The Collaborative Ocular Melanoma Study (COMS) randomized trial of pre-enucleation radiation of large choroidal melanoma III: local complications and observations following enucleation COMS report no. 11. *Am J Ophthalmol.* 1998; 126: 362–372.
61. Straatsma BR, Fine SL, Earle JD, Hawkins BS, Diener-West M, McLaughlin JA. Enucleation versus plaque irradiation for choroidal melanoma. *Ophthalmology.* 1988; 95: 1000–1004.
62. Diener-West M, Earle JD, Fine SL, Hawkins BS, Moy CS, Reynolds SM, Schachat AP, Straatsma BR, The Collaborative Ocular Melanoma Study Group. The COMS randomized trial of iodine 125 brachytherapy for choroidal melanoma, III: initial mortality findings. COMS Report No. 18. *Arch Ophthalmol.* 2001; 119: 969–982.
63. Seddon JM, Gragoudas ES, Albert DM, Hsieh CC, Polivogianis L, Friedenberg GR. Comparison of survival rates for patients with uveal melanoma after treatment with proton beam irradiation or enucleation. *Am J Ophthalmol.* 1985; 99: 282–290.
64. Guthoff R, Frischmuth J, Jensen OA, Bjerrum K, Prause JU. Das Aderhautmelanom. Eine retrospektive randomisierte Vergleichsstudie Ruthenium-Bestrahlung vs Enukleation. *Klin Monatsbl Augenheilkd.* 1992; 200: 257–261.
65. Augsburger JJ, Gamel JW, Shields JA. Cobalt plaque radiotherapy versus enucleation for posterior uveal melanoma: comparison of survival by prognostic index groups. *Trans Am Ophthalmol Soc.* 1989; 87: 348–359.
66. Augsburger JJ, Correa ZM, Freire J, Brady LW. Long-term survival in choroidal and ciliary body melanoma after enucleation versus plaque radiation therapy. *Ophthalmology.* 1998; 105: 1670–1678.
67. Augsburger JJ, Schneider S, Freire J, Brady LW. Survival following enucleation versus plaque radiotherapy in statistically matched subgroups of patients with choroidal melanomas: results in patients treated between 1980 and 1987. *Graefes Arch Clin Exp Ophthalmol.* 1999; 237: 558–567.

68. Singh AD, Topham A. Survival rates with uveal melanoma in the United States: 1973–1997. *Ophthalmology.* 2003; 110: 962–965.
69. Cohen VM, Carter MJ, Kemeny A, Radatz M, Rennie IG. Metastasis-free survival following treatment for uveal melanoma with either stereotactic radiosurgery or enucleation. *Acta Ophthalmol Scand.* 2003; 81: 383–388.
70. Summanen P, Immonen I, Kivelä T, Tommila P, Heikkonen J, Tarkkanen A. Visual outcome of eyes with malignant melanoma of the uvea after ruthenium plaque radiotherapy. *Ophthalmic Surg Lasers.* 1995; 26: 449–460.
71. Finger PT. Radiation therapy for choroidal melanoma. *Surv Ophthalmol.* 1997; 42: 215–232.
72. Shields CL, Shields JA, Cater J, Gunduz K, Miyamoto C, Micaily B, Brady LW. Plaque radiotherapy for uveal melanoma: long-term visual outcome in 1106 consecutive patients. *Arch Ophthalmol.* 2000; 118: 1219–1228.
73. Gragoudas ES, Lane AM, Regan S, Li W, Judge HE, Munzenrider JE, Seddon JM, Egan KM. A randomized controlled trial of varying radiation doses in the treatment of choroidal melanoma. *Arch Ophthalmol.* 2000; 118: 773–778.
74. Summanen P, Immonen I, Kivelä T, Tommila P, Heikkonen J, Tarkkanen A. Radiation related complications after ruthenium plaque radiotherapy of uveal melanoma. *Br J Ophthalmol.* 1996; 80: 732–739.
75. Harbour JW, Char DH, Kroll S, Quivey JM, Castro J. Metastatic risk for distinct patterns of postirradiation local recurrence of posterior uveal melanoma. *Ophthalmology.* 1997; 104: 1785–1792.
76. Egan KM, Ryan LM, Gragoudas ES. Survival implications of enucleation after definitive radiotherapy for choroidal melanoma: an example of regression on time-dependent covariates. *Arch Ophthalmol.* 1998; 116: 366–370.
77. Luyten GP, Mooy CM, Eijkenboom WM, Stijnen T, Hellemons LP, Luider TM, De Jong PT. No demonstrated effect of pre-enucleation irradiation on survival of patients with uveal melanoma. *Am J Ophthalmol.* 1995; 119: 786–791.
78. The Collaborative Ocular Melanoma Study Group. The Collaborative Ocular Melanoma Study (COMS) randomized trial of pre-enucleation radiation of large choroidal melanoma II: initial mortality findings. COMS report no. 10. *Am J Ophthalmol.* 1998; 125: 779–796.
79. Oosterhuis JA, Journee-De Korver HG, Kakebeeke-Kemme HM, Bleeker JC. Transpupillary thermotherapy in choroidal melanomas. *Arch Ophthalmol.* 1995; 113: 315–321.
80. Oosterhuis JA, Journee-De Korver HG, Keunen JE. Transpupillary thermotherapy: results in 50 patients with choroidal melanoma. *Arch Ophthalmol.* 1998; 116: 157–162.
81. Shields CL, Shields JA, De Potter P, Kheterpal S. Transpupillary thermotherapy in the management of choroidal melanoma. *Ophthalmology.* 1996; 103: 1642–1650.
82. Shields CL, Shield JA, Perez N, Singh AD, Cater J. Primary transpupillary thermotherapy for small choroidal melanoma in 256 consecutive cases: outcomes and limitations. *Ophthalmology.* 2002; 109: 225–234.
83. Peyman GA, Apple DJ. Local excision of choroidal malignant melanoma. *Arch Ophthalmol.* 1974; 92: 216–218.
84. Foulds WS, Damato BE. Alternatives to enucleation in the management of choroidal melanoma. *Aust N Z J Ophthalmol.* 1986; 14: 19–27.
85. Shields JA, Shields CL, Shah P, Sivalingam V. Partial lamellar sclerouvectomy for ciliary body and choroidal tumors. *Ophthalmology.* 1991; 98: 971–983.
86. Damato BE. Local resection of uveal melanoma. *Bull Soc Belge Ophtalmol.* 1993; 248: 11–17.

87. Damato B, Groenewald C, McGalliard J, Wong D. Endoresection of choroidal melanoma. *Br J Ophthalmol.* 1998; 82: 213–218.
88. Favilla I, Favilla ML, Gosbell AD, Barry WR, Ellims P, Hill JS, Byrne JR. Photodynamic therapy: a 5-year study of its effectiveness in the treatment of posterior uveal melanoma, and evaluation of haematoporphyrin uptake and photocytotoxicity of melanoma cells in tissue culture. *Melanoma Res.* 1995; 5: 355–364.
89. Marchini G, Gerosa M, Piovan E, Pasoli A, Babighian S, Rigotti M, Rossato M, Bonomi L. Gamma Knife stereotactic radiosurgery for uveal melanoma: clinical results after 2 years. *Stereotact Funct Neurosurg.* 1996; 66 Suppl 1: 208–213.
90. Augsburger JJ, Gamel JW, Lauritzen K, Brady LW. Cobalt-60 plaque radiotherapy vs enucleation for posterior uveal melanoma. *Am J Ophthalmol.* 1990; 109: 585–592.
91. Eskelin S, Pyrhönen S, Summanen P, Hahka-Kemppinen M, Kivelä T. Tumor doubling times in metastatic malignant melanoma of the uvea: tumor progression before and after treatment. *Ophthalmology.* 2000; 107: 1443–1449.
92. Albert DM, Niffenegger AS, Willson JK. Treatment of metastatic uveal melanoma: review and recommendations. *Surv Ophthalmol.* 1992; 36: 429–438.
93. Pyrhönen S. The treatment of metastatic uveal melanoma. *Eur J Cancer.* 1998; 34: S27–S30.
94. Fournier GA, Albert DM, Arrigg CA, Cohen AM, Lamping KA, Seddon JM. Resection of solitary metastasis. Approach to palliative treatment of hepatic involvement with choroidal melanoma. *Arch Ophthalmol.* 1984; 102: 80–82.
95. Salmon RJ, Levy C, Plancher C, Dorval T, Desjardins L, Leyvraz S, Pouillart P, Schlienger P, Servois V, Asselain B. Treatment of liver metastases from uveal melanoma by combined surgery-chemotherapy. *Eur J Surg Oncol.* 1998; 24: 127–130.
96. Aoyama T, Mastrangelo MJ, Berd D, Nathan FE, Shields CL, Shields JA, Rosato EL, Rosato FE, Sato T. Protracted survival after resection of metastatic uveal melanoma. *Cancer.* 2000; 89: 1561–1568.
97. Kivelä T, Suciu S, Hansson J, Kruit WH, Vuoristo MS, Kloke O, Gore M, Hahka-Kemppinen M, Parvinen LM, Kumpulainen E, Humblet Y, Pyrhönen S. Bleomycin, vincristine, lomustine and dacarbazine (BOLD) in combination with recombinant interferon alpha-2b for metastatic uveal melanoma. *Eur J Cancer.* 2003; 39: 1115–1120.
98. Becker JC, Kampgen E, Brocker E. Classical chemotherapy for metastatic melanoma. *Clin Exp Dermatol.* 2000; 25: 503–508.
99. Van der Pol JP, Blom DJ, Flens MJ, Luyten GP, De Waard S, Koornneef L, Scheper RJ, Jager MJ. Multidrug resistance-related proteins in primary choroidal melanomas and in vitro cell lines. *Invest Ophthalmol Vis Sci.* 1997; 38: 2523–2530.
100. Pfohler C, Cree IA, Ugurel S, Kuwert C, Haass N, Neuber K, Hengge U, Corrie PG, Zutt M, Tilgen W, Reinhold U. Treosulfan and gemcitabine in metastatic uveal melanoma patients: results of a multicenter feasibility study. *Anticancer Drugs.* 2003; 14: 337–340.
101. Shammas HF, Blodi FC. Prognostic factors in choroidal and ciliary body melanomas. *Arch Ophthalmol.* 1977; 95: 63–69.
102. Seddon JM, Albert DM, Lavin PT, Robinson N. A prognostic factor study of disease-free interval and survival following enucleation for uveal melanoma. *Arch Ophthalmol.* 1983; 101: 1894–1899.
103. Gamel JW, McLean IW, McCurdy JB. Biologic distinctions between cure and time to death in 2892 patients with intraocular melanoma. *Cancer.* 1993; 71: 2299–2305.
104. Kujala E, Mäkitie T, Kivelä T. Very long-term prognosis of patients with malignant uveal melanoma. *Invest Ophthalmol Vis Sci.* 2003; 44: 4651–4659.

105. Shields JA, Augsburger JJ, Donoso LA, Bernardino VJ, Portenar M. Hepatic metastasis and orbital recurrence of uveal melanoma after 42 years. *Am J Ophthalmol.* 1985; 100: 666–668.
106. Midena E, De Belvis V, Dei Tos AP, Antonini C. Isolated brain metastasis of malignant choroidal melanoma 27 years after enucleation. *Arch Ophthalmol.* 1999; 117: 1553–1556.
107. Char DH. Metastatic choroidal melanoma. *Am J Ophthalmol.* 1978; 86: 76–80.
108. Zimmerman LE, McLean IW, Foster WD. Does enucleation of the eye containing a malignant melanoma prevent or accelerate the dissemination of tumour cells. *Br J Ophthalmol.* 1978; 62: 420–425.
109. McLean IW, Foster WD, Zimmerman LE, Martin DG. Inferred natural history of uveal melanoma. *Invest Ophthalmol Vis Sci.* 1980; 19: 760–770.
110. Zimmerman LE, McLean IW. Metastatic disease from untreated uveal melanomas. *Am J Ophthalmol.* 1979; 88: 524–534.
111. Raivio I. Uveal melanoma in Finland. An epidemiological, clinical, histological and prognostic study. *Acta Ophthalmol (Suppl).* 1977; 1–64.
112. Manschot WA, Lee WR, Van Strik R. Uveal melanoma: updated considerations on current management modalities. *Int Ophthalmol.* 1995; 19: 203–209.
113. Manschot WA, Van Strik R. Is irradiation a justifiable treatment of choroidal melanoma? Analysis of published results. *Br J Ophthalmol.* 1987; 71: 348–352.
114. Manschot WA. The natural history of uveal melanomas and its therapeutic consequences. *Doc Ophthalmol.* 1980; 50: 83–99.
115. Augsburger JJ, Gamel JW. Clinical prognostic factors in patients with posterior uveal malignant melanoma. *Cancer.* 1990; 66: 1596–1600.
116. Kroll S, Char DH, Quivey J, Castro J. A comparison of cause-specific melanoma mortality and all-cause mortality in survival analyses after radiation treatment for uveal melanoma. *Ophthalmology.* 1998; 105: 2035–2045.
117. Barr CC, McLean IW, Zimmerman LE. Uveal melanoma in children and adolescents. *Arch Ophthalmol.* 1981; 99: 2133–2136.
118. Singh AD, Shields CL, Shields JA, Sato T. Uveal melanoma in young patients. *Arch Ophthalmol.* 2000; 118: 918–923.
119. Folberg R, Rummelt V, Parys-Van Ginderdeuren R, Hwang T, Woolson RF, Pe'er J, Gruman LM. The prognostic value of tumor blood vessel morphology in primary uveal melanoma. *Ophthalmology.* 1993; 100: 1389–1398.
120. Egan KM, Quinn JL, Gragoudas ES. Childbearing history associated with improved survival in choroidal melanoma. *Arch Ophthalmol.* 1999; 117: 939–942.
121. Coleman K, Baak JP, Van Diest P, Mullaney J, Farrell M, Fenton M. Prognostic factors following enucleation of 111 uveal melanomas. *Br J Ophthalmol.* 1993; 77: 688–692.
122. Foss AJE, Alexander RA, Jefferies LW, Hungerford JL, Harris AL, Lightman S. Microvessel count predicts survival in uveal melanoma. *Cancer Res.* 1996; 56: 2900–2903.
123. Seregard S, Spångberg B, Juul C, Oskarsson M. Prognostic accuracy of the mean of the largest nucleoli, vascular patterns, and PC-10 in posterior uveal melanoma. *Ophthalmology.* 1998; 105: 485–491.
124. Anastassiou G, Schilling H, Stang A, Djakovic S, Heiligenhaus A, Bornfeld N. Expression of the cell adhesion molecules ICAM-1, VCAM-1 and NCAM in uveal melanoma: A clinicopathological study. *Oncology.* 2000; 58: 83–88.
125. Seddon JM, MacLaughlin DT, Albert DM, Gragoudas ES, Ference M. Uveal melanomas presenting during pregnancy and the investigation of oestrogen receptors in melanomas. *Br J Ophthalmol.* 1982; 66: 695–704.
126. Lambert SR, Char DH, Howes EJ, Crawford JB, Wells J. Spontaneous regression of a choroidal melanoma. *Arch Ophthalmol.* 1986; 104: 732–734.

127. De Waard-Siebinga I, Hilders CG, Hansen BE, Van Delft JL, Jager MJ. HLA expression and tumor-infiltrating immune cells in uveal melanoma. *Graefes Arch Clin Exp Ophthalmol.* 1996; 234: 34–42.
128. Durie FH, Campbell AM, Lee WR, Damato BE. Analysis of lymphocytic infiltration in uveal melanoma. *Invest Ophthalmol Vis Sci.* 1990; 31: 2106–2110.
129. Tobal K, Deuble K, McCartney A, Lightman S. Characterization of cellular infiltration in choroidal melanoma. *Melanoma Res.* 1993; 3: 63–65.
130. Durie FH, George WD, Campbell AM, Damato BE. Analysis of clonality of tumour infiltrating lymphocytes in breast cancer and uveal melanoma. *Immunol Lett.* 1992; 33: 263–269.
131. The Collaborative Ocular Melanoma Study Group. Histopathologic characteristics of uveal melanomas in eyes enucleated from the Collaborative Ocular Melanoma Study. COMS report no. 6. *Am J Ophthalmol.* 1998; 125: 745–766.
132. Mäkitie T, Summanen P, Tarkkanen A, Kivelä T. Tumor-infiltrating macrophages ($CD68^{+}$ cells) and prognosis in malignant uveal melanoma. *Invest Ophthalmol Vis Sci.* 2001; 42: 1414–1421.
133. Clarijs R, Schalkwijk L, Ruiter DJ, De Waal RM. EMAP-II expression is associated with macrophage accumulation in primary uveal melanoma. *Invest Ophthalmol Vis Sci.* 2003; 44: 1801–1806.
134. Sunderkötter C, Steinbrink K, Goebeler M, Bhardwaj R, Sorg C. Macrophages and angiogenesis. *J Leukoc Biol.* 1994; 55: 410–422.
135. Mantovani A. Tumor-associated macrophages in neoplastic progression: a paradigm for the in vivo function of chemokines. *Lab Invest.* 1994; 71: 5–16.
136. Ma D, Niederkorn JY. Transforming growth factor-beta down-regulates major histocompatibility complex class I antigen expression and increases the susceptibility of uveal melanoma cells to natural killer cell-mediated cytolysis. *Immunology.* 1995; 86: 263–269.
137. All-Ericsson C, Girnita L, Seregard S, Bartolazzi A, Jager MJ, Larsson O. Insulin-like growth factor-1 receptor in uveal melanoma: a predictor for metastatic disease and a potential therapeutic target. *Invest Ophthalmol Vis Sci.* 2002; 43: 1–8.
138. Dithmar S, Crowder J, Jager MJ, Vigniswaran N, Grossniklaus HE. [HLA class I antigen expression correlates with histological cell type in uveal melanoma]. *Ophthalmologe.* 2002; 99: 625–628.
139. Jager MJ, Hurks HM, Levitskaya J, Kiessling R. HLA expression in uveal melanoma: there is no rule without some exception. *Hum Immunol.* 2002; 63: 444–451.
140. Blom DJ, Mooy CM, Luyten GP, Kerkvliet S, Ouwerkerk I, Zwinderman AH, Schrier PI, Jager MJ. Inverse correlation between expression of HLA-B and c-myc in uveal melanoma. *J Pathol.* 1997; 181: 75–79.
141. Jager MJ, Völker-Dieben HJ, De Wolff-Rouendaal D, Kakebeeke-Kemme H, D'Amaro J. Possible relation between HLA and ABO type and prognosis of uveal melanoma. *Doc Ophthalmol.* 1992; 82: 43–47.
142. Toth-Molnar E, Hammer H, Olah J. Cutaneous dysplastic naevi in uveal melanoma patients: markers for prognosis? *Melanoma Res.* 2000; 10: 36–39.
143. Shors AR, Iwamoto S, Doody DR, Weiss NS. Relationship of uveal and cutaneous malignant melanoma in persons with multiple primary tumors. *Int J Cancer.* 2002; 102: 266–268.
144. Egan KM, Gragoudas ES, Seddon JM, Walsh SM. Smoking and the risk of early metastases from uveal melanoma. *Ophthalmology.* 1992; 99: 537–541.
145. Seregard S, Kock E. Prognostic indicators following enucleation for posterior uveal melanoma. A multivariate analysis of long-term survival with minimized loss to follow-up. *Acta Ophthalmol Scand.* 1995; 73: 340–344.

146. Li W, Gragoudas ES, Egan KM. Metastatic melanoma death rates by anatomic site after proton beam irradiation for uveal melanoma. *Arch Ophthalmol.* 2000; 118: 1066–1070.
147. Rummelt V, Folberg R, Woolson RF, Hwang T, Pe'er J. Relation between the microcirculation architecture and the aggressive behavior of ciliary body melanomas. *Ophthalmology.* 1995; 102: 844–851.
148. Mäkitie T, Summanen P, Tarkkanen A, Kivelä T. Microvascular loops and networks as prognostic indicators in choroidal and ciliary body melanomas. *J Natl Cancer Inst.* 1999; 91: 359–367.
149. Sisley K, Rennie IG, Parsons MA, Jacques R, Hammond DW, Bell SM, Potter AM, Rees RC. Abnormalities of chromosomes 3 and 8 in posterior uveal melanoma correlate with prognosis. *Genes Chromosomes Cancer.* 1997; 19: 22–28.
150. Dithmar S, Diaz CE, Grossniklaus HE. Intraocular melanoma spread to regional lymph nodes: report of two cases. *Retina.* 2000; 20: 76–79.
151. Affeldt JC, Minckler DS, Azen SP, Yeh L. Prognosis in uveal melanoma with extrascleral extension. *Arch Ophthalmol.* 1980; 98: 1975–1979.
152. Pach JM, Robertson DM, Taney BS, Martin JA, Campbell RJ, O'Brien PC. Prognostic factors in choroidal and ciliary body melanomas with extrascleral extension. *Am J Ophthalmol.* 1986; 101: 325–331.
153. Gunduz K, Shields CL, Shields JA, Cater J, Brady L. Plaque radiotherapy for management of ciliary body and choroidal melanoma with extraocular extension. *Am J Ophthalmol.* 2000; 130: 97–102.
154. McLean IW, Foster WD, Zimmerman LE. Uveal melanoma: location, size, cell type, and enucleation as risk factors in metastasis. *Hum Pathol.* 1982; 13: 123–132.
155. Miller MV, Herdson PB, Hitchcock GC. Malignant melanoma of the uveal tract — a review of the Auckland experience. *Pathology.* 1985; 17: 281–284.
156. McLean MJ, Foster WD, Zimmerman LE. Prognostic factors in small malignant melanomas of choroid and ciliary body. *Arch Ophthalmol.* 1977; 95: 48–58.
157. Mehaffey MG, Folberg R, Meyer M, Bentler SE, Hwang T, Woolson R, Moore KC. Relative importance of quantifying area and vascular patterns in uveal melanomas. *Am J Ophthalmol.* 1997; 123: 798–809.
158. The Collaborative Ocular Melanoma Study Group. Mortality in patients with small choroidal melanoma. COMS report no. 4. The Collaborative Ocular Melanoma Study Group. *Arch Ophthalmol.* 1997; 115: 886–893.
159. Sobin LH, Wittekind Ch. *TNM Classification of Malignant Tumours.* 5th ed. New York: J. Wiley & Sons, Inc.; 1997.
160. Sobin LH, Wittekind Ch. *TNM Classification of Malignant Tumours.* 6th ed. New York: Wiley-Liss; 2002.
161. McLean IW, Foster WD, Zimmerman LE, Gamel JW. Modifications of Callender's classification of uveal melanoma at the Armed Forces Institute of Pathology. *Am J Ophthalmol.* 1983; 96: 502–509.
162. Gamel JW, McLean IW. Quantitative analysis of the Callender classification of uveal melanoma cells. *Arch Ophthalmol.* 1977; 95: 686–691.
163. Mäkitie T, Summanen P, Tarkkanen A, Kivelä T. Microvascular density in predicting survival of patients with choroidal and ciliary body melanoma. *Invest Ophthalmol Vis Sci.* 1999; 40: 2471–2480.
164. Moshari A, McLean IW. Uveal melanoma: mean of the longest nucleoli measured on silver-stained sections. *Invest Ophthalmol Vis Sci.* 2001; 42: 1160–1163.
165. Seddon JM, Polivogianis L, Hsieh CC, Albert DM, Gamel JW, Gragoudas ES. Death from uveal melanoma. Number of epithelioid cells and inverse SD of nucleolar area as prognostic factors. *Arch Ophthalmol.* 1987; 105: 801–806.

166. Char DH, Kroll SM, Miller T, Castro J, Quivey J. Irradiated uveal melanomas: cytopathologic correlation with prognosis. *Am J Ophthalmol.* 1996; 122: 509–513.
167. Bechrakis NE, Sehu KW, Lee WR, Damato BE, Foerster MH. Transformation of cell type in uveal melanomas: a quantitative histologic analysis. *Arch Ophthalmol.* 2000; 118: 1406–1412.
168. Fuchs U, Kivelä T, Summanen P, Immonen I, Tarkkanen A. An immunohistochemical and prognostic analysis of cytokeratin expression in malignant uveal melanoma. *Am J Pathol.* 1992; 141: 169–181.
169. McLean IW, Keefe KS, Burnier MN. Uveal melanoma: comparison of the prognostic value of fibrovascular loops, mean of the ten largest nucleoli, cell type, and tumor size. *Ophthalmology.* 1997; 104: 777–780.
170. Kinnaert E, Morandini R, Simon S, Hill HZ, Ghanem G, Van Houtte P. The degree of pigmentation modulates the radiosensitivity of human melanoma cells. *Radiat Res.* 2000; 154: 497–502.
171. Folberg R, Pe'er J, Gruman LM, Woolson RF, Jeng G, Montague PR, Moninger TO, Yi H, Moore KC. The morphologic characteristics of tumor blood vessels as a marker of tumor progression in primary human uveal melanoma: a matched case-control study. *Hum Pathol.* 1992; 23: 1298–1305.
172. Rummelt V, Gardner LM, Folberg R, Beck S, Knosp B, Moninger TO, Moore KC. Three-dimensional relationships between tumor cells and microcirculation with double cyanine immunolabeling, laser scanning confocal microscopy, and computer-assisted reconstruction: an alternative to cast corrosion preparations. *J Histochem Cytochem.* 1994; 42: 681–686.
173. Rummelt V, Folberg R, Rummelt C, Gruman LM, Hwang T, Woolson RF, Yi H, Naumann GO. Microcirculation architecture of melanocytic nevi and malignant melanomas of the ciliary body and choroid: a comparative histopathologic and ultrastructural study. *Ophthalmology.* 1994; 101: 718–727.
174. Rummelt V, Axmacher K, Folberg R, Naumann GOH. Microcirculation patterns as prognostic factor in conjunctival melanoma. *Invest Ophthalmol Vis Sci [ARVO Abstr].* 1997; 38: S807.
175. Warso MA, Maniotis AJ, Chen X, Majumdar D, Patel MK, Shilkaitis A, Gupta TK, Folberg R. Prognostic significance of periodic acid-Schiff-positive patterns in primary cutaneous melanoma. *Clin Cancer Res.* 2001; 7: 473–477.
176. Hess AR, Seftor EA, Gardner LM, Carles-Kinch K, Schneider GB, Seftor RE, Kinch MS, Hendrix MJ. Molecular regulation of tumor cell vasculogenic mimicry by tyrosine phosphorylation: role of epithelial cell kinase (Eck/EphA2). *Cancer Res.* 2001; 61: 3250–3255.
177. Weidner N, Semple JP, Welch WR, Folkman J. Tumor angiogenesis and metastasis-correlation in invasive breast carcinoma. *N Engl J Med.* 1991; 324: 1–8.
178. Weidner N. Intratumor microvessel density as a prognostic factor in cancer. *Am J Pathol.* 1995; 147: 9–19.
179. Weidner N. Angiogenesis as a predictor of clinical outcome in cancer patients. *Hum Pathol.* 2000; 31: 403–405.
180. Graham CH, Rivers J, Kerbel RS, Stankiewicz KS, White WL. Extent of vascularization as a prognostic indicator in thin (<0.76 mm) malignant melanomas. *Am J Pathol.* 1994; 145: 510–514.
181. Busam KJ, Berwick M, Blessing K, Fandrey K, Kang S, Karaoli T, Fine J, Cochran AJ, White WL, Rivers J. Tumor vascularity is not a prognostic factor for malignant melanoma of the skin. *Am J Pathol.* 1995; 147: 1049–1056.

182. De Waal RM, Van Altena MC, Erhard H, Weidle UH, Nooijen PT, Ruiter DJ. Lack of lymphangiogenesis in human primary cutaneous melanoma. Consequences for the mechanism of lymphatic dissemination. *Am J Pathol.* 1997; 150: 1951–1957.
183. Folberg R, Mehaffey M, Gardner LM, Meyer M, Rummelt V, Pe'er J. The microcirculation of choroidal and ciliary body melanomas. *Eye.* 1997; 11: 227–238.
184. Folberg R, Hendrix MJC, Maniotis AJ. Vasculogenic mimicry and tumor angiogenesis. *Am J Pathol.* 2000; 156: 361–381.
185. Foss AJE, Alexander RA, Hungerford JL, Harris AL, Cree IA, Lightman S. Reassessment of the PAS patterns in uveal melanoma. *Br J Ophthalmol.* 1997; 81: 240–246.
186. Schaling DF, Van der Pol JP, Schlingemann RO, Parys-Van Ginderdeuren R, Ruiter DJ, Jager MJ. Vascular density and vascular patterns in the prognosis of choroidal melanoma. *Thesis D.F. Schaling: Radionuclides and radiolabelled antibodies in choroidal melanoma (diagnosis and therapy).* Leiden: Rijksuniversiteit te Leiden; 1996: 43–54.
187. Lane AM, Egan KM, Yang J, Saornil MA, Alroy J, Albert D, Gragoudas ES. An evaluation of tumour vascularity as a prognostic indicator in uveal melanoma. *Melanoma Res.* 1997; 7: 237–242.
188. Chen X, Maniotis AJ, Majumdar D, Pe'er J, Folberg R. Uveal melanoma cell staining for CD34 and assessment of tumor vascularity. *Invest Ophthalmol Vis Sci.* 2002; 43: 2533–2539.
189. Al Jamal RT, Mäkitie T, Kivelä T. Nucleolar diameter and microvascular factors as independent predictors of mortality from malignant melanoma of the choroid and ciliary body. *Invest Ophthalmol Vis Sci.* 2003; 44: 2381–2389.
190. Hendrix MJ, Seftor EA, Hess AR, Seftor RE. Molecular plasticity of human melanoma cells. *Oncogene.* 2003; 22: 3070–3075.
191. Hendrix MJ, Seftor EA, Seftor REB, Kirschmann DA, Gardner LM, Boldt HC, Meyer M, Pe'er J, Folberg R. Regulation of uveal melanoma interconverted phenotype by hepatocyte growth factor/scatter factor (HGF/SF). *Am J Pathol.* 1998; 152: 855–863.
192. Hendrix MJ, Seftor EA, Seftor RE, Gardner LM, Boldt HC, Meyer M, Pe'er J, Folberg R. Biologic determinants of uveal melanoma metastatic phenotype: role of intermediate filaments as predictive markers. *Lab Invest.* 1998; 78: 153–163.
193. Mooy CM, Luyten GP, De Jong PT, Jensen OA, Luider TM, Van der Ham F, Bosman FT. Neural cell adhesion molecule distribution in primary and metastatic uveal melanoma. *Hum Pathol.* 1995; 26: 1185–1190.
194. Foss AJ, Alexander RA, Guille MJ, Hungerford JL, McCartney AC, Lightman S. Estrogen and progesterone receptor analysis in ocular melanomas. *Ophthalmology.* 1995; 102: 431–435.
195. Mäkitie T, Tarkkanen A, Kivelä T. Comparative immunohistochemical oestrogen receptor analysis in primary and metastatic uveal melanoma. *Graefes Arch Clin Exp Ophthalmol.* 1998; 236: 415–419.
196. Ma D, Niederkorn JY. Role of epidermal growth factor receptor in the metastasis of intraocular melanomas. *Invest Ophthalmol Vis Sci.* 1998; 39: 1067–1075.
197. Hurks HM, Metzelaar-Blok JA, Barthen ER, Zwinderman AH, Wolff-Rouendaal D, Keunen JE, Jager MJ. Expression of epidermal growth factor receptor: risk factor in uveal melanoma. *Invest Ophthalmol Vis Sci.* 2000; 41: 2023–2027.
198. Scholes AG, Hagan S, Hiscott P, Damato BE, Grierson I. Overexpression of epidermal growth factor receptor restricted to macrophages in uveal melanoma. *Arch Ophthalmol.* 2001; 119: 373–377.

199. Väisänen A, Kallioinen M, von Dickhoff K, Laatikainen L, Hoyhtya M, Turpeenniemi-Hujanen T. Matrix metalloproteinase-2 (MMP-2) immunoreactive protein — A new prognostic marker in uveal melanoma? *J Pathol.* 1999; 188: 56–62.
200. Van der Velden PA, Zuidervaart W, Hurks MH, Pavey S, Ksander BR, Krijgsman E, Frants RR, Tensen CP, Willemze R, Jager MJ, Gruis NA. Expression profiling reveals that methylation of TIMP3 is involved in uveal melanoma development. *Int J Cancer.* 2003; 106: 472–479.
201. Mooy CM, Luyten GP, De Jong PT, Luider TM, Stijnen T, Van der Ham F, Van Vroonhoven CC, Bosman FT. Immunohistochemical and prognostic analysis of apoptosis and proliferation in uveal melanoma. *Am J Pathol.* 1995; 147: 1097–1104.
202. Karlsson M, Boeryd B, Carstensen J, Franlund B, Gustafsson B, Kagedal B, Sun XF, Wingren S. Correlations of Ki-67 and PCNA to DNA ploidy, S-phase fraction and survival in uveal melanoma. *Eur J Cancer.* 1996; 32A: 357–362.
203. Seregard S, Oskarsson M, Spångberg B. PC-10 as a predictor of prognosis after antigen retrieval in posterior uveal melanoma. *Invest Ophthalmol Vis Sci.* 1996; 37: 1451–1458.
204. Coupland SE, Anastassiou G, Stang A, Schilling H, Anagnostopoulos I, Bornfeld N, Stein H. The prognostic value of cyclin D1, p53, and MDM2 protein expression in uveal melanoma. *J Pathol.* 2000; 191: 120–126.
205. Ghazvini S, Kroll S, Char DH, Frigillana H. Comparative analysis of proliferating cell nuclear antigen, bromodeoxyuridine, and mitotic index in uveal melanoma. *Invest Ophthalmol Vis Sci.* 1995; 36: 2762–2767.
206. Coupland SE, Bechrakis N, Schuler A, Anagnostopoulos I, Hummel M, Bornfeld N, Stein H. Expression patterns of cyclin D1 and related proteins regulating G1-S phase transition in uveal melanoma and retinoblastoma. *Br J Ophthalmol.* 1998; 82: 901–970.
207. Gamel JW, McCurdy JB, McLean IW. A comparison of prognostic covariates for uveal melanoma. *Invest Ophthalmol Vis Sci.* 1992; 33: 1919–1922.
208. Sørensen FB, Gamel JW, Jensen OA, Ladekarl M, McCurdy J. Prognostic value of nucleolar size and size pleomorphism in choroidal melanomas. *APMIS.* 1993; 101: 358–368.
209. Coleman K, Baak JP, van Diest PJ, Mullaney J. Prognostic value of morphometric features and the callender classification in uveal melanomas. *Ophthalmology.* 1996; 103: 1634–1641.
210. McLean IW, Sibug ME, Becker RL, McCurdy JB. Uveal melanoma: the importance of large nucleoli in predicting patient outcome — An Automated image analysis study. *Cancer.* 1997; 79: 982–988.
211. Pe'er J, Rummelt V, Mawn L, Hwang T, Woolson RF, Folberg R. Mean of the ten largest nucleoli, microcirculation architecture, and prognosis of ciliochoroidal melanomas. *Ophthalmology.* 1994; 101: 1227–1235.
212. Meecham WJ, Char DH. DNA content abnormalities and prognosis in uveal melanoma. *Arch Ophthalmol.* 1986; 104: 1626–1629.
213. Toti P, Greco G, Mangiavacchi P, Bruni A, Palmeri ML, Luzi P. DNA ploidy pattern in choroidal melanoma: correlation with survival. A flow cytometry study on archival material. *Br J Ophthalmol.* 1998; 82: 1433–1437.
214. Hodge WG, Duclos AJ, Rocha G, Antecka E, Baines MG, Corriveau C, Brownstein S, Deschenes J. DNA index and S phase fraction in uveal malignant melanomas. *Br J Ophthalmol.* 1995; 79: 521–526.
215. Horsthemke B, Prescher G, Bornfeld N, Becher R. Loss of chromosome 3 alleles and multiplication of chromosome 8 alleles in uveal melanoma. *Genes Chromosomes Cancer.* 1992; 4: 217–221.

216. Prescher G, Bornfeld N, Hirche H, Horsthemke B, Jockel KH, Becher R. Prognostic implications of monosomy 3 in uveal melanoma. *Lancet.* 1996; 347: 1222–1225.
217. Myatt N, Aristodemou P, Neale MH, Foss AJ, Hungerford JL, Bhattacharya S, Cree A. Abnormalities of the transforming growth factor-beta pathway in ocular melanoma. *J Pathol.* 2000; 192: 511–518.
218. Ma D, Luyten GP, Luider TM, Jager MJ, Niederkorn JY. Association between NM23-H1 gene expression and metastasis of human uveal melanoma in an animal model. *Invest Ophthalmol Vis Sci.* 1996; 37: 2293–2301.
219. Greco IM, Calvisi G, Ventura L, Cerrito F. An immunohistochemical analysis of nm23 gene product expression in uveal melanoma. *Melanoma Res.* 1997; 7: 231–236.
220. Chana JS, Cree IA, Foss AJ, Hungerford JL, Wilson GD. The prognostic significance of c-myc oncogene expression in uveal melanoma. *Melanoma Res.* 1998; 8: 139–144.
221. Chana JS, Wilson GD, Cree IA, Alexander RA, Myatt N, Neale M, Foss AJ, Hungerford JL. c-myc, p53, and Bcl-2 expression and clinical outcome in uveal melanoma. *Br J Ophthalmol.* 1999; 83: 110–114.
222. Jay V, Yi Q, Hunter WS, Zielenska M. Expression of bcl-2 in uveal malignant melanoma. *Arch Pathol Lab Med.* 1996; 120: 497–498.
223. Brantley MA, Jr., Harbour JW. Deregulation of the Rb and p53 pathways in uveal melanoma. *Am J Pathol.* 2000; 157: 1795-1801.
224. Kishore K, Ghazvini S, Char DH, Kroll S, Selle J. p53 gene and cell cycling in uveal melanoma. *Am J Ophthalmol.* 1996; 121: 561–567.
225. Schurmans LRHM, Blom DJR, De Waard-Siebinga I, Keunen JEE, Prause JU, Jager MJ. Effects of transpupillary thermotherapy on immunological parameters and apoptosis in a case of primary uveal melanoma. *Melanoma Res.* 1999; 9: 297–302.
226. Shaif-Muthana M, McIntyre C, Sisley K, Rennie I, Murray A. Dead or alive: immunogenicity of human melanoma cells when presented by dendritic cells. *Cancer Res.* 2000; 60: 6441–6447.
227. Kim K, Pang KM, Evans M, Hay ED. Overexpression of beta-catenin induces apoptosis independent of its transactivation function with LEF-1 or the involvement of major G1 cell cycle regulators. *Mol Biol Cell.* 2000; 11: 3509–3523.

JACOB PE'ER

# 2. Uveal Nevi versus Uveal Melanomas

## INTRODUCTION

As compared to cutaneous and conjunctival melanocytic lesions, very little is known about the histogenesis and evolution of uveal melanocytic lesions, other than uveal melanoma which necessitates enucleation of the affected eye. The precursor lesions to cutaneous and conjunctival melanomas are well known, and nevi and pre-cancerous melanocytic lesions such as primary acquired melanosis in these sites have been extensively studied.[1–4] Unfortunately, it is difficult to study nevi and possible pre-malignant conditions in the uvea, because, unlike the skin and conjunctiva which are accessible to biopsy for establishing clinicopathologic correlations of early precursor stages, it is not feasible to obtain tissue from early uveal precursor lesions, except from the rare eyes studied clinically that are subsequently obtained at post-mortem examination.[5]

Currently, all animal models of uveal melanoma are established by injecting melanoma cells into various parts of animals' eyes. These models do not enable the study of the natural evolution of uveal melanoma from their precursors, such as nevi and atypical melanocytic lesions. About ten years ago, we tried to induce primary uveal melanocytic lesions in the eyes of Dutch pigmented rabbits, using a two-stage carcinogenesis protocol involving initiation by topical application of DMBA followed by topical applications of croton oil.[6] By this method we induced clinically detectable pigmented fundus lesions. Histologically, a spectrum of melanocytic proliferations developed, including benign nevi, nevi with varying grades of cytologic atypia, and clusters of confluent atypical melanocytes that may represent early melanomas. Although in this model we did not succeed in developing a real melanoma mass, we proposed the existence of a spectrum of melanocytic uveal lesions including intermediate atypical melanocytic uveal precursor lesions that are not known in humans.

## FEATURES OF CHOROIDAL NEVI

An uveal nevus was defined as an aggregate of variably pigmented melanocytic cells arranged in a mass or nodule that replaces the normal uveal architecture.

The type of cells comprising a uveal nevus varies, and are generally classified as plump polyhedral, slender spindle, plump spindle or fusiform, dendritic, or balloon cells.[7]

Dr. Donald Gass in his Jackson Memorial lecture[5] in 1976 suggested the following features of choroidal nevi: (1) they are not present at birth and are infrequently found in children under 12 years of age; (2) they arise probably from very small cell nests as hyperplastic lesions that exhibit growth primarily but not exclusively in late childhood and early adulthood; (3) their growth may not occur in a linear fashion but may be subject to periods of acceleration in response to humoral or other factors; (4) although they usually attain an average size of 0.5 to 2 disk diameters and are flat or slightly elevated, a small percentage may achieve a larger size that may be mistaken for a malignant melanoma; (5) they frequently cause overlying pigmented epithelial and retinal degenerative changes, such as drusen, atrophy of the pigment epithelium and other retinal layers, serous detachment of the pigment epithelium and retina, choroidal neovascularization and hemorrhagic detachment of the overlying retina; and (6) the Callender classification includes choroidal nevi as well as malignant melanomas.

A major part of this book is devoted to prognostic parameters of uveal melanoma. The comparison between clinical and histologic features of melanomas and nevi is difficult because of a lack of pathologic specimens of uveal nevi. I'll try to compare at least part of the clinical and histopathologic parameters in order to find the similarities and the differences between these two types of melanocytic uveal lesions.

## CLINICAL INFORMATION

Naumann and colleagues[7] found a median age of 44.5 years and mean age of 59.2 years in patients with diagnosed posterior uveal nevi, similar to the age of patients with posterior uveal melanoma at the time of diagnosis. The vast majority of the patients with nevi were Caucasians, similar to the melanoma patients. Six percent of the nevi were located in the ciliary body, as compared to about 10% of the uveal melanomas. Of course, the involvement of the ciliary body in these cases does not have prognostic significance. The majority of the uveal nevi were smaller than 5 mm in diameter and less than 2 mm in thickness, as opposed to melanomas that are usually significantly larger; and actually when a suspected lesion is smaller than the above-mentioned sizes, it is considered to be a nevus.

As mentioned above,[5] clinical features that are considered by some experts to be of prognostic importance, such as the existence of drusen, retinal detachment, RPE changes, choroidal neovascularization or hemorrhagic retinal detachment, can be found in uveal nevi. Even growth of a melanocytic uveal lesion is not a pathognomonic sign for melanoma.

## HISTOLOGY AND VASCULAR PATTERNS

Histologically, the cell types in choroidal nevi are variable, as mentioned above. Gass[5] suggests the spindle cell type A, and even type B, can be found in uveal nevi, but of course we do not expect to find epithelioid cells in these lesions. Also, mitotic figures that are not frequently observed even in melanomas, are not expected to be found in nevi. Two studies by Marcus et al.[8,9] showed significantly less silver-stained nucleolar organizer region dots per cell in posterior uveal and in iris nevi as compared to melanomas in similar locations. They concluded that this method may help in differentiating benign uveal melanocytic lesions from malignant melanomas.

Folberg et al. described 10 years ago nine microcirculation patterns in histologic sections of posterior uveal melanoma:[10,11] normal vessels, avascular (silent) zones, straight vessels, parallel vascular channels without and with cross-linking, arcs without and with branching, closed loops surrounding clusters of tumor cells, and networks of loops, defined as a focus of at least three back-to-back loops. The last six vascular patterns, especially the last two, were found to be associated with death from metastatic melanomas. This association has been confirmed by other independent groups of researchers.[12–15]

Rummelt et al.[16] described the vascular patterns of ciliary body and choroidal nevi and compared them to those of posterior uveal melanomas. They found that the only vascular patterns identified in nevi are 'normal' vessels, zones of avascularity—namely 'silent', straight and parallel vessels. Not one of the closed vascular patterns was found in the nevi. None of the patients with nevi died of metastatic disease. Among the melanoma patients who had the same vascular profile as nevi, only 14% died of metastatic disease, whereas 32% of patients whose melanomas had patterns that carry a bad prognosis died of metastatic melanoma. According to these findings, they graded the melanocytic uveal lesion into nevi that are benign, melanomas that have the same vascular profile as nevi as having intermediate biologic behavior, and melanomas with closed vascular patterns as strongly associated with death due to metastatic disease.

## IRIS MELANOMA

Iris melanomas are known to have very benign biological behavior, and only less than 4% of them will metastasize.[17] Histologically, a higher proportion of iris melanomas than posterior uveal melanomas are composed of spindle cells rather than epithelioid cells or mixed cell population.[18] Thus, iris melanomas are more comparable to posterior uveal nevi than to posterior uveal melanomas. Chowers et al.[19] compared the tumor cell proliferation as measured histologically by staining of tumor cells by MIB-1 antibody and histologic microcirculation patterns between melanomas confined to the iris and melanomas involving either the ciliary body or choroid. They found that histologic microcirculation patterns associated with death from metastatic disease in posterior uveal melanomas were not found at all in any of the iris melanomas. The only vascular patterns found in iris melanomas were 'normal', 'silent', and straight, as in posterior uveal nevi. The mean MIB-1 positive cell count per high-power field was $1.9 \pm 0.4$ in iris melanomas, as compared to $19.9 \pm 3.5$ in choroidal and $27 \pm 5.3$ in ciliary body melanomas ($p = 0.003$). Both features are consistent with the relatively benign nature of iris lesions, which is quite comparable to uveal nevi.

## SUMMARY AND CONCLUSION

Due to the lack of accessible tissue of uveal nevi, especially from the posterior uvea, it is difficult to assess the nature of these benign lesions and their possible evolution to melanomas. Their clinical appearance and complications may confuse them in some cases with uveal melanomas, but their clinical behavior and histologic findings are of a benign nature. Some of their histologic features, such as microcirculatory patterns, are similar to iris melanomas that are of known relatively benign biologic behavior.

## REFERENCES


1. Clark WH Jr, From L, Bernardino EH, Mihm MC. The histogenesis and biologic behavior of primary human malignant melanomas of the skin. *Cancer Res.* 1969;29: 705–727.
2. Clark WH Jr, Elder DE, Guerry D IV, Epstein MN, Greene MH, Van Horn M. A study of tumor progression: the precursor lesions of superficial spreading and nodular melanoma. *Hum Pathol.* 1984;15:1147–1165.
3. Folberg R, McLean IW, Zimmerman LE. Primary acquired melanosis of the conjunctiva. *Hum Pathol.* 1985;16:129–135.
4. Folberg R, McLean IW. Primary acquired melanosis and melanoma of the conjunctiva: terminology, classification and biologic behavior. *Hum Pathol.* 1986;17:652–654.
5. Gass JDM. Problems in the differential diagnosis of choroidal nevi and malignant melanomas. The XXXII Edward Jackson Memorial Lecture. *Am J Ophthalmol.* 1977;83: 299–323.
6. Pe'er J, Folberg R, Massicotte SJ, Baron J, Parys-Van Ginderdeuren R, Zimmerman B, Meyer ML, Worsey H. Clinicopathologic spectrum of primary uveal melanocytic lesions in an animal model. *Ophthalmology.* 1992;99:977–986.
7. Naumann G, Yanoff M, Zimmerman LE. Histogenesis of malignant melanomas of the uvea. I. Histopathologic characteristics of nevi of the choroid and ciliary body. *Arch Ophthalmol.* 1966;76:784–796.
8. Marcus DM, Minkovitz JB, Wardwell SD, Albert DM. The value of nucleolar organizer regions in uveal melanoma. The Collaborative Ocular Melanoma Study Group. *Am J Ophthalmol.* 1990;110:527–534.
9. Marcus DM, Mawn LA, Egan KM, Albert DM. Nucleolar organizer regions in iris nevi and melanomas. *Am J Ophthalmol.* 1992;114:202–207.
10. Folberg R, Pe'er J, Gruman LM, Woolson RF, Jeng G, Montague PR, Moninger TO, Yi H, Moore KC. The morphologic characteristics of tumor blood vessels as a marker of tumor progression in primary human uveal melanoma: a matched case-control study. *Hum Pathol.* 1992;23:1298–1305.
11. Folberg R, Rummelt V, Parys-Van Ginderdeuren R, Hwang T, Woolson RF, Pe'er J, Gruman LM. The prognostic value of tumor blood vessel morphology in primary uveal melanoma. *Ophthalmology.* 1993;100:1389–1398.
12. Sakamoto T, Sakamoto M, Yoshikawa H, Hata Y, Ishibashi T, Ohnishi Y, Inomata H. Histologic findings and prognosis of uveal malignant melanoma in Japanese patients. *Am J Ophthalmol.* 1996;121:276–283.
13. McLean IW, Keefe KS, Burnier MN. Uveal melanoma: comparison of the prognostic value of fibrovascular loops, mean of the ten largest nucleoli, cell type and tumor size. *Ophthalmology.* 1997;104:777–780.

14. Seregard S, Spangberg B, Juul C, Oskarsson M. Prognostic accuracy of the mean of the largest nucleoli, vascular patterns, and PC-10 in posterior uveal melanoma. *Ophthalmology.* 1998;105:485–491.
15. Makitie T, Summanen P, Tarkkannen A, Kivela T. Microvascular loops and networks as prognostic indicators in choroidal and ciliary body melanomas. *J Natl Cancer Inst.* 1999;91:359–367.
16. Rummelt V, Folberg R, Rummelt C, Gruman LM, Hwang T, Woolson RF, Yi H, Naumann GO. Microcirculation architecture of melanocytic nevi and malignant melanomas of the ciliary body and choroid. A comparative histopathologic and ultrastructural study. *Ophthalmology.* 1994;101:718–727.
17. Geisse LJ, Robertson DM. Iris melanomas. *Am J Ophthalmol.* 1985;99:638–648.
18. Davidorf FH. The melanoma controversy. A comparison of choroidal, cutaneous, and iris melanomas. *Surv Ophthalmol.* 1981;25:373–377.
19. Chowers I, Folberg R, Livni N, Pe'er, J. Comparison of microcirculation patterns and MIB-1 immunoreactivity in iris and posterior uveal melanoma. *Ophthalmology.* 2001; 108:367–371.

ARUN D. SINGH

# 3. Genetic Predisposition in Uveal Melanoma

## INTRODUCTION

Uveal melanoma usually occurs sporadically without any obvious genetic or environmental predisposing factors.[1] However, in rare patients, there is a suggestion of ill understood genetic factors. Almost 100 years ago Silcock first reported occurrence of uveal melanoma in a mother and her two daughters.[2] Since then few reports have discussed the role of genetic factors in uveal melanoma.[3,4]

In general, patients with an inherited cancer predisposition syndrome tend to have familial occurrence of cancer, develop cancer at an earlier age, have bilateral involvement of paired organs, multiple primary tumors, and phenotypic associations.[5] Occurrence of uveal melanoma in each settings such as familial uveal melanoma, uveal melanoma in young individuals, bilateral primary uveal melanoma, multi-focal primary uveal melanoma, and phenotypic associations with oculo (dermal) melanocytosis, familial atypical mole and melanoma syndrome, and neurofibromatosis type 1 have been described (Table 3.1). The purpose of this chapter is to present a comprehensive review of genetic factors predisposing to uveal melanoma.

Table 3.1. Clinical subtypes of uveal melanoma.

| Feature | Subtype of uveal melanoma |
|---|---|
| Familial occurrence | Familial uveal melanoma |
| Occurrence at an earlier age | Uveal melanoma in young individual |
| Bilateral involvement | Bilateral primary uveal melanoma |
| Multiple primary tumor | Multi-focal primary uveal melanoma |
| Phenotypic associations | |
| Ocular | Oculo (dermal) melanocytosis |
| Systemic | Familial atypical mole and melanoma syndrome |
| | Neurofibromatosis type 1 |

## FAMILIAL UVEAL MELANOMA

The occurrence of familial uveal melanoma is very rare, comprising only 0.6% of all uveal melanoma patients.[6] A review of published kindreds with familial uveal melanoma reveals that involvement over many generations, typical of autosomal dominant inheritance, is extremely rare and usually is limited to only two relatives in a family.[6,7] The expected features of a genetic predisposition such as earlier age at diagnosis, bilateral involvement, multiple primary tumors, and phenotypic associations are not clearly evident in familial uveal melanoma.[8,9]

The probability of two affected members in a family (Pfum) = $[(Puvm)(x)]^2$ can be derived from the prevalence of uveal melanoma (Puvm) adjusted for family size ($x$).[9] The likelihood of familial uveal melanoma (Pfum) in the family studied by us was calculated to be 1 in 10 million = $[(7.4 \times 10^{-5})(5)]^2$, where $7.4 \times 10^{-5}$ is the estimated prevalence of uveal melanoma and 5 is the number of the first degree relatives of the proband.[9] Considering the low prevalence of uveal melanoma in the general population, the likelihood of uveal melanoma occurring in a family setting is very remote.[8,9]

## UVEAL MELANOMA IN YOUNG INDIVIDUALS

Approximately 1% of all uveal melanomas occur in patients less than 20 years of age.[10] Most of the pediatric uveal melanomas occur around puberty although they can even be present at birth. The clinical features of pediatric uveal melanoma are similar to those of adult uveal melanoma. Uveal melanomas in young patients have been successfully treated with enucleation, local resection, episcleral radioactive plaque application and photocoagulation, the modalities used to treat uveal melanoma in adults. The data regarding systemic prognosis suggest that the long-term prognosis (15 years) is no worse than in adults (30% mortality) and the short term prognosis (up to 5 years) may be even better than in adults.[10]

Occurrence of a tumor at an early age, among other features, is suggestive of an inherited cancer predisposition. Verdaguer reported the presence of ocular melanocytosis, a condition predisposing to uveal melanoma in four out of seven young patients with choroidal melanoma.[11] Greer in his case report of a congenital uveal melanoma noted 'numerous pigmented cutaneous nevi in the infant and the mother.'[12] A case of iris melanoma in a ten-year-old boy who had features suggestive of familial atypical mole and melanoma syndrome has also been reported.[13] Young patients with uveal melanoma represent a heterogeneous group displaying various associations, especially with oculo (dermal) melanocytosis. Oculo (dermal) melanocytosis is nine times more common in young patients with uveal melanoma than uveal melanoma in the general population.[10] Children with uveal melanoma provide a unique opportunity to investigate the presence of a genetic predisposition.

## BILATERAL UVEAL MELANOMA

Primary uveal melanoma is rarely bilateral.[14] Since the report of Shine in 1930 approximately 44 well documented cases of bilateral primary uveal melanoma have been reported worldwide.[14,15] Bilateral primary uveal melanoma should be distinguished from benign diffuse uveal melanocytic proliferation (BDUMP) syndrome which is characterized by a benign paraneoplastic proliferation of uveal melanocytes in association with a systemic malignancy.[16] Shammas and Watzke estimated that in the United States only one case of bilateral uveal melanoma will occur every 18 years.[17] In the absence of any identifiable predisposing factors, the occurrence of bilateral primary uveal melanoma has been assumed to be a rare random event.

In a series of bilateral primary uveal melanoma patients that were analyzed for the role of genetic predisposition, there was no apparent clinical evidence to indicate inherited cancer predisposition.[14] Bilateral ocular melanocytosis was thought to be contributory in two patients. No association between bilateral primary uveal melanoma with familial atypical mole and melanoma syndrome, familial uveal melanoma, neurofibromatosis type 1, or Li–Fraumeni syndrome was observed.

## MULTI-FOCAL UVEAL MELANOMA

Typically, uveal melanoma is a solitary tumor. Multi-focal melanoma, a rare variant of uveal melanoma is extremely rare. In the majority of the reported cases no predisposition has been observed[18] where as some cases had underlying oculo (dermal) melanocytosis.[19]

## PHENOTYPIC ASSOCIATIONS

### OCULAR

*Oculo (dermal) melanocytosis*

Oculo (dermal) melanocytosis represents congenital hyperpigmentation of skin, episclera, uvea, orbit and meninges.[20] It is estimated to occur about 35 times more often in patients with uveal melanoma than in general Caucasian population.[20] Melanoma can also arise from other hyperpigmented sites such as orbit and meninges. In the majority of cases oculo (dermal) melanocytosis is unilateral and uveal melanoma develops ipsilateral to the side of hyperpigmentation.

It is estimated that about 1 in 400 patients with ODM followed for life will develop uveal melanoma.[21] Excessive melanocytes in the uveal tract in ODM may provide the biologic basis for susceptibility to the development of uveal melanoma. Patients with ODM should be monitored ophthalmoscopically.

### SYSTEMIC

*Familial atypical multiple mole and melanoma syndrome*

The syndrome of autosomal dominant predisposition to cutaneous melanoma was previously described by various names such as BK mole syndrome,[22] and dysplastic nevus syndrome.[23] Familial atypical multiple mole and melanoma (FAMMM) syndrome is now considered the preferred terminology.[24] According to the National Institutes of Health (US) consensus panel it is defined by the occurrence of a large number of atypical (often more than 50) irregular and multicolored cutaneous nevi, cutaneous melanoma in one or more first or second degree relatives and the presence of certain distinct histologic features such as melanocytic nuclear pleomorphism, hyperchromatism, melanocytic hyperplasia, architectural disorder with asymmetry, subepidermal fibroplasia, and frequent dermal lymphocytic infiltration.[24]

Several cases of uveal melanoma have been reported in patients with FAMMM syndrome.[25] The lifetime chance of coexistence of primary uveal melanoma and primary cutaneous melanoma is remote (estimated to be 1 in 160,000) and therefore, such an occurrence is thought to represent an association between the two entities.[25,26] This hypothesis is appealing because cutaneous and uveal melanocytes share similar embryologic, morphologic and antigenic properties. An increased number of uveal nevi in patients with the FAMMM syndrome and the occurrence of cutaneous melanoma and uveal melanoma in different members of a family with FAMMM syndrome supports an association between FAMMM syndrome and uveal melanoma.[27–29] In a prospective study of 207 consecutive patients with ocular melanoma (uveal, conjunctival and eyelid melanoma) a greater than expected prevalence of cutaneous melanoma (five patients) was observed. Two of these five patients had features of FAMMM syndrome. The authors concluded that FAMMM syndrome predisposes to both cutaneous and ocular melanoma.[30]

On the other hand, the coexistence of uveal melanoma and FAMMM syndrome has been suggested to be coincidental.[31,32] The Connecticut Tumor Registry Data revealed only one case of uveal melanoma (representing the expected prevalence) in a population of 13,841 individuals with cutaneous melanoma.[33]

Some of the discrepancy in different studies could be attributed to the lack of uniform criteria used for diagnosis of the FAMMM syndrome. With the use of a uniform definition as proposed by the NIH consensus panel this will be eliminated in the future. Long-term prospective studies are necessary to investigate the relationship between FAMMM syndrome and uveal melanoma because the interval between the diagnosis of these two entities may be as long as 10 years.[25] With increased awareness we may see a stronger association between FAMMM syndrome and primary uveal melanoma.

*Neurofibromatosis type 1*

NF1 is a common autosomal dominant hamartomatous disorder, and is considered to be a neurocristopathy.[34] Uveal melanoma, also of neural crest origin, is the most common primary malignant intraocular tumor in adults. The association of NF1 and uveal melanoma is controversial. To our knowledge, only 18 cases of uveal melanoma including three cases of iris melanoma have been reported in association with NF1.[35] On the basis of the prevalence of NF1 (1 in 3000) and the prevalence of uveal melanoma (1 in 13,500) it can be estimated that approximately seven patients with NF1 in the United States would have an associated uveal melanoma by chance alone. We conclude that despite the theoretical possibility of a causal association between uveal melanoma and NF1, it may still be regarded as coincidental in the absence of any strong evidence to the contrary.[35]

*Li–Fraumeni syndrome*

The presence of breast cancer in a family with uveal melanoma led Jay and McCartney to speculate on the presence of the Li–Fraumeni syndrome.[36] The Li–Fraumeni syndrome is an autosomal dominant trait which predisposes to soft tissue sarcoma, brain tumors, leukemia, breast cancer and other cancers in many members of a family.[37,38] Although patients with familial uveal melanoma have been calculated to have a four times increased likelihood for developing a second primary malignancy as compared to the general population,[6] an association of familial uveal melanoma with a generalized inherited predisposition to cancer remains to be firmly established.

## CONCLUSIONS

Of all conditions discussed above, only oculo (dermal)melanocytosis represents a genetic predisposition to uveal melanoma. All cases of familial uveal melanoma, bilateral primary uveal melanoma or uveal melanoma occurring in the presence of a clinical syndrome such as familial atypical mole and melanoma syndrome should be documented with a complete family history and investigated further.

## REFERENCES


1. Egan KM, Seddon JM, Glynn RJ, Gragoudas ES, Albert DM. Epidemiologic aspects of uveal melanoma. *Surv Ophthalmol.* 1988;32:239–251.
2. Silcock AQ. Hereditary sarcoma of the eyeball. *Trans Pathol Soc Lond.* 1892;43:140–141.
3. Singh AD, Wang MX, Donoso LA, Shields CL, De Potter P, Shields JA. Genetic aspects of uveal melanoma: a brief review. *Sem Oncol.* 1996;23:768–772.
4. Houlston RS, Damato BE. Genetic predisposition to ocular melanoma. *Eye.* 1999;13: 43–46.
5. Ponder BAJ. Inherited cancer syndromes. In: Carney D, Sikora K, eds. *Genes and Cancer.* New York: John Wiley and Sons, 1990;99–106.
6. Singh AD, Shields CL, De Potter P, Shields JA, Trock B, Cater J, Pastore D. Familial uveal melanoma I: Clinical observations on 56 patients. *Arch Ophthalmol.* 1996;114:392–399.
7. Young LHY, Egan KM, Walsh SM, Gragoudas ES. Familial uveal melanoma. *Am J Ophthalmol.* 1994;117:516–520.
8. Singh AD, Wang MX, Donoso LA, Shields CL, De Potter P, Shields JA, Elston RC, Fijal B. Familial uveal melanoma III: Is the occurrence of familial uveal melanoma coincidental? *Arch Ophthalmol.* 1996;114:1101–1104.
9. Singh AD, Demirci H, Smith AF, Shields CL, Shields JA. Concurrent Choroidal Melanoma in Son and Father. *Am J Ophthalmol.* 2000;130:679–680.
10. Singh AD, Shields CL, Shields JA, Sato T. Uveal melanoma in young patients. *Arch Ophthalmol.* 2000;118:918–923.
11. Verdaguer J Jr. Prepuberal and puberal melanomas in ophthalmology. *Am J Ophthalmol.* 1965;60:1002–1011.
12. Greer CH. Congenital melanoma of the anterior uvea. *Arch Ophthalmol.* 1966;76:77–78.
13. Singh AD, Shields JA, Eagle RC, Shields CL, Marmor M, De Potter P. Iris melanoma in a ten-year-old boy with familial atypical mole and melanoma (FAM-M) syndrome. *Ophthalmic Genet.* 1994;15:145–149.
14. Singh AD, Shields CL, Shields JA, De Potter P, Cater JR. Bilateral Primary Uveal Melanoma: Bad Luck or Bad genes? *Ophthalmology.* 1996;103:256–262.
15. Shine FW. Report of a case of bilateral sarcoma of the uveal tract. *N Y Eye Ear Infirm Clin Rep.* 1930;1:31–33.
16. Barr CC, Zimmerman LE, Curtin VT, Font RL. Bilateral diffuse melanocytic uveal tumors associated with systemic malignant neoplasms. A recently recognized syndrome. *Arch Ophthalmol.* 1982;100:249–255.

17. Shammas HF, Watzke RC. Bilateral choroidal melanomas. Case report and incidence. *Arch Ophthalmol.* 1977;95:617–623.
18. Dithmar S, Volcker HE, Grossniklaus HE. Multifocal intraocular malignant melanoma: report of two cases and review of the literature. *Ophthalmology.* 1999; 106:1345–1348.
19. Seregard S, Ladenvall G, Kock E. Multiple melanocytic tumours in a case of ocular melanocytosis. *Acta Ophthalmol* 1993;71:562–565.
20. Gonder JR, Ezell PC, Shields JA, Augsburger JJ. Ocular melanocytosis. A study to determine the prevalence rate of ocular melanocytosis. *Ophthalmology.* 1982;89:950–952.
21. Singh AD, De Potter P, Fijal B, Shields CL, Shields CL, Elston RC. Lifetime Prevalence of uveal melanoma in caucasian patients with oculo (dermal) melanocytosis. *Ophthalmology.* 1998;105:195–198.
22. Clark Jr WH, Reimer RR, Greene M, Ainsworth AM, Mastrangelo MJ. Origin of familial malignant melanomas from heritable melanocytic lesions: 'The B-K Mole syndrome'. *Arch Dermatol.* 1978;114:732–738.
23. Greene MH, Clark Jr WH, Tucker MA, Elder DE, Kraemer KH, Fraser MC, Bondi EE, Guerry D. Precursor nevi in cutaneous malignant melanoma: A proposed nomenclature. *Lancet.* 1980;2:1024.
24. NIH Consensus conference. Diagnosis and treatment of early melanoma. *JAMA.* 1992; 268:1314–1319.
25. Singh AD, Shields CL, Shields JA, Eagle RC, De Potter P. Uveal melanoma and familial atypical mole and melanoma (FAM-M) syndrome. *Ophthalmic Genet.* 1995; 16:53–61.
26. Rodriguez-Sains RS. The familial occurrence of cutaneous melanoma, intraocular melanoma, and the dysplastic nevus syndrome. *Am J Ophthalmol.* 1984;97:114–115.
27. Oosterhuis JA, Went LN, Rumke P, Neering H, Lynch HT, Fusaro RM, Pester J. Tumor spectrum in the FAMMM syndrome. *Br J Cancer.* 1981;44:553–560.
28. Jensen OA, Movin M, Muller J. Malignant melanoma of the choroid in an infant with the dysplastic nevus syndrome. *Acta Ophthalmol.* 1987;65:91–100.
29. Rodriguez-Sains RS. Ocular findings in patients with dysplastic nevus syndrome. *Ophthalmology.* 1986;93:661–665.
30. Bataille V, Pinney E, Hungerford JL, Cuzik J, Bishop DT, Newton JA. Five cases of coexistent primary ocular and cutaneous melanoma. *Arch Dermatol.* 1993;129:198–201.
31. Greene MH, Sanders RJ, Chu FC, Clark Jr WH, Elder DE, Cogan DG. The familial occurrence of cutaneous melanoma, intraocular melanoma, and the dysplastic nevus syndrome. *Am J Ophthalmol.* 1983;96:238–245.
32. Taylor MR, Guerry D, Bondi EE, Shields JA, Augsburger JJ, Lusk EJ, Elder DE, Clark Jr WH, Van Horn M. Lack of association between intraocular melanoma and cutaneous dysplastic nevi. *Am J Ophthalmol.* 1984;98:478–482.
33. Greene MH, Sanders RJ, Chu FC, Clark Jr WH, Elder DE, Cogan DG. The familial occurrence of cutaneous melanoma, intraocular melanoma, and the dysplastic nevus syndrome. *Am J Ophthalmol.* 1984;97:115–117.
34. Bolande RP. Neurofibromatosis—the quintessential neurocristopathy: Pathogenetic concepts and relationships. *Adv Neurol.* 1981;29:67–75.
35. Honavar S, Singh AD, Shields CL, Eagle RC, Shields JA. Iris melanoma and neurofibromatosis type 1: Are they associated? *Surv Ophthalmol.* 2000;45:231–236.
36. Jay M, McCartney A. Familial malignant melanoma of the uvea and p53: A Victorian detective story. *Surv Ophthalmol.* 1993;37:457–462.
37. Li FP, Fraumeni JF. Soft tissue sarcomas, breast cancer and other neoplasms: a familial syndrome? *Ann Intern Med.* 1969;71:747–752.
38. Garber JE, Goldstein AM, Kantor AF, et al. Follow-up study of twenty-four families with Li–Fraumeni syndrome. *Cancer Res.* 1991;51:6094–6097.

J. WILLIAM HARBOUR

# 4. Oncogenes and Tumor Suppressor Genes in Uveal Melanoma

## INTRODUCTION

During embryonic development, cells become imprinted with a genetic and epigenetic program that determines their allotted number of cell divisions, their differentiated function, and their ultimate destination in the organism. A number of molecular safeguards, which we recognize as tumor suppressor mechanisms, ensure that each cell behaves according to its determined fate. In a fundamental sense, tumor suppressor genes regulate the orderly progression of cells towards their ultimate fate, whereas mutational inactivation of these genes (or activation of proto-oncogenes) leads to deregulated cell fate and thus cancer. These mutations are thought to be the initiating events in cancer, causing cells to resist growth inhibitory signals, to escape from their differentiation program, to proliferate beyond their intended number of cell divisions, or to resist apoptosis.[1] Subsequent to these events, the nascent tumor increasingly becomes genetically unstable and acquires additional properties associated with cancer progression, such as the ability to attract a blood supply, migrate through tissues, and evade the immune system. Many of these properties seem to recapitulate the activities of embryonal cells; thus tumorigenesis may involve the aberrant re-activation of genetic programs employed by embryonic precursor cells. As will be seen in this and subsequent chapters, research groups around the world have contributed greatly to our understanding of how these mutations may be involved in the pathogenesis of uveal melanoma. This chapter will focus on the molecular abnormalities that have been identified in the cell cycle and apoptotic pathways in uveal melanoma.

## CELL CYCLE

Mutations that deregulate the cell cycle are hallmarks of neoplastic cells.[1] Hence, an investigation of the genetic abnormalities involving the cell cycle pathway is mandatory for understanding the molecular pathogenesis of uveal melanoma.

## CORE CELL CYCLE PATHWAY

At the core of cell cycle regulatory machinery is the retinoblastoma protein (Rb)—the first tumor suppressor gene to be identified. Rb and the related proteins p107 and p130 share a conserved pocket domain that binds various proteins involved in cell cycle control.[2] Under growth inhibitory conditions, hypophosphorylated (active) Rb arrests the cell cycle in G1 phase by binding E2F transcription factors, which tether Rb to the promoters of cell cycle genes. Rb then recruits chromatin remodeling enzymes and other regulatory proteins to block transcription by altering chromatin structure.[3] Under proliferative conditions, Rb is inactivated by hyperphosphorylation, allowing E2Fs to be released and the cell cycle to progress. Rb can also arrest cells in S and G2 phases when activated by various checkpoints, such as in response to DNA damage.[4] Since the activity of Rb depends on its phosphorylation state, the kinases that phosphorylate Rb are important regulators of the cell cycle. Kinases known to phosphorylate Rb include cyclin dependent kinase-4/6 (CDK4/6) and CDK2. These CDKs are only active when complexed with coenzymes called cyclins; cyclin D associates with CDK4/6 and cyclin E associates with CDK2. In most situations, CDK activity is regulated by the availability of cyclins. For example, Ras stimulates cell division in part by upregulating cyclin D, which then activates CDK4/6.[5] Adding another layer of complexity to this 'Rb pathway', there are CDK inhibitors such as p16 (which inhibits CDK4/6) and p21/p27 (which inhibit both CDK4/6 and CDK2).[6] p16 is a tumor suppressor that becomes expressed under conditions favoring permanent cell cycle arrest (e.g., senescence and differentiation).[7] p21 is upregulated under specific circumstances, such as by p53 in response to DNA damage.[8]

In recent years, our understanding of the Rb cell cycle pathway in uveal melanoma has greatly improved. Although a detailed mutational analysis of the Rb gene has not been reported in uveal melanoma, the status of the gene can be inferred from studies of Rb expression in these tumors.[9,10] In one immunohistochemical analysis of 33 primary uveal melanomas, the vast majority of tumors displayed strong Rb staining, although a significant proportion of the Rb molecules in these tumors was functionally inactive as a consequence of phosphorylation on specific amino acid residues.[9] Unlike retinoblastomas, therefore, uveal melanomas rarely mutate the Rb gene, but rather, they functionally inactivate Rb by hyperphosphorylation. What upstream mutation in the Rb pathway may explain this Rb hyperphosphorylation? Mutation of p16 is one common tumor mechanism for functionally inactivating Rb.[6] Although p16 mutations play an important role in cutaneous melanoma,[11] most reports to date suggest that both germline and somatic p16 mutations are rare in uveal melanoma.[9,12,13] However, a recent study lends support to the idea that at least some uveal melanomas may inactivate p16 by methylating the promoter.[14] More work is needed to determine the pathogenetic significance of this finding in uveal melanoma. Another common mechanism for hyperphosphorylating Rb is by overexpression of cyclin D.[6] Several studies have found strong cyclin D expression in a significant proportion of uveal melanomas (up to 65%) by immunohistochemistry and western blot.[9,15,16] These results suggest that Rb is functionally inactivated in most uveal melanomas, either by mutation of p16, overexpression of cyclin D, or perhaps other upstream mutations. Since the cell cycle is closely linked to pathways controlling cell proliferation and senescence, we will next explore how abnormalities in these pathways may contribute to cell cycle deregulation in uveal melanomas.

## PROLIFERATIVE SIGNALING PATHWAYS

Cell proliferation is required for normal development, wound healing, tissue replenishment and other processes. However, proliferation is tightly regulated in order to maintain tissue homeostasis. Most normal cells progressively lose their proliferative potential as they become more differentiated, with terminally differentiated and senescent cells being mitotically inactive. In some cells, such as neurons, this cell cycle exit appears to be irreversible, whereas other cell types can re-enter the cell cycle if activated by appropriate growth stimuli. For example, adult uveal melanocytes have a very low proliferative rate *in vivo*, but they easily can be coaxed to undergo cell division in culture with adequate growth factors. Cell cycle activity is regulated by a complex interplay of growth-promoting and growth-inhibiting signals that interact to balance proliferation with differentiation and senescence. In this section, we will investigate how mutations in proliferative signaling pathways may deregulate the Rb cell cycle pathway in uveal melanoma.

### *Ras pathway*

The Ras GTP-binding proteins play a central role in mitogen-induced cell proliferation by coupling growth factor receptors to activation of a kinase cascade, including Raf, MEK and ERK protein kinases.[5] Activation of the Ras pathway promotes cell division by inducing cells to enter S phase of the cell cycle. Rb is a major target of Ras signaling; Ras causes an upregulation of cyclin D and downregulation of CDK inhibitors, with consequent hyperphosphorylation of Rb.[17] Two groups have examined Ras genes in uveal melanoma, and both found no mutations in c-Ha-ras1, c-Ki-ras2, or N-ras.[18,19] Therefore, Ras mutations appear to be rare in uveal melanoma, but further work is needed to rule out mutations elsewhere in the Ras signal transduction pathway in this tumor.

### *Myc pathway*

The Myc genes are involved in cell proliferation and are deregulated in approximately 30% of human cancers.[20] The major Myc family member, c-Myc, is an immediate early serum response gene involved in the G1-to-S phase transition.[21] Loss of c-Myc by genetic knockout leads to dramatic decrease in tissue growth rates,[22] whereas overexpression of c-Myc participates in cell growth and neoplastic transformation.[21] c-Myc is most often deregulated in cancer by overexpression of the protein, such as by gene amplification or translocation. There is increasing evidence that c-Myc is a frequent target of mutations in uveal melanoma. Royds et al. reported immunohistochemical staining for c-Myc in 24 uveal melanomas, and they found a correlation between c-Myc expression and proliferative index.[23] Chana et al. examined 71 uveal melanomas by flow cytometry and found that 70% of tumors expressed c-Myc in a majority of cells.[24] Providing more direct evidence for Myc mutations in uveal melanoma, the group of Merbs found an increased copy number of c-Myc in 72% and gene amplification in 42% of 43 uveal melanomas using fluorescence *in situ* hybridization.[25] Additionally, one of the most common cytogenetic abnormalities in uveal melanoma is an increase in copies of chromosome 8 (especially 8q), which may be pathogenetically linked to the presence of the c-Myc gene at 8q24.[26,27]

## SENESCENCE

Senescence is an important tumor suppressor mechanism for opposing the proliferative signals discussed above, and limiting the number of divisions that a cell may undergo. Cells that are allowed to divide indefinitely are at risk for sustaining mutations that could lead to malignant transformation. Furthermore, virtually all malignant cells are 'immortalized' and can divide indefinitely. Therefore, escape from senescence is a ubiquitous feature of cancer cells.[1] There are probably several molecular processes that underlie the phenomenon of senescence, but some general conclusions can be drawn. First, hypophosphorylated (active) Rb is required for senescence.[28] Specifically, in melanocytes undergoing senescence, there is increased expression of CDK inhibitors, which leads to accumulation of hypophosphorylated Rb, and decreased activity of E2F proliferative factors.[29] Therefore, inactivation of Rb by hyperphosphorylation, as occurs in uveal melanoma, may defeat the senescence program.

Another key regulator of senescence in human cells is the length of telomeres (the end segments of chromosomes). With each cell division, telomeres become shorter because they are not completely replicated. When telomeres erode to a certain length, a DNA damage checkpoint is triggered through the p53 and Rb pathways, leading to cell cycle arrest.[30] In order to escape this senescence checkpoint, many tumors overexpress telomerase, a reverse transcriptase that can avert the senescence checkpoint by maintaining longer telomere length.[30] To investigate whether telomerase activity may be deregulated in uveal melanomas, Heine et al.[30a] studied 14 uveal melanomas for telomerase activity. By TRAP assay and *in situ* hybridization, moderate to high telomerase expression was observed in all cases, suggesting that telomerase deregulation is a common abnormality in uveal melanoma. Telomerase upregulation and inactivation of the Rb pathway appear to function in concert to escape senescence, which leads to increasing genomic instability, accumulation of additional mutations, and evolution towards a more malignant phenotype.[31]

## APOPTOSIS

In multicellular organisms, apoptosis (programmed cell death) is critical for eliminating abnormal cells and avoiding neoplastic transformation.[32] Apoptosis can be triggered in response to inappropriate cell proliferation, DNA damage, and other oncogenic insults.[1] Virtually all 'successful' tumors must evolve means of defeating the apoptotic defense mechanism; thus apoptotic defects are ubiquitous in clinically detectable tumors. We will consider the role of two components of the apoptotic response in uveal melanoma: the p53-mediated surveillance mechanism and the intrinsic apoptotic machinery.

## SURVEILLANCE MECHANISM

The p53 tumor suppressor is a unique regulatory protein that has the ability to trigger cell cycle arrest and/or apoptosis in response to DNA damage, hyperproliferative conditions, hypoxia and other cellular insults.[33] This tumor suppressor function of p53 appears to explain why it is the most commonly mutated gene in human cancer.[34] Interestingly, however, p53 mutations appear to be rare in uveal melanoma.[35–37] This suggests that there may be mutations elsewhere in the p53 pathway that functionally inactivate p53. HDM2 binds p53 and blocks its function, thereby serving as a natural inhibitor that keeps p53 in check under normal conditions. In some cancers, HDM2 is overexpressed as a mutational mechanism of suppressing p53 activity.[38] Two groups examined the immunohistochemical expression of HDM2 in uveal melanoma and found strong expression of HDM2 in up to 97% of uveal melanomas.[37,39] Further work is needed to determine the mutational basis for HDM2 overexpression in uveal melanoma (e.g., gene amplification, transcriptional deregulation, protein stabilization). To confirm whether HDM2 overexpression is pathogenetically relevant in uveal melanoma, we used a synthetic peptide to inhibit HDM2 in uveal melanoma cells and found that indeed inhibition of HDM2 rapidly induced apoptosis, suggesting that overexpression of HDM2 is important for tumor maintenance.[44]

## APOPTOTIC MACHINERY

The core machinery of the intrinsic apoptotic pathway includes a family of proteins with homology to Bcl-2.[40] This 'Bcl-2 pathway' consists of anti-apoptotic proteins (e.g., Bcl-2 and Bcl-$X_L$) and pro-apoptotic proteins (e.g., Bax and Bad), which interact in a complex manner to determine whether the apoptotic program will be executed. The upstream regulators of this pathway include p53, as well as other regulatory factors such as p73.[41] The downstream effectors of the apoptotic program include mitochondrial release of cytochrome C, caspase activation, chromosomal DNA disruption, and other morphological events associated with apoptosis.[40] While this pathway has not been studied extensively in uveal melanoma, one consistent finding among several labs has been a high rate of Bcl-2 overexpression in this tumor.[24,37,42] In fact, Bcl-2 overexpression is probably the most common molecular abnormality described thus far in uveal melanoma. A major consequence of Bcl-2 overexpression may be to titrate and functionally inactivate the pro-apoptotic components of the pathway, effectively neutralizing p53 and other apoptotic signals.

# CONCLUSIONS

Current evidence does not favor the existence of a single uveal melanoma gene, but rather, this eye tumor appears to result from an accumulation of genetic abnormalities that disrupt key cell cycle and apoptotic checkpoints. The lack of a single, rate-limiting genetic mutation could explain the rarity of familial uveal melanoma.[43] The requirement for multiple stochastic mutational events may explain why most uveal melanomas occur later in life. It seems likely that many of the cytogenetic alterations that occur in uveal melanoma (discussed in subsequent chapters) begin to accumulate subsequent to this initial stage in tumorigenesis where the basic tumor suppressor checkpoints have been defeated. An important question is whether the nonrandom cytogenetic changes in uveal melanoma (e.g., loss of chromosome 3, gain of chromosomes 6 and 8) target specific oncogenes and/or tumor suppressor genes, or whether they are simply markers for malignant evolution. With the recent solution of the human genome, an intensive effort to answer this question is now feasible.

Further work is needed to translate these advances in our basic knowledge into clinically useful technologies. For example, we have found that uveal melanoma cells require the overexpression of HDM2 to avoid apoptosis, so an effective therapeutic strategy may be to block this protein (J.W. Harbour, unpublished data). As we learn more about the molecular pathogenesis of uveal melanoma, other novel therapeutic targets may become apparent.

## ACKNOWLEDGEMENTS

Dr. Harbour is supported by grants from the NIH and Research to Prevent Blindness, Inc.

## REFERENCES

1. Hanahan D, Weinberg RA. The hallmarks of cancer. *Cell.* 2000;100:57–70.
2. Harbour JW, Dean DC. The Rb/E2F pathway: expanding roles and emerging paradigms. *Genes Dev.* 2000;14:2545–2562.
3. Zhang HS, Gavin M, Dahiya A, Postigo AA, Ma D, Luo RX, Harbour JW, Dean DC. Exit from G1 and S phase of the cell cycle is regulated by repressor complexes containing HDAC-Rb-hSWI/SNF and Rb-hSWI/SNF. *Cell.* 2000;101:79–89.
4. Harrington EA, Bruce JL, Harlow E, Dyson N. pRB plays an essential role in cell cycle arrest induced by DNA damage. *Proc Natl Acad Sci USA.* 1998;95:11945–11950.
5. Mittnacht S, Paterson H, Olson MF, Marshall CJ. Ras signalling is required for inactivation of the tumour suppressor pRb cell-cycle control protein. *Curr Biol.* 1997;7:219–221.
6. Sherr CJ. Cancer cell cycles. *Science.* 1996;274:1672–1677.
7. Dai CY, Enders GH. p16 INK4a can initiate an autonomous senescence program. *Oncogene.* 2000;19:1613–1622.
8. Brugarolas J, Moberg K, Boyd SD, Taya Y, Jacks T, Lees JA. Inhibition of cyclin-dependent kinase 2 by p21 is necessary for retinoblastoma protein-mediated G1 arrest after gamma-irradiation. *Proc Natl Acad Sci USA.* 1999;96:1002–1007.
9. Brantley MA Jr., Harbour JW. Inactivation of retinoblastoma protein in uveal melanoma by phosphorylation of sites in the COOH-terminal region. *Cancer Res.* 2000;60: 4320–4323.
10. Massaro-Giordano M, Baldi G, De Luca A, Baldi A, Giordano A. Differential expression of the retinoblastoma gene family members in choroidal melanoma: prognostic significance. *Clin Cancer Res.* 1999;5:1455–1458.
11. Kamb A, Gruis NA, Weaver-Feldhaus J, Liu Q, Harshman K, Tavtigian SV, Stockert E, Day RS 3rd, Johnson BE, Skolnick MH. A cell cycle regulator potentially involved in genesis of many tumor types. *Science.* 1994;264:436–440.
12. Singh AD, Croce CM, Wary KK, Shields JA, Donoso LA, Shields CL, Huebner K, Ohta M. Familial uveal melanoma: absence of germline mutations involving the cyclin-dependent kinase-4 inhibitor gene (p16). *Ophthalmic Genet.* 1996;17:39–40.

13. Merbs SL, Sidransky D. Analysis of p16 (CDKN2/MTS-1/INK4A) alterations in primary sporadic uveal melanoma. *Invest Ophthalmol Vis Sci.* 1999;40:779–783.
14. Van der Velden PA, Metzelaar-Blok JA, Bergman W, Hurks HMH, Frants RR, Gruis NA, Jager MJ. Promoter hypermethylation: a common cause of reduced p16(INK4a) expression in uveal melanoma. *Cancer Res.* 2001;61:5303–5306.
15. Coupland SE, Bechrakis N, Schuler A, Anagnostopoulos I, Hummel M, Bornfeld N, Stein H. Expression patterns of cyclin D1 and related proteins regulating G1-S phase transition in uveal melanoma and retinoblastoma. *Br J Ophthalmol.* 1998;82: 961–970.
16. Mouriaux F, Casagrande F, Pillaire MJ, Manenti S, Malecaze F, Darbon JM. Differential expression of G1 cyclins and cyclin-dependent kinase inhibitors in normal and transformed melanocytes. *Invest Ophthalmol Vis Sci.* 1998;39:876–884.
17. Peeper DS, Upton TM, Ladha MH, Neuman E, Zalvide J, Bernards R, DeCaprio JA, Ewen ME. Ras signalling linked to the cell-cycle machinery by the retinoblastoma protein. *Nature.* 1997;386:177–181.
18. Soparker CN, O'Brien JM, Albert DM. Investigation of the role of the ras protooncogene point mutation in human uveal melanomas. *Invest Ophthalmol Vis Sci.* 1993;34: 2203–2209.
19. Mooy CM, Van der Helm MJ, Van der Kwast TH, De Jong PT, Ruiter DJ, Zwarthoff EC. No N-ras mutations in human uveal melanoma: the role of ultraviolet light revisited. *Br J Cancer.* 1991;64:411–413.
20. Henriksson M, Luscher B. Proteins of the Myc network: essential regulators of cell growth and differentiation. *Adv Cancer Res.* 1996;68:109–182.
21. Evan GI, Littlewood TD. The role of c-myc in cell growth. *Curr Opin Genet Dev.* 1993; 3:44–49.
22. Davis AC, Wims M, Spotts GD, Hann SR, Bradley A. A null c-myc mutation causes lethality before 10.5 days of gestation in homozygotes and reduced fertility in heterozygous female mice. *Genes Dev.* 1993;7:671–682.
23. Royds JA, Sharrard RM, Parsons MA, Lawry J, Rees R, Cottam D, Wagner B, Rennie IG. C-myc oncogene expression in ocular melanomas. *Graefes Arch Clin Exp Ophthalmol.* 1992;230:366–371.
24. Chana JS, Wilson GD, Cree IA, Alexander RA, Myatt N, Neale M, Foss AJ, Hungerford JL. C-myc, p53, and Bcl-2 expression and clinical outcome in uveal melanoma. *Br J Ophthalmol.* 1999;83:110–114.
25. Parrella P, Caballero OL, Sidransky D, Merbs SL. Detection of c-myc amplification in uveal melanoma by fluorescent *in situ* hybridization. *Invest Ophthalmol Vis Sci.* 2001;42:1679–1684.
26. Horsthemke B, Prescher G, Bornfeld N, Becher R. Loss of chromosome 3 alleles and multiplication of chromosome 8 alleles in uveal melanoma. *Genes Chromosomes Cancer.* 1992;4:217–221.
27. Prescher G, Bornfeld N, Becher R. Nonrandom chromosomal abnormalities in primary uveal melanoma. *J Natl Cancer Inst.* 1990;82:1765–1769.
28. Stein GH, Beeson M, Gordon L. Failure to phosphorylate the retinoblastoma gene product in senescent human fibroblasts. *Science.* 1990;249:666–669.
29. Haddad MM, Xu W, Schwahn DJ, Liao F, Medrano EE. Activation of a cAMP pathway and induction of melanogenesis correlate with association of p16(INK4) and p27(KIP1) to CDKs, loss of E2F-binding activity, and premature senescence of human melanocytes. *Exp Cell Res.* 1999;253:561–572.
30. Sherr CJ, DePinho RA. Cellular senescence: mitotic clock or culture shock? *Cell.* 2000;102:407–410.

30a. Heine B, Coupland SE, Kneiff S, Demel G, Bornfeld N, Hummel M, Stein H. Telomerase expression in uveal melanoma. *Br J Opthalmol.* 2000;84:217–223.
31. Kiyono T, Foster SA, Koop JI, McDougall JK, Galloway DA, Klingelhutz AJ. Both Rb/p16INK4a inactivation and telomerase activity are required to immortalize human epithelial cells. *Nature.* 1998;396:84–88.
32. Jacobson MD, Weil M, Raff MC. Programmed cell death in animal development. *Cell.* 1997;88:347–354.
33. Prives C, Hall PA. The p53 pathway. *J Pathol.* 1999;187:112–126.
34. Harris CC, Hollstein M. Clinical implications of the p53 tumor-suppressor gene. *N Eng J Med.* 1993;329:1318–1327.
35. Jay V, Yi Q, Hunter WS, Zielenska M. p53 expression in uveal malignant melanomas. *Pathology.* 1996;28:306–308.
36. Kishore K, Ghazvini S, Char DH, Kroll S, Selle J. p53 gene and cell cycling in uveal melanoma. *Am J Ophthalmol.* 1996;121:561–567.
37. Brantley MA Jr., Harbour JW. Deregulation of the Rb and p53 pathways in uveal melanoma. *Am J Pathol.* 2000;157:1795–1801.
38. Florenes VA, Maelandsmo GM, Forus A, Andreassen A, Myklebost O, Fodstad O. MDM2 gene amplification and transcript levels in human sarcomas: relationship to TP53 gene status. *J Natl Cancer Inst.* 1994;86:1297–1302.
39. Coupland SE, Anastassiou G, Stang A, Schilling H, Anagnostopoulos I, Bornfeld N, Stein H. The prognostic value of cyclin D1, p53, and MDM2 protein expression in uveal melanoma. *J Pathol.* 2000;191:120–126.
40. Gross A, McDonnell JM, Korsmeyer SJ. BCL-2 family members and the mitochondria in apoptosis. *Genes Dev.* 1999;13:1899–1911.
41. Irwin M, Marin MC, Phillips AC, Seelan RS, Smith DI, Liu W, Flores ER, Tsai KY, Jacks T, Vousden KH, Kaelin WG Jr. Role for the p53 homologue p73 in E2F-1-induced apoptosis. *Nature.* 2000;407:645–648.
42. Jay V, Yi Q, Hunter WS, Zielenska M. Expression of bcl-2 in uveal malignant melanoma. *Arch Pathol Lab Med.* 1996;120:497–498.
43. Singh AD, Shields CL, De Potter P, Shields JA, Trock B, Cater J, Pastore D. Familial uveal melanoma. Clinical observations on 56 patients. *Arch Ophthalmol.* 1996;114:392–399.
44. Harbour JW, Worley L, Ma D, Cohen M. Transducible peptide therapy for uveal melanoma and retinoblastoma. *Arch Opthalmol.* 2002;120:1341–1346.

NELLEKE A. GRUIS

# 5. CDKN2A (p16) and Uveal Melanoma

## INTRODUCTION

Uveal melanoma is the most common malignancy of the eye, but unlike melanoma of the skin, little is known about the underlying genetic defects. In general, uveal melanoma is rarely hereditary and has not been linked consistently to mutations in tumor suppressor genes. Recently, the close link between oncogenesis and cell cycle regulation has drawn attention to several regulators of the Rb and p53 pathways as potential candidate genes for uveal melanoma. For example, methylation of the cyclin dependent kinase inhibitor, p16 (CDKN2A) gene seems to be a common event in uveal melanoma. p16 hypermethylation might be related to the metastatic potential since methylation turns out to be associated with a poor prognosis in patients. Apart from p16, expression of other genes seems to be influenced by methylation in uveal melanoma. Therefore, micro-array analysis turns out to be a promising tool to investigate additional genes or genetic pathways involved in the genesis and progression of uveal melanoma.

## p16, A CELL CYCLE REGULATOR INVOLVED IN MANY TUMOR TYPES

Both genetic studies of cutaneous melanoma prone families and molecular analysis of regulators of cell cycle checkpoints identified the CDKN2A (p16) gene as a tumor suppressor gene on the short arm of chromosome 9 (9p21).[1–4] The CDKN2A gene is a key player in cell cycle regulation.[3] The gene encodes the p16 protein that binds and inhibits cyclin dependent kinase (CDK) 4 and 6, an inhibition that prevents complex formation of CDK4 with cyclin D1.[3,5] The CDK4/cyclin D complex normally supports the transition from G1 to S phase in the cell cycle by phosphorylation and inactivation of the retinoblastoma gene product.[5]

Since its discovery as an inhibitor of cyclin-dependent kinases 4 and 6, the tumor suppressor p16 has gained widespread importance in cancer.[6] The high frequency of deletions of the CDKN2A gene in cell lines of several tumor types first suggested an important role for p16 in carcinogenesis.[2,7–9] Moreover, a high frequency of CDKN2A gene alterations was found in primary tumors, while recent studies have identified CDKN2A promoter methylation as a major mechanism of tumor-suppressor-gene silencing.[10,11] Additional insight into p16's role in cancer has come from the genetic analysis of precancerous lesions and various tissue culture models. It is now believed that loss of p16 is an early and often critical event in tumor progression. Consequently, p16 is a major tumor-suppressor gene whose frequent loss occurs early in many human cancers.

The CDKN2A inactivation rate in cutaneous melanoma cell lines is high (about 80%). Also in cutaneous melanoma homozygous deletions, point mutations or gene silencing by promoter methylation contribute to this high percentage of CDKN2A gene inactivation.[12,13] On the contrary, CDKN2A inactivation in fresh primary melanomas reaches only 30%.[14–17] Contamination of the tumor with normal material, undetected mutations outside the coding region, tissue culture artifacts and selective growth of subpopulations of cultured cells have been put forward to account for these discrepancies. Most of the point mutations identified in melanoma cell lines turn out to be typical of ultraviolet induced carcinogenesis.[18] C → T and CC → TT transitions indicate a direct role for ultraviolet radiation (UVR)-induced pyrimidine dimers in the formation of some tumors, confirming the importance of this major environmental risk factor for cutaneous melanoma.[19]

## CDKN2A, THE MAJOR MELANOMA GENE

Support for the role of the CDKN2A in cutaneous melanoma predisposition was additionally provided by the identification of germline mutations in affected members of melanoma kindreds all over the world.[20–23] Of all melanoma families, 50% turned out to be linked to chromosome 9p. Germline mutations in CDKN2A are typically point mutations, insertions or small intragenic deletions within the first or second exon and are present in approximately 40% of the 9p-linked melanoma families studied.[24] The chance to observe germline mutations in CDKN2A increases with the number of melanoma cases within the family. It turned out that in families with five or more melanoma cases the chance to identify CDKN2A mutations is 37% whereas in families with only two cases the chance was only 11%.[25] Despite the fact that germline mutations in the coding sequence of CDKN2A have been identified in about 40% of melanoma prone families, most of these mutations have not been formally tested for loss of function.

Of potential importance regarding the role of p16 in the development of melanoma was the discovery of two individuals within one of the Dutch melanoma kindreds with germline deletions in both copies of CDKN2A.[21] Surprisingly, one of these human 'knock-outs' did not develop melanoma prior to her death at the age of 55 from an adenocarcinoma. The presence of three very mildly atypical nevi was the only sign possibly related to FAMMM. Her progeny had the classic FAMMM phenotype, with melanomas and atypical nevi present in two of her three children. On the contrary, the other homozygous individual developed atypical moles in very large numbers at the age of eleven. Already at the age of 15, he developed a melanoma *in situ* and an invasive melanoma. Our observation of normal development in the absence of functional p16 implies that p16 is not sufficient to develop melanoma. Either other endogenous or exogenous factors or the presence of functionally redundant genes seems to be required for phenotypic expression.

## ADDITIONAL CELL CYCLE REGULATORS AS CANDIDATE GENES FOR MELANOMA

Besides CDKN2A, two other tumor suppressor genes have been identified in the 9p21 region, that has been recognized as the site of a locus for predisposition to melanoma. In conjunction with the cloning of the CDKN2A, a gene with 93% sequence homology to the CDKN2A gene was cloned 30 kb downstream of CDKN2A.[2] This CDKN2B gene encodes p15, another inhibitor of CDK4. CDKN2B is often co-deleted together with the CDKN2A gene in many tumor cell lines including melanoma.[12,26] The latter suggests that p15 may be a tumor suppressor as well. Ectopic expression of p15 inhibits growth of tumor-derived cell lines, although, lack of p15 mutations in tumor cell lines and in 9p21-linked melanoma kindreds suggests a role for p15 in growth regulation, but a limited role for p15 in tumor progression.[27,28]

Furthermore there is a gene encoding p14ARF.[29] p14ARF is encoded by an alternative exon 1 (1β) and exon 2 of the CDKN2A gene. Exon 1β lies 12 kb upstream of CDKN2A exon 1α. Under the transcriptional control of its own promoter, exon 1β is spliced to CDKN2A exon 2 in an alternate reading frame (ARF) to that of the p16 protein.[29,30] As a consequence of the alternate reading frames, the proteins p16 and p14ARF share no homology at the amino acid level, although both proteins, including p15 are considered cell cycle regulators. Both p15 and p16 sact in the retinoblastoma (Rb) pathway as inhibitors of CDK4/CDK6. The p14ARF protein acts in both the p53 and Rb pathways via a protein common to both pathways, human MDM2.[31–33] By binding to p53, MDM2 targets p53 for degradation by the ubiquitin pathway.[34] p14ARF binds to MDM2, sequestering it in the nucleolus and preventing binding to p53, which results in p53 activation and arrest of both G1 and G2. Binding of the p14ARF N-terminal domain to p53 (encoded by CDKN2A exon 1β) seems to be necessary and sufficient to induce cell cycle arrest.[35] These results place p14ARF in an independent pathway upstream of p53 and imply that CDKN2A encodes two proteins that are involved in tumor suppression (Fig. 5.1).

Until now, no germline mutations have been observed in the CDKN2B gene or in the first exon (exon 1β) of p14ARF in melanoma families.[27,36,37] Germline mutations observed in CDKN2A exon 2 might both affect p16 and p14ARF function due to the dual utilization of this exon.[36] Mutations in exon 2 of the CDKN2A gene are predicted to affect the amino acid sequence of p14ARF as well as p16. The impact of these mutations with regard to the function of p14ARF is unclear, as the cell cycle inhibitory functions of the protein are located in the N-terminal region coded by p14ARF-specific exon 1β.[35] Germline deletions of the 9p21 region containing the genes CDKN2A, CDKN2B and CDKN2A exon 1β have been reported in families predisposed to melanoma and neural system tumors, commonly astrocytoma.[38,39] These large deletions suggest that contiguous loss of

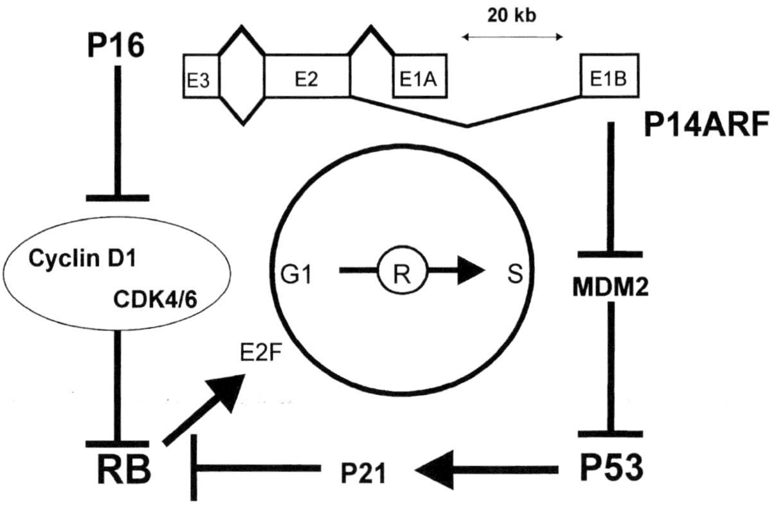


Fig. 5.1. Key players in the G1/S restriction point. The CDKN2A product p16 is an inhibitor of the Rb pathway, whereas its alternative reading frame product p14ARF leads to arrest of the cell cycle via the p53 pathway.

both the p16 and p14ARF tumor suppressor genes is a predisposing factor in these families. Recently, a melanoma-astrocytoma family was described with a germline deletion of the p14ARF-specific exon 1β of the CDKN2A gene. This deletion does not affect the coding or minimal promoter sequences of either the CDKN2A or CDKN2B genes.[40] These results suggest p14ARF to be the critical gene related to this syndrome, rather than contiguous loss of both the CDKN2A and CDKN2B genes.[40]

p16 regulates passage through the G1 checkpoint of the cell cycle by CDK4/cyclinD1 and CDK6/cylin D1 kinases that phosphorylate the retinoblastoma protein. This negative regulatory pathway suggests several other candidates for examination in not 9p-linked melanoma kindreds. Today, in two unrelated melanoma families who do not carry p16 germline mutations, an Arg24Cys mutation in the CDK4 gene has been observed, that averts binding of the p16 protein to CDK4.[41] In one other 9p-linked melanoma kindred an Arg24His mutation was observed.[42] Despite the strong evidence that CDK4 can be considered a second familial melanoma gene, the very low frequency of CDK4 mutations in melanoma kindreds suggests that additional genes play a role in the development of familial melanoma.

## GENES INVOLVED IN UVEAL MELANOMA

The principal aim of genetic studies of uveal melanoma is to identify genes involved in the malignant transformation of melanocytes and in melanoma tumor progression. An approach to reach this aim is to perform cytogenetic studies of tumors to identify frequently rearranged regions of the genome, which presumably mark the location of genes involved in the progression of the tumor. In uveal melanoma several specific chromosomal abnormalities have been described. Loss of chromosome band 1p36, monosomy 3, abnormalities on chromosome 6 and gain of the q arm of chromosome 8 have been observed in many tumors.[43,44] Most of these cytogenetic abnormalities turn out to be valuable predictors of diagnosis and prognosis.[44–46] Since loss or amplification of whole chromosomes or chromosome arms hamper the identification of loci that are specifically involved in uveal melanoma development, comparative genomic hybridization turned out to be a more accurate technique to identify small genetic regions of interest (see Chapters 7 and 8, this book).[43,47,48] Despite the fact that very specific genetic regions of interest have been recognized in uveal melanoma, no specific uveal melanoma genes have been identified in these regions so far. In absence of genes specifically involved in uveal melanoma, genes involved in cutaneous melanoma, e.g., CDKN2A, have been followed up as candidate genes for uveal melanoma.

## CDKN2A INVOLVEMENT IN UVEAL MELANOMA

Ohta was the first to determine the involvement of the melanoma susceptibility gene CDKN2A in dissected melanomas of uveal origin.[49] No mutations could be detected in the coding region of the CDKN2A gene. The latter observation has been repeatedly confirmed by others.[50,51] Besides the lack of somatic mutations involving the CDKN2A gene in uveal melanoma, the absence of germline mutations in familial uveal melanoma patients[49–51] provided even more evidence that the cutaneous melanoma predisposition gene CDKN2A does not predispose to uveal melanoma.

Merbs and Sidransky[52] defined more clearly the role of the CDKN2A gene in uveal melanoma by determining the contribution of all known mechanisms of CDKN2A inactivation in uveal melanoma. Genetic analysis of the CDKN2A gene was performed in 33 primary sporadic ciliochoroidal and choroidal melanomas. All tumors were analysed by fourteen highly polymorphic microsatellite markers surrounding the CDKN2A locus to detect loss of heterozygosity. Sequence analysis of the CDKN2A gene was performed on those tumors with 9p21 loss of heterozygosity (LOH). LOH was found in eight of 33 (24%) uveal melanomas. There was no evidence of a second region of LOH that did not include the CDKN2A locus. Four tumors showed hemizygous losses including markers both distal and proximal to p16. Homozygous deletion of the CDKN2A gene was detected in four tumors. Sequence analysis revealed no p16 mutations in the tumors with hemizygous loss of CDKN2A. To investigate methylation as an alternative mechanism of inactivation of CDKN2A, methylation-specific polymerase chain reaction was performed on all tumor DNA samples. Methylation of the 5′ CpG island of CDKN2A was found in one tumor with 9p21 LOH and in another without LOH. CDKN2A inactivation by promoter methylation turned out to be present in two of the 33 (6%) uveal melanomas studied.

## p16 METHYLATION AND TUMOR PROGRESSION

That the role of CDKN2A and especially the role of CDKN2A gene silencing by promoter methylation in uveal melanoma is much more important than previously anticipated, has been shown by van der Velden et al., who described CDKN2A promoter hypermethylation in 32% of primary uveal melanoma and 50% of uveal melanoma cell lines.[53] CDKN2A promoter methylation was accompanied by loss of p16 expression in all uveal melanoma cell lines with a hypermethylated CDKN2A promoter. The expression of p14ARF was however retained. Five out of seven patients with CDKN2A promoter methylation in the primary tumor died of metastatic disease, compared to two out of 15 patients with a non-methylated primary tumor, suggesting that CDKN2A might be involved in the development of metastatic disease as well.

## METHYLATION RELATED PROGRESSION MARKERS OF UVEAL MELANOMA

Van der Velden et al.[53] furthermore showed that treatment of methylated uveal melanoma cell lines with de demethylating agent 5-aza-2′-deoxycytidine resulted in demethylation of CDKN2A and in re-expression of p16 messenger RNA, which was maintained upon withdrawal of the 5-aza-2′-deoxycytidine. Since demethylation of the CDKN2A promoter has such a dominant effect on the expression, it seems that apart from promoter methylation there is no other major genetic or epigenetic inhibitor of expression present in the uveal melanoma cell lines to prevent CDKN2A expression.

In order to identify additional genes to the CDKN2A gene that are involved in uveal melanoma tumor growth and metastasis, new technology like gene expression profiling will be an eye opener.[54,55] Gene expression profiles are obtained by hybridizing isolated messenger RNA from tissue or cell lines to arrays of hundreds or thousands of known cDNAs. The amount of labeled-RNA bound to a gene spot on the array reflects the expression level of that specific gene in the cell line or tissue. To identify molecules involved in dissemination of uveal melanoma, Van der Velden et al. performed microarray analysis in a tumor progression model comprising a primary uveal melanoma and two liver metastases from the same patient.[56] An important finding was the five-fold decreased expression of TIMP3 in the metastatic cell lines, a molecule involved in extracellular matrix degradation. TIMP3 expression, like the expression of CDKN2A,[53] was regulated by methylation. The results were confirmed in primary uveal melanoma and suggests a role for TIMP3 in uveal melanoma development.

## CONCLUSIONS

The field of cutaneous melanoma genetics has progressed considerably since the identification of the melanoma susceptibility gene CDKN2A. In uveal melanoma no involvement of a major gene has been observed yet, although a different look at inactivating mechanisms of candidate genes might alter insight in the importance of these genes in uveal melanoma. In addition, new technology such as gene expression profiling by micro-array analysis will increase our interest in potential new candidate genes for uveal melanoma. This technique will not only enable us to identify new genes but may also provide insight into the genetic pathways in which those genes are involved.

## REFERENCES


1. Kamb A, Shattuck-Eidens D, Eeles R, Liu Q, Gruis NA, Ding W, Hussey C, Tran T, Miki Y, Weaver-Feldhaus J, et al. Analysis of the p16 gene (CDKN2) as a candidate for the chromosome 9p melanoma susceptibility locus. *Nat Genet.* 1994;8:23–26.
2. Kamb A, Gruis NA, Weaver-Feldhaus J, Liu Q, Harshman K, Tavtigian SV, Stockert E, Day RS 3rd, Johnson BE, Skolnick MH. A cell cycle regulator potentially involved in genesis of many tumor types. *Science.* 1994;264:436–440.
3. Serrano M, Hannon GJ, Beach D. A new regulatory motif in cell-cycle control causing specific inhibition of cyclin D/CDK *Nature.* 1993;366:704–707.
4. Nobori T, Miura K, Wu DJ, Lois A, Takabayashi K, Carson DA. Deletions of the cyclin-dependent kinase-4 inhibitor gene in multiple human cancers. *Nature.* 1994;368: 753–756.
5. Lukas J, Parry D, Aagaard L, Mann DJ, Bartkova J, Strauss M, Peters G, Bartek J. Retinoblastoma-protein-dependent cell-cycle inhibition by the tumour suppressor p16. *Nature.* 1995;375:503–506.
6. Rocco JW, Sidransky D. p16(MTS-1/CDKN2/INK4a) in cancer progression. *Exp Cell Res.* 2001;264:42–55.
7. Gruis NA, Weaver-Feldhaus J, Liu Q, Frye C, Eeles R, Orlow I, Lacombe L, Ponce-Castaneda V, Lianes P, Latres E, et al. Genetic evidence in melanoma and bladder cancers that p16 and p53 function in separate pathways of tumor suppression. *Am J Pathol.* 1995;146:1199–1206.
8. Weaver-Feldhaus J, Gruis NA, Neuhausen S, Le Paslier D, Stockert E, Skolnick MH, Kamb A. Localization of a putative tumor suppressor gene by using homozygous deletions in melanomas. *Proc Natl Acad Sci USA.* 1994;91:7563–7567.
9. Liu Q, Neuhausen S, McClure M, Frye C, Weaver-Feldhaus J, Gruis NA, Eddington K, Allalunis-Turner MJ, Skolnick MH, Fujimura FK, et al. CDKN2 (MTS1) tumor suppressor gene mutations in human tumor cell lines. *Oncogene.* 1995;11:2455.
10. Xing EP, Nie Y, Song Y, Yang GY, Cai YC, Wang LD, Yang CS. Mechanisms of inactivation of p14ARF, p15INK4b, and p16INK4a genes in human esophageal squamous cell carcinoma. *Clin Cancer Res.* 1999;5:2704–2713.
11. Xing EP, Nie Y, Wang LD, Yang GY, Yang CS. Aberrant methylation of p16INK4a and deletion of p15INK4b are frequent events in human esophageal cancer in Linxian, China. *Carcinogenesis.* 1999;20:77–84.
12. Walker GJ, Flores JF, Glendening JM, Lin AH, Markl ID, Fountain JW. Virtually 100% of melanoma cell lines harbor alterations at the DNA level within CDKN2A, CDKN2B, or one of their downstream targets. *Genes Chromosomes Cancer.* 1998;22: 157–163.
13. Herman JG, Merlo A, Mao L, Lapidus RG, Issa JP, Davidson NE, Sidransky D, Baylin SB. Inactivation of the CDKN2/p16/MTS1 gene is frequently associated with aberrant DNA methylation in all common human cancers. *Cancer Res.* 1995;55: 4525–4530.
14. Kumar R, Lundh Rozell B, Louhelainen J, Hemminki K. Mutations in the CDKN2A (p16INK4a) gene in microdissected sporadic primary melanomas. *Int J Cancer.* 1998;75:193–198.
15. Ruiz A, Puig S, Lynch M, Castel T, Estivill X. Retention of the CDKN2A locus and low frequency of point mutations in primary and metastatic cutaneous malignant melanoma. *Int J Cancer.* 1998;76:312–316.
16. Healy E, Sikkink S, Rees JL. Infrequent mutation of p16INK4 in sporadic melanoma. *J Invest Dermatol.* 1996;107:318–321.

17. Funk JO, Schiller PI, Barrett MT, Wong DJ, Kind P, Sander CA. p16INK4a expression is frequently decreased and associated with 9p21 loss of heterozygosity in sporadic melanoma. *J Cutan Pathol.* 1998;25:291–296.
18. Pollock PM, Yu F, Qiu L, Parsons PG, Hayward NK. Evidence for u.v. induction of CDKN2 mutations in melanoma cell lines. *Oncogene.* 1995;11:663–668.
19. Wang SQ, Setlow R, Berwick M, Polsky D, Marghoob AA, Kopf AW, Bart RS. Ultraviolet A and melanoma: a review. *J Am Acad Dermatol.* 2001;44:837–846.
20. Harland M, Meloni R, Gruis N, Pinney E, Brookes S, Spurr NK, Frischauf AM, Bataille V, Peters G, Cuzick J, Selby P, Bishop DT, Bishop JN. Germline mutations of the CDKN2 gene in UK melanoma families. *Hum Mol Genet.* 1997;6:2061–2067.
21. Gruis NA, Van der Velden PA, Sandkuijl LA, Prins DE, Weaver-Feldhaus J, Kamb A, Bergman W, Frants RR. Homozygotes for CDKN2 (p16) germline mutation in Dutch familial melanoma kindreds. *Nat Genet.* 1995;10:351–353.
22. Hussussian CJ, Struewing JP, Goldstein AM, Higgins PA, Ally DS, Sheahan MD, Clark WH Jr., Tucker MA, Dracopoli NC. Germline p16 mutations in familial melanoma. *Nat Genet.* 1994;8:15–21.
23. Pollock PM, Spurr N, Bishop T, Newton-Bishop J, Gruis N, Van der Velden PA, Goldstein AM, Tucker MA, Foulkes WD, Barnhill R, Haber D, Fountain J, Hayward NK. Haplotype analysis of two recurrent CDKN2A mutations in 10 melanoma families: evidence for common founders and independent mutations. *Hum Mutat.* 1998;11:424–431.
24. Foulkes WD, Flanders TY, Pollock PM, Hayward NK. The CDKN2A (p16) gene and human cancer. *Mol Med.* 1997;3:5–20.
25. Hayward N. New developments in melanoma genetics. *Curr Oncol Rep.* 2000;2:300–306.
26. Hamada K, Kohno T, Kawanishi M, Ohwada S, Yokota J. Association of CDKN2A (p16)/CDKN2B(p15) alterations and homozygous chromosome arm 9p deletions in human lung carcinoma. *Genes Chromosomes Cancer.* 1998;22:232–240.
27. Liu L, Goldstein AM, Tucker MA, Brill H, Gruis NA, Hogg D, Lassam NJ. Affected members of melanoma-prone families with linkage to 9p21 but lacking mutations in CDKN2A do not harbor mutations in the coding regions of either CDKN2B or p19ARF. *Genes Chromosomes Cancer.* 1997;19:52–54.
28. Stone S, Dayananth P, Jiang P, Weaver-Feldhaus JM, Tavtigian SV, Cannon-Albright L, Kamb A. Genomic structure, expression and mutational analysis of the P15 (MTS2) gene. *Oncogene.* 1995;11:987–991.
29. Stone S, Jiang P, Dayananth P, Tavtigian SV, Katcher H, Parry D, Peters G, Kamb A. Complex structure and regulation of the P16 (MTS1) locus. *Cancer Res.* 1995;55:2988–2994.
30. Mao L, Merlo A, Bedi G, Shapiro GI, Edwards CD, Rollins BJ, Sidransky D. A novel p16INK4A transcript. *Cancer Res.* 1995;55:2995–2997.
31. Stott FJ, Bates S, James MC, McConnell BB, Starborg M, Brookes S, Palmero I, Ryan K, Hara E, Vousden KH, Peters G. The alternative product from the human CDKN2A locus, p14(ARF), participates in a regulatory feedback loop with p53 and MDM2. *EMBO J.* 1998;17:5001–5014.
32. Kamijo T, Zindy F, Roussel MF, Quelle DE, Downing JR, Ashmun RA, Grosveld G, Sherr CJ. Tumor suppression at the mouse INK4a locus mediated by the alternative reading frame product p19ARF. *Cell.* 1997;91:649–659.
33. Kamijo T, Weber JD, Zambetti G, Zindy F, Roussel MF, Sherr CJ. Functional and physical interactions of the ARF tumor suppressor with p53 and Mdm2. *Proc Natl Acad Sci USA.* 1998;95:8292–8297.
34. Weber JD, Taylor LJ, Roussel MF, Sherr CJ, Bar-Sagi D. Nucleolar Arf sequesters Mdm2 and activates p53. *Nat Cell Biol.* 1999;1:20–26.

35. Quelle DE, Cheng M, Ashmun RA, Sherr CJ. Cancer-associated mutations at the INK4a locus cancel cell cycle arrest by p16INK4a but not by the alternative reading frame protein p19ARF. *Proc Natl Acad Sci USA* 1997;94:669–673.
36. FitzGerald MG, Harkin DP, Silva-Arrieta S, MacDonald DJ, Lucchina LC, Unsal H, O'Neill E, Koh J, Finkelstein DM, Isselbacher KJ, Sober AJ, Haber DA. Prevalence of germ-line mutations in p16, p19ARF, and CDK4 in familial melanoma: analysis of a clinic-based population. *Proc Natl Acad Sci USA*. 1996;93:8541–8545.
37. Platz A, Hansson J, Mansson-Brahme E, Lagerlof B, Linder S, Lundqvist E, Sevigny P, Inganas M, Ringborg U. Screening of germline mutations in the CDKN2A and CDKN2B genes in Swedish families with hereditary cutaneous melanoma. *J Natl Cancer Inst.* 1997;89:697–702.
38. Bahuau M, Vidaud D, Jenkins RB, Bieche I, Kimmel DW, Assouline B, Smith JS, Alderete B, Cayuela JM, Harpey JP, Caille B, Vidaud M. Germ-line deletion involving the INK4 locus in familial proneness to melanoma and nervous system tumors. *Cancer Res.* 1998;58:2298–2303.
39. Tachibana I, Smith JS, Sato K, Hosek SM, Kimmel DW, Jenkins RB. Investigation of germline PTEN, p53, p16(INK4A)/p14(ARF), and CDK4 alterations in familial glioma. *Am J Med Genet.* 2000;92:136–141.
40. Randerson-Moor JA, Harland M, Williams S, Cuthbert-Heavens D, Sheridan E, Aveyard J, Sibley K, Whitaker L, Knowles M, Bishop JN, Bishop DT. A germline deletion of p14(ARF) but not CDKN2A in a melanoma-neural system tumour syndrome family. *Hum Mol Genet.* 2001;10:55–62.
41. Zuo L, Weger J, Yang Q, Goldstein AM, Tucker MA, Walker GJ, Hayward N, Dracopoli NC. Germline mutations in the p16INK4a binding domain of CDK4 in familial melanoma. *Nat Genet.* 1996;12:97–99.
42. Soufir N, Avril MF, Chompret A, Demenais F, Bombled J, Spatz A, Stoppa-Lyonnet D, Benard J, Bressac-de Paillerets B. Prevalence of p16 and CDK4 germline mutations in 48 melanoma-prone families in France. The French Familial Melanoma Study Group. *Hum Mol Genet.* 1998;7:209–216.
43. Naus NC, van Drunen E, de Klein A, Luyten GP, Paridaens DA, Alers JC, Ksander BR, Beverloo HB, Slater RM. Characterization of complex chromosomal abnormalities in uveal melanoma by fluorescence in situ hybridization, spectral karyotyping, and comparative genomic hybridization. *Genes Chromosomes Cancer.* 2001;30: 267–273.
44. Sisley K, Parsons MA, Garnham J, Potter AM, Curtis D, Rees RC, Rennie IG. Association of specific chromosome alterations with tumour phenotype in posterior uveal melanoma. *Br J Cancer.* 2000;82:330–338.
45. Sisley K, Rennie IG, Parsons MA, Jacques R, Hammond DW, Bell SM, Potter AM, Rees RC. Abnormalities of chromosomes 3 and 8 in posterior uveal melanoma correlate with prognosis. *Genes Chromosomes Cancer.* 1997;19:22–28.
46. Prescher G, Bornfeld N, Hirche H, Horsthemke B, Jockel KH, Becher R. Prognostic implications of monosomy 3 in uveal melanoma. *Lancet.* 1996;347:1222–1225.
47. Kallioniemi A, Kallioniemi OP, Sudar D, Rutovitz D, Gray JW, Waldman F, Pinkel D. Comparative genomic hybridization for molecular cytogenetic analysis of solid tumors. *Science.* 1992;258:818–821.
48. Tschentscher F, Prescher G, Horsman DE, White VA, Rieder H, Anastassiou G, Schilling H, Bornfeld N, Bartz-Schmidt KU, Horsthemke B, Lohmann DR, Zeschnigk M. Partial deletions of the long and short arm of chromosome 3 point to two tumor suppressor genes in uveal melanoma. *Cancer Res.* 2001;61:3439–3442.

49. Ohta M, Berd D, Shimizu M, Nagai H, Cotticelli MG, Mastrangelo M, Shields JA, Shields CL, Croce CM, Huebner K. Deletion mapping of chromosome region 9p21–p22 surrounding the CDKN2 locus in melanoma. *Int J Cancer* 1996;65:762–767.
50. Singh AD, Croce CM, Wary KK, Shields JA, Donoso LA, Shields CL, Huebner K, Ohta M. Familial uveal melanoma: absence of germline mutations involving the cyclin-dependent kinase-4 inhibitor gene (p16). *Ophthalmic Genet.* 1996;17:39–40.
51. Singh AD, Wang MX, Donoso LA, Shields CL, De Potter P, Shields JA. Genetic aspects of uveal melanoma: a brief review. *Semin Oncol.* 1996;23:768–772.
52. Merbs SL, Sidransky D. Analysis of p16 (CDKN2/MTS-1/INK4A) alterations in primary sporadic uveal melanoma. *Invest Ophthalmol Vis Sci.* 1999;40:779–783.
53. Van Der Velden PA, Metzelaar-Blok JA, Bergman W, Hurks HMH, Frants RR, Gruis NA, Jager MJ. Promoter hypermethylation: A common cause of reduced p16(INK4a) expression in uveal melanoma. *Cancer Res.* 2001;61:5303–5306.
54. Khan J, Bittner ML, Chen Y, Meltzer PS, Trent JM. DNA microarray technology: the anticipated impact on the study of human disease. *Biochim Biophys Acta* 1999;1423: M17–28.
55. DeRisi J, Penland L, Brown PO, Bittner ML, Meltzer PS, Ray M, Chen Y, Su YA, Trent JM. Use of a cDNA microarray to analyse gene expression patterns in human cancer. *Nat Genet.* 1996;14:457–460.
56. Van der Velden PA, Zuidervaart W, Hurks HMH, Pavey S, Ksander BR, Krijgsman E, Frants RR, Tensen CP, Willemze R, Jager MJ, Gruis NA. Expression profiling reveals that methylation of TIMP3 is involved in uveal melanoma development. *Int. J. Cancer.* 2003;106:472–479.

M.A. BLASI* AND P. GRAMMATICO

# 6. Inheritance and p16

## INTRODUCTION

It is becoming well understood that the development of cancer is not simply a result of random events or environmental hazards, but can depend on an individual's genetic composition as well. Approximately 10% of individuals who develop cutaneous melanoma, for example, carry an inborn susceptibility for that type of cancer.[1] Identification of the specific genes involved has obvious implications both for detection of susceptible individuals and for the development of new treatments.

## CONCEPTS IN CARCINOGENESIS

The concept of tumor suppressor genes is a fundamental tenet in the current understanding of malignant transformation. The existence of suppressor genes was originally postulated from the experimental observation that somatic hybridisation between a normal cell and a cancer cell yields a hybrid of profoundly depressed tumorigenic potential.[2] This effect led to the assumption that tumor suppressor genes restrain aberrant cell growth, and escape from growth control may result from inactivation of suppressor-gene function by a genetic lesion. Thus the products of these genes may function antithetically to the products of oncogenes, which promote malignant cell growth.

Oncogenes, which may exhibit gain-of-function mutations, and their normal cellular counterparts, proto-oncogenes, are often growth factors or growth factor receptors. By comparison, tumor suppressor genes occur in two alternative alleles: the wild type that inhibits tumor development, and a mutant allele that is defective in suppressor function. Normal (wild type) suppressor genes are generally dominant in their effects, in that one normal copy is sufficient to suppress malignant growth, whereas disease-conferring alleles have undergone recessive loss-of-function mutations. Sporadic transformation of a cell requires mutation or deletion of the normal allele on both homologous chromosomes at the tumor suppressor locus that is relevant to oncogenesis of the specific tumor target tissue.[3]

* To whom correspondence should be addressed.

The normal regulation of cell growth and differentiation appears to require the concerted action of growth-inhibiting tumor suppressors and growth-promoting oncogenes. Progression to full malignancy in tumor systems, in contrast, could involve multiple stochastic events of random progression.

The current paradigm of familial predisposition to cancer, that developed originally from studies of retinoblastoma, holds that two successive and coordinate genetic lesions are required to initiate carcinogenesis. The basic model postulates that a defective allele at the critical locus is inherited, substantially increasing the probability of inactivation of that suppressor locus, because only a single subsequent somatic mutational event is then capable of inactivating the other gene copy in tumor target tissue.[4] Delay in onset of the secondary somatic events, that complete the inactivation of the suppressor locus, to the second and third decades of life is necessary to ensure the reproductive fitness of those inheriting the mutant allele, thereby propagating the familial nature of cancer predisposition.[3]

## GENETIC SUSCEPTIBILITY TO CUTANEOUS MELANOMA

Cutaneous melanoma, once a rare disease, is now one of the fastest growing cancers in incidence throughout the world. The cause of cutaneous melanoma is not understood. A number of risk factors for the development of the disease have been identified, one of which is sun exposure. Several lines of evidence support the contribution of sun exposure to the risk of development of melanoma, but the definition of the precise features of this exposure (total exposure, occupational exposure, intensity of exposure) that determine the risk has been somewhat problematic. It is clear, however, that one of the factors that modify the risk of developing melanoma is skin colour.[5] Variation in human skin pigmentation is due to varied amounts of eumelanin (brown/black) and pheomelanin (red) produced by melanocytes. Melanin pigment protects the skin from the damaging effects of ultraviolet radiation. Dark-skinned populations show a substantially lower incidence of melanoma than fair-skinned populations exposed to similar levels of incident sunlight. Thus the demonstration that exogenous solar radiation augments the risk for the development of the disease in some individuals, and that the magnitude of this effect is modified by heritable skin type, together suggest that identifiable genetic predisposing factors exist and correlate to skin colour genes.[5]

The melanocortin-1 receptor (MC1-R) is a regulator of eumelanin and pheomelanin production after binding of the melanocyte-stimulating hormone (MSH). In humans, variants of the MC1-R gene are of key significance in determining the pigmentary phenotype and response to ultraviolet radiation.[6] Although molecular details of MC1-R signaling are not fully understood, the preliminary new insights in MC1-R signal transduction assume that the receptor is involved not only in pigment production but also in additional signaling pathways which evoke different biological responses.[6]

The second risk factor that suggests a genetic predisposition for cutaneous melanoma is family history. Approximately 10% of patients with melanoma describe a history of an affected family member. The susceptibility to melanoma is inherited with an autosomal dominant model and variable penetrance.[7] A portion of these cases occur in the absence of an identifiable predisposing dermatologic condition. However, some cases occur in the setting of the familial atypical multiple mole and melanoma (FAMMM) syndrome, also known as the dysplastic nevus syndrome (DNS), a condition characterized by the early development of large numbers of atypical moles. This disease is inherited as an autosomal dominant trait, although the precise pattern of inheritance remains a source of dispute.[5] In addition, there is general disagreement regarding the precise definition of a dyplastic nevus. There is clinical variability in the size and number of dysplastic lesions that may be present. Furthermore, histopathologic ambiguity also exists. The current working definition of a dysplastic nevus requires both a size of 5 mm or more and the presence of a macular component in the lesion (the 'obligatory criteria') plus at least two of the following features: (1) variable pigmentation; (2) irregular, asymmetric outline; or (3) indistinct borders.[8] Regardless of controversy surrounding the dysplastic nevus, quantitatively abnormal and clinically atypical nevus phenotypes have consistently been related to an increased risk of cutaneous melanoma.[9]

## CLINICAL FEATURES OF HEREDITARY AND SPORADIC CUTANEOUS MELANOMA

Familial cases tend to be younger. In males, the median age is 36 years in hereditary melanoma and 57 years in sporadic melanoma, in females, 29 versus 50 years, respectively. In 10% of hereditary cases and 2% of sporadic ones the diagnosis is made before age 20. The male/female ratio is 1.4 for hereditary melanoma and 1.2 for sporadic disease.

Hereditary melanoma syndrome includes a striking predisposition toward multiple primary melanomas, 30% versus 4% in sporadic cases. The former shows a higher number of atypical nevi (majority of cases) than the latter (about 30% of cases).

Histologic detection of a nevus at the edge of a melanoma has been found in 85% of familial cases and 50% of sporadic melanomas.[9]

## MELANOMA SUSCEPTIBILITY LOCI

Formal genetic analysis is required to prove the existence of a mendelian basis for a particular disease. For melanoma, this work began in the late 1970s, and several loci were examined for linkage to melanoma predisposition.[9]

### CMM1

Several families were described in which a higher risk of familial melanoma was associated with FAMMM syndrome. The investigators proposed that dysplastic nevi were both markers that identified those family members who were at increased risk of cutaneous malignant melanoma (CMM) and precursor lesions from which the majority of newly diagnosed melanomas evolved. These findings were thought to be analogous to those previously made in families with colonic polyposis and colorectal cancer.[10] The hunt for melanoma susceptibility loci was initially hampered by the belief that an atypical nevus and CMM may represent pleiotrophic manifestations of the same defect.[11] In initial studies regarding familial melanoma, individuals affected with CMM and those affected with dysplastic nevi but not CMM were included together in linkage analyses. In this way, chromosome 1 was the first region implicated in familial melanoma when statistically significant evidence for a melanoma susceptibility locus (CMM1) on chromosome 1p36 was reported.[12] This locus was proposed to confer susceptibility to both CMM and atypical nevi; however, the results could not be replicated in other cohorts of melanoma families. Both etiologic and diagnostic heterogeneity have been suggested as explanations for this discrepancy. However, the validity of this finding has since been debated because there is no significant linkage to 1p when only the individuals with CMM are analyzed.[11] This of course does not exclude the possibility that in the analysed kindreds a 1p locus contributes to melanoma susceptibility, but its general importance remains unclear at this time.

### CMM2

Recent observations have shifted the focus of familial melanoma research to a second gene site, located on chromosome 9p (Fig. 6.1). This region was first implicated by loss of heterozygosity (LOH) studies and cytogenetically detectable rearrangements in melanoma cell lines and uncultured tumors at 9p21–22. Given the evidence that chromosome 9p harboured a tumor suppressor gene involved in melanoma development, several markers mapping to chromosome 9p were analysed in families demonstrating melanoma predisposition. Soon after, the CMM2 gene was identified as cyclin dependent kinase inhibitor 2A (CDKN2A), a member of a new class of molecules that play a central role in controlling the progression through the cell cycle.[13,14] Although this gene has been given a wide variety of names including MTS1, CDK4I, INK4A, the p16 gene, and p16$^{INK4a}$, the official designation of this gene by the Human Gene Nomenclature Committee is CDKN2A.[11] CDKN2A consists of three coding exons, exon 1 containing 125 bp, exon 2 with 307 bp, and exon 3 with 12 bp, and encodes the cell cycle inhibitor, p16. The p16 protein functions as a negative regulator of the cyclin D1/CDK4/p16/pRb signaling pathway, the major growth control pathway controlling entry of the cell into the cell cycle.

For cells to progress through G1 into S phase they must pass what is known as the late G1 restriction point, where cyclin D/CDK4 must phosphorylate the retinoblastoma protein, Rb. During G0/G1 the Rb protein exists in a DNA-bound protein complex, where it is bound to the transactivation domain of the E2F transcription factors, preventing transactivation of E2F target genes. The phosphorylation of pRb results in the disassociation of this protein complex and the release of E2F transcription factors in such a way that they can transactivate the necessary genes required for entry into S phase. Overexpression studies have revealed that p16 negatively regulates this pathway by binding to CDKN2A and cyclin D complexes (or CDK6 and cyclin D) and blocking the kinase activity of this enzyme, thereby inhibiting progression through the cell cycle. In the absence of a functional p16 protein, pRb is hyperphosphorylated by CDK4, and the E2F transcription factors, normally sequestered by the unphosphorylated pRb,

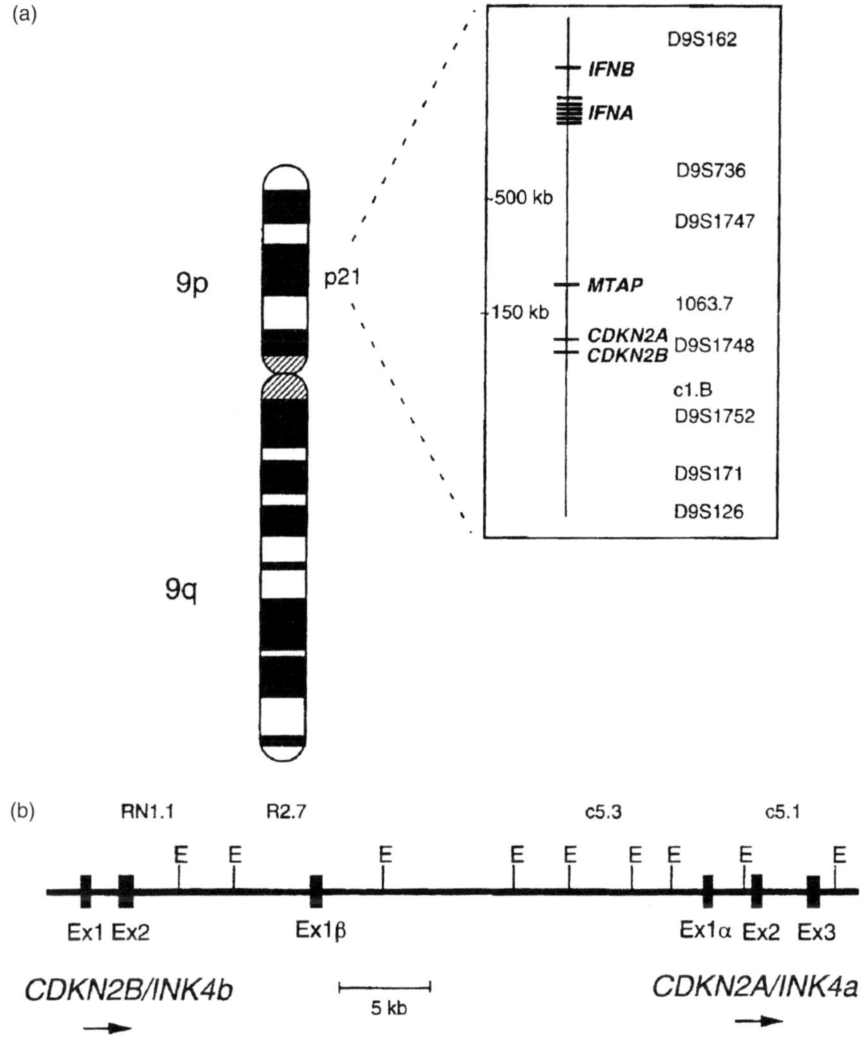


Fig. 6.1. (a) Location of CDKN2A and CDKN2B on chromosome 9. (b) Location of CDKN2 exons.

constantly activate the genes involved in entry of the cell into S phase, leading to uncontrolled cellular growth.[11]

Recently it has been suggested that there is an additional role for p16 in a separate signalling pathway acting at the G2/M restriction point, and more importantly, that there are clues to one of the cellular functions of p16 in the melanocyte.[15] Melanoma cell lines carrying mutations in either CDKN2A or CDK4 failed to exhibit G2 delay in response to ultraviolet radiation, suggesting that the effects of p16 on the G2 delay were mediated through CDK4. The investigators demonstrated an increase in the levels of p16/CDK4/cyclin D complexes in ultraviolet irradiated cells, which led to inhibition of CDK4 activity in ultraviolet irradiated G2-delayed cells that was dependent on the binding of p16. These data suggest that p16 may have dual functions in the cell cycle, and provide tantalizing clues as to how inactivation of CDKN2A could lead to melanoma. The authors postulate that inactivation of CDKN2A disrupts a p16-dependent G2 cell cycle checkpoint, and cells progress through the cell cycle without repairing ultraviolet-light-induced DNA damage, leading to an acquisition of genetic defects.

Although the discovery of the p16 gene was a major breakthrough for melanoma genetics, there is wide variation in the frequency of germline CDKN2A mutations identified in individuals who report a family history of melanoma. It is estimated that only 20% of melanoma families world-wide are linked to p16 mutations.[9] A review of the relevant literature reveals that although loss of heterozygosity (LOH) on chromosome 9 is observed in 30–70% of all uncultured melanomas, mutations in CDKN2A have been observed only in 5–10% of samples. Several explanations for this paradox have been put forward including the following: (1) failure to identify 100% of the coding region mutations because of technical limitations and/or their presence outside a coding region; (2) transcriptional silencing of CDKN2A by methylation of the CpG island spanning the promoter and exon 1 α of the gene; (3) the inactivation of CDKN2A by homozygous deletion; (4) the existence of another tumor suppressor gene within this region that accounts for 9p21 LOH in a subset of tumors.[16]

Actually, the presence of melanoma families linked to 9p but not carrying CDKN2A mutations has induced investigators to search for one or more tumor suppressor gene loci mapping to chromosome 9p. Recently published LOH data support previous reports that additional tumor suppressor gene loci involved in melanoma progression map both centromeric and telomeric to CDKN2A.[16]

A wide variety of tumors have been shown to carry alterations in CDKN2A and this locus seems to be an important one in the development of pancreatic carcinoma. A study aimed to assess the risk of developing pancreatic cancer in FAMMM families with a 19 pb deletion in exon 2 of the p16 gene (p16-Leiden) showed that the estimated cumulative risk in putative mutation carriers, by age 75, was 17%.[17]

## CMM3

A third melanoma gene candidate has emerged from studies of a melanoma cell line in which a mutation in the cyclin-dependent kinase 4 (CDK4) gene was found. As noted above, this protein, mapped to chromosome 12q14 is one step down-stream from CDKN2A in its cell cycle pathway. This melanoma susceptibility gene accounts for only a tiny fraction of all hereditary melanomas. The described CDK4 mutations result in activation of this protein by interfering with its binding to, and thus inhibition by, p16. Therefore, CDK4 functions as a dominant oncogene, not a tumor suppressor gene.[9]

## EXON 1β OF CDKN2A

CDKN2A is unique among human genes in that it has the capacity to encode two different proteins. Two alternative first exons, denoted E1α and E1β, are used

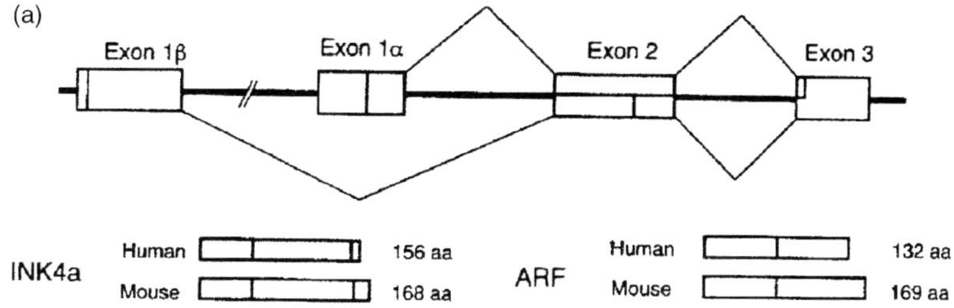


Fig. 6.2. Location of exons, and resulting proteins, of INK4a and ARF.

upstream of exon 2. The α transcript encodes the p16 protein. The β transcript, however, uses an initiation codon that results in translation of the exon 2 and 3 sequence in an alternative reading frame (Fig. 6.2). The polypeptide that results from the translation of the alternative reading frame has been designated p19$^{ARF}$ in the mouse and p14$^{ARF}$ in humans.[18] p19$^{ARF}$ has no amino acid homology to p16. It was found to induce p-53 dependent cell cycle arrest. Although many of the original investigations into the functions of this protein were performed with p19$^{ARF}$ in murine cells, subsequent experiments have confirmed similar functions of p14$^{ARF}$ in human cells.[11] A recent paper has presented a model summarizing the way in which ARF functions to induce cell cycle arrest.[19]

As mentioned previously, disregulation of the Rb pathway results in the generation of a hyperproliferative signal by E2F which, in turn, has been shown to induce transcription of ARF. ARF is believed to function by sequestering MDM2 in the nucleus, preventing the nucleocytoplasmic shuttling of the MDM2–p53 complex, which is essential for MDM2 to target p53 to the cytoplasmic proteosome for degradation. Loss of p14$^{ARF}$ results in rapid destruction of p53, leading to reduction of the p53-associated apoptotic response.[11]

Many families that demonstrate linkage or haplotype sharing on chromosome 9p21 do not have mutations in CDKN2A. Because p14$^{ARF}$ was found to act as a tumor suppressor gene, exon 1β has also been screened for mutations in melanoma families. To date, no mutations that specifically target exon 1β have been found. Although some mutations in exon 2 of CDKN2A could also affect the function of p14$^{ARF}$, the absence of exon 1β mutations, combined with the identification of germline mutations in exon 1α of the CDKN2A gene, indicates that p16 is the primary target of these mutations in exon 2 of CDKN2A.[11]

## GENES OF SPORADIC MELANOMA

Sporadic cutaneous melanoma accounts for approximately 90% of all melanoma cases, but the molecular genetics of melanoma development have been slow to emerge. Cytogenetic and LOH studies have revealed six chromosomes–chromosomal regions (1p, 6p, 7p, 9p, 10, and 11q) likely to harbour genes involved in melanoma development.[11] Candidate genes have been identified from only two of these regions: (1) CDKN2A, mapping to chromosome 9p21; and (2) PTEN, mapping to chromosome 10q23. It is unknown whether the latter chromosomal regions also hold additional genes involved in melanoma pathogenesis, however, increasing amount of data shows that this may be the case.[11]

## CDKN2A

It is estimated that only 0.02% of sporadic melanomas may be attributed to p16 mutations.[20] The low prevalence of p16 mutations suggests that other melanoma genes remain to be discovered or that p16 may still be involved via complex gene–gene or gene–environment interactions. Studies investigating p16 expression in sporadic melanoma tumors have shown that this gene still has an important role during tumor progression with loss of expression in more advanced stage of the disease often associated with LOH at the 9p21 locus.[21,22]

## PTEN

Chromosome 10 was first implicated in melanoma pathogenesis by the presence of cytogenetically detectable rearrangements, normally translocations or deletions, in melanocytic lesions and uncultured melanomas.[11] Most of LOH studies were unable to narrow down the region of interest, because loss of the entire chromosome was the most common event. LOH on chromosome 10q is a feature of a wide variety of different cancers, and the PTEN gene was identified as a tumor suppressor gene mapping to chromosome 10q23 involved in multiple cancer types including glioblastoma, and cancer of the breast, kidney, and prostate.[23]

The protein PTEN is unusual in that it possesses both lipid phosphatase activity and protein phosphatase activity. Moreover PTEN seems to function in two separate signal transduction pathways. Cell survival and proliferation require the presence of appropriate growth factors and anchorage to the extracellular matrix. Recent data suggest that PTEN plays a role in regulating cell survival and cell proliferation by regulating the levels of the lipid second messenger PI-3,4,5-$P_3$ in response to growth factor stimulation. In addition, PTEN has been implicated in modulating cell migration and invasion by negatively regulating the signals generated at focal adhesions through the direct dephosphorylation and inhibition of focal adhesion kinase.[24]

However, the role of PTEN/MMAC1 gene in the pathogenesis and progression of cutaneous melanoma is still controversial. In fact, while some authors[25] have described the presence of both LOH and mutations in primary and metastatic melanoma, suggesting that PTEN/MMAC1 alteration could represent an important step in the development and progression of this tumor, other investigators,[26] in a study carried on 25 primary melanoma and 25 metastatic melanoma, proposed a mutation of PTEN/MMAC1 as a non-essential event in the early stages of melanoma.

# p16/CDKN2A AND UVEAL MELANOMA

Uveal melanomas differ substantially in their incidence and biological behaviour from cutaneous melanomas.[27] Main differences between the two tumors include the following: (1) the role of sunlight as a risk factor is controversial in uveal melanoma; (2) there has been no evidence for an increase in ocular melanoma incidence over the last 20 years, even in countries such as Australia in which a clear increase in cutaneous melanoma has been observed;[27] (3) there is no clear inheritable predisposing condition for uveal melanoma.

Little is known about the genetic alterations that are involved in the development of uveal melanoma and the progression to metastatic disease. A number of chromosomal loci have been implicated based on cytogenetic studies, including sites on chromosomes 3, 6 and 8.[28] Given the common origin of cutaneous and uveal melanoma from melanocytes of the neural crest, the coexistence of cutaneous and ocular melanoma that supports a predisposition to both types of tumor,[1] and cytogenetic defects in chromosome 9, found in approximately 30% of choroidal melanoma,[29] p16/CDKN2A could represent the common gene for uveal melanoma susceptibility. No mutations of this gene were detected in several studies,[30,32] although these studies were based on analyses of small groups of patients, but an interesting report showed that p16 inactivation for homozygous deletion or methylation occurs in 27% of uveal melanomas, representing the most common molecular genetic alteration identified thus far in uveal melanoma.[33] Positive immunostaining for p16 was reported as well, but no correlation with clinicopathologic parameters was observed.[34,35] A large study including a total of 385 uveal melanoma patients found only one Gly35Ala substitution in exon 1α of $p16^{INK4A}$ and no mutations in $p14^{ARF}$ or p15.[36] No mutations were found in BRCA2 either.

Uveal melanoma may arise from a series of genetic changes which are likely different from those contributing to the onset of cutaneous melanoma, and currently there is no significant evidence implicating CDKN2A in the aetiology of uveal melanoma.

## REFERENCES


1. Bataille V. Genetics of familial and sporadic melanoma. *Clin Exp Dermatol.* 2000;25:464–470.
2. Harris H, Miller OJ, Klein G, Worst P, Tachibana T. Suppression of malignancy by cell fusion. *Nature.* 1969;223:363–368.
3. Piepkorn MW. Genetic basis of susceptibility to melanoma. *J Am Acad Dermatol.* 1994;31:1022–1039.
4. Knudson Ag. Mutation and cancer: statistical study of retinoblastoma. *Proc Natl Acad Sci USA.* 1971;68:820–823.
5. Haluska FG, Hodi FS. Molecular genetics of familial cutaneous melanoma. *J Clin Oncol.* 1998;16:670–682.
6. Van der Velden PA, Sandkuijl LA, Bergman W, Pavel S, Van Mourik L, Frants RR, Gruis NA. Melanocortin-1 receptor variant R151C modifies melanoma risk in Dutch families with melanoma. *Am J Hum Genet.* 2001;69:774–779.
7. Ruiz A, Puig S, Malvehy J, Lazaro C, Lynch M, Gimenez-Arnau AM, Puig L, Sanchez-Conejo J, Estivill X, Castel T. CDKN2A mutations in spanish cutaneous malignant melanoma families and patients with multiple melanomas and other neoplasia. *J Med Genet.* 1999;36:490–493.
8. Tucker MA, Halpern A, Holly EA, Hartge P, Elder DE, Sagebiel RV, Guerry D 4th, Clark WH Jr. Clinically recognized dysplastic nevi: a central risk factor for cutaneous melanoma. *JAMA.* 1997;277:1439–1444.

9. Greene MH. The genetics of hereditary melanoma and nevi 1998 update. *Cancer.* 1999;86:2464–2477.
10. Greene MH, Clark WH Jr, Tucker MA, Kraemer KH, Elder DE, Fraser MC. High risk of malignant melanoma in melanoma-prone families with dysplastic nevi. *Ann Intern Med.* 1985;102:458–465.
11. Pollock PM, Trent JM. The genetics of cutaneous melanoma. *Clin Lab Med.* 2000;20(4):667–690.
12. Bale SJ, Dracopoli NC, Tucker MA, Clark WH Jr, Fraser MC, Stanger BZ, Green P, Donis-Keller H, Housman DE, Greene MH. Mapping the gene for hereditary cutaneous malignant melanoma-dysplastic nevus to chromosome 1p. *N Engl J Med.* 1989;320:1367–1372.
13. Kamb A, Gruis NA, Weaver-Feldhaus J, Liu Q, Harshman K, Tautigian SV, Stockert E, Day RS 3rd, Johnson BE, Skolnick MH. A cell cycle regulator potentially involved in genesis of many tumor types. *Science.* 1994;264:436–440.
14. Nobori T, Miura K, Wu DJ, et al. Deletions of the cyclin-dependent kinase-4 inhibitor gene in multiple human cancers. *Nature.* 1994;368:753–756.
15. Gabrielli BG, Sarcevic B, Sinnamon J, Walker G, Castellano M, Wang XQ, Ellem KA. A cyclin D-CDK4 activity required for G2 phase cell cycle progression is inhibited in ultraviolet radiation-induced G2 phase delay. *J Biol Chem.* 1999;274:13961–13969.
16. Pollock PM, Welch J, Hayward NK. Evidence for three tumor suppressor loci on chromosome 9p involved in melanoma development. *Cancer Res.* 2001;61:1154–1161.
17. Vasen HFA, Gruis NA, Frants RR, Van der Velden PA, Hille ET, Bergman W. Risk of developing pancreatic cancer in families with FAMMM associated with a specific 19 deletion of p16 (p16-Leiden). *Int J Cancer.* 2000;87:809–811.
18. Quelle DE, Zindy F, Ashmun RA, Sherr CJ. Alternative reading frames of the INK4a tumor suppressor gene encode two unrelated proteins capable of inducing cell cycle arrest. *Cell.* 1995;83:993–1000.
19. Piepkorn M. Melanoma genetics: an update with focus on the CDKN2A(p16)ARF tumor suppressor. *J Am Acad Dermatol.* 2000;42:705–722.
20. Aitken J, Welch J, Duffy D, Milligan A, Green A, Martin N, Hayward N. CDKN2 variants in a population-based sample of Queensland families with melanoma. *J Nat Cancer Inst.* 1999;91:446–452.
21. Healy E, Belgaid C, Takata M, Harrison D, Zhu NW, Burd DA, Rigby HS, Matthews JN, Rees JL. Prognostic significance of allelic losses in primary melanoma. *Oncogene.* 1998;16:2213–2218.
22. Grover R, Chana JS, Wilson GD, Richman PI, Sanders R. Analysis of p16 protein expression in sporadic malignant melanoma. *Melanoma Res.* 1998;8:267–272.
23. Li J, Yen C, Liaw D, et al. PTEN, a putative protein tyrosine phosphatase gene mutated in human brain, breast, and prostate cancer. *Science.* 1977;275:1943–1947.
24. Besson A, Robbins SM, Yong VW. PTEN/MMAC1/TEP1 in signal transduction and tumorigenesis. *Eur J Biochem.* 1999;263:605–611.
25. Birck A, Ahrenkiel V, Zeuthen J, Hou-Jensen K, Guldberg P. Mutations and allelic loss of the PTEN/MMAC1 gene in primary and metastatic melanoma biopsies. *J Invest Dermatol.* 2000;114:277–280.
26. Poetsch M, Dittberner T, Woenckhaus C. PTEN/MMAC1 in malignant melanoma and its importance for tumour progression. *Cancer Genet Cytogenet.* 2001;125:21–26.
27. Houlston RS, Damato BE. Genetic predisposition to ocular melanoma. *Eye.* 1999; 13:43–46.
28. Singh AD, Donoso LA. Genetic aspects of uveal melanoma. *Int Ophthalmol Clin.* 1993;33:47–52.

29. Singh AD, Boghosian-Sell L,Wary KK, Shields CL, De Potter P, Donoso LA, Shields JA, Cannissard LA. Cytogenetic findings in primary uveal melanomas. *Cancer Genet Cytogenet.* 1994;72:109–115.
30. Wang X, Egan KM, Gragoudas ES, Kelsey KT. Constitutional alterations in p16 in patients with uveal melanoma. *Melanoma Res.* 1996;6:405–410.
31. Singh AD, Croce CM, Wary KK, Shields JA, Donoso LA, Shields CL, Huebner K, Ohta M. Familial uveal melanoma: absence of germline mutations involving the cyclin-dependent kinase-4 inhibitor gene (p16). *Ophthalmic Genet.* 1996;17:39–40.
32. Blasi MA, Binni F, De Bernardo C, et al. Analysis of CDKN2A constitutional mutations in 15 patients affected by uveal melanoma. *Invest Ophthalmol Vis Sci.* (Abstract) 2000;41:S382.
33. Merbs SL, Sidransky D. Analysis of p16 (CDKN2/MTS-1/INK4A) alterations in primary sporadic uveal melanoma. *Invest Ophthalmol Vis Sci.* 1999;40:779–783.
34. Coupland SE, Bechrakis N, Schuler A, Anagnostopoulos I, Hummel M, Bornfeld N, Stein H. Expression patterns of cyclin D1 and related proteins regulating G1-S phase transition in uveal melanoma and retinoblastoma. *Br J Ophthalmol.* 1998;82:961–970.
35. Mouriaux F, Maurage CA, Labalette P, Salbonniere B, Malecaze F, Darbon JM. Cyclin-dependent kinase inhibitory protein expression in human choroidal melanoma tumors. *Invest Ophthalmol Vis Sci.* 2000; 41: 2837–2843.
36. Hearle N, Damato BE, Humphreys J, Wixey J, Green H, Stone J, Easton DF, Houlston RS. Contribution of germine mutatins in BRCA2, P16INK4A, P14ARF and p15 to uveal melanoma. *Inv Ophthalmol Vis Sci.* 2003;44:458–462.

KAREN SISLEY AND NICOLE NAUS

# 7. The Relevance of Chromosome Abnormalities in Posterior Uveal Melanoma

## INTRODUCTION

Uveal melanoma research has mainly concentrated on the identification of prognostic factors for metastatic disease. These prognostic factors can be divided into clinical parameters, such as tumor diameter and location, histopathological and genetic parameters. In this chapter we will discuss the genetic parameters only.

Cancer itself can be considered as a genetic disease, the identification of genetic changes therefore provides seminal information on how tumors initiate, develop and propagate. An effective starting point is to study the chromosomes. This procedure, known as cytogenetics, provides information about the extent of genetic damage throughout the genome, including the gains and losses of whole chromosomes, deletions, translocations and other structural rearrangements. For over forty years, cytogenetics has played an important role in the study of cancer, with its coming of age rapidly following the identification of the first chromosome abnormality associated with cancer, that of the Philadelphia chromosome of Chronic Myeloid Leukaemia.[1] Following this initial observation, many other cytogenetic alterations have been identified in the haematological malignancies, and these abnormalities are of direct clinical relevance, impinging both on the diagnosis and prognosis of these cancers.[2] In contrast, data from cytogenetic analysis of solid tumors are restricted due to technical difficulties associated with obtaining good quality metaphase spreads.

Solid tumors frequently have highly complex chromosome alterations, and are often very heterogeneous with no two cells exactly alike,[3] and they appear to have a tendency to acquire additional chromosome changes as they progress.[4–6] It can therefore be considered that some abnormalities are specifically related to the development of the tumor or its progression to a more aggressive form, whilst others are coincidental.[4–6] All these factors make the identification of specific relevant changes in solid tumors an arduous procedure.

Uncharacteristically, posterior uveal melanomas have shown themselves to be highly amenable to cytogenetic study. Their suitability arises mainly because of two reasons. Initially they can be readily grown in culture, at least in the short-term, and

Table 7.1. Overview of chromosomal aberrations in uveal melanoma (% of cases).

| Reference | No. | Method | Loss of 1p36 | Monosomy 3 | Gain of 6p | Gain of 8(q) |
|---|---|---|---|---|---|---|
| Sisley et al. 1997[13] | 42 | cytogenetics | 29 | 50 | 19 | 54 |
| Prescher et al. 1996[12] | 54 | cytogenetics/CGH | nr | 57 | nr | nr |
| White et al. 1998[20] | 54 | cytogenetics | nr | 50 | 46* | 48 |
| Parella et al. 1999[14] | 50 | microsatellite | 33 | 59 | 28 | 60 |
| McNamara 1997[15a] | 17 | FISH | nr | 12 | nr | nr |

*Abnormalities of chromosome 6.
Abbreviations: (nr) not reported; (FISH) Fluorescent *in situ* Hybridisation; (CGH) Comparative Genomic Hybridization.

it is possible under the right conditions to culture over 80% of all tumors received. Such high levels of success increase the likelihood of obtaining sufficient numbers of good quality chromosome spreads for analysis. Secondly, they are intrinsically more suited to the identification of specific chromosome abnormalities, as they frequently contain few alterations. It is therefore fundamentally easier to identify chromosome changes that are consistently present in these melanomas, with such alterations therefore considered as non-random. Non-random changes are less likely to be coincidental, but probably are specifically related to the cancer in question, either as primary changes related to its development, or as secondary abnormalities associated with the malignant progression of that particular tumor. In the 15 years or so, since the first reported case on uveal melanoma, our knowledge of the cytogenetics of these tumors has advanced dramatically, although in hindsight some of the non-random chromosome alterations now considered to be characteristic of this melanoma, were evident from the very first study.

In 1985 cytogenetic analysis of a single uveal melanoma, albeit metastatic, reported changes of chromosomes 6 and 8.[7] These observations were followed 3 years later by a second report, again on a single tumor, in which the sole abnormality was trisomy of chromosome 6p.[8] After a slow start the beginning of the last decade proved to be a turning point, with a total of 21 new cases presented independently by three groups.[9–11] Soon it became apparent that certain chromosomes were more commonly implicated than others, and consistent anomalies of chromosomes 1, 3, 6 and 8 were found.[9–11] Continued study combining the techniques of cytogenetics with Fluorescence *in situ* Hybridization (FISH) and Comparative Genomic Hybridization (CGH), has confirmed the non-random status of these chromosome changes, and extended the number of cases beyond 200 (Table 7.1; see also Chapter 8, this book). Of all the chromosome alterations reported by far the most frequent change, occurring to date in approximately 50% of all analysed melanomas, is the loss of one copy, or monosomy, of chromosome 3 (Fig. 7.1).[12–15]

## MONOSOMY 3

The loss of an entire chromosome, with the regularity observed in posterior uveal melanoma, is a relatively uncommon event amongst other solid tumors,[3] although

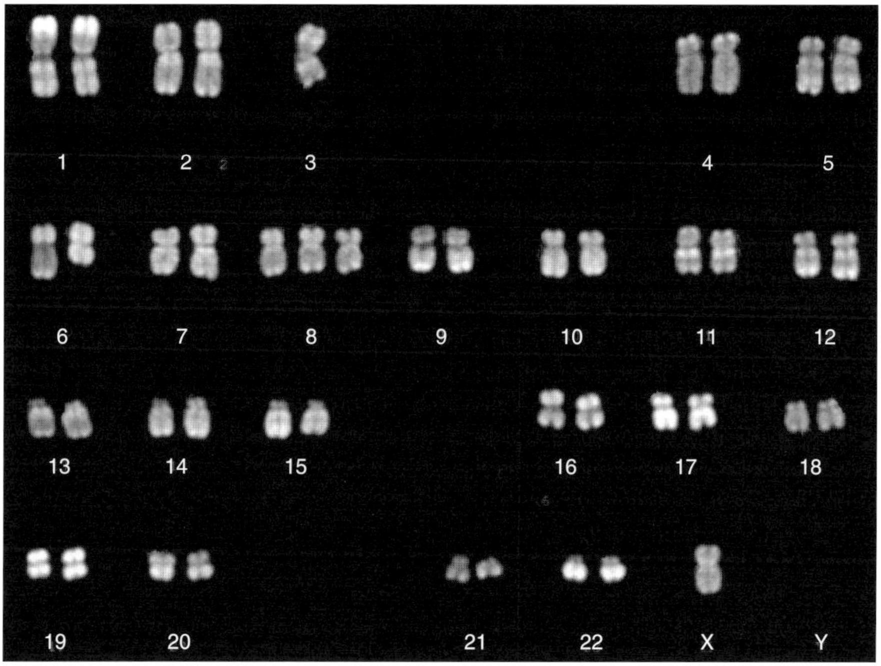


Fig. 7.1. Karyogram of a choroidal melanoma. This tumor showed a −3, i(6)(p), +8, typically found in uveal melanoma. This case shows also a loss of the Y chromosome.

it is possible that in some cancers such losses are later masked by subsequent genetic rearrangements. In uveal melanomas the consistent finding of monosomy 3 is emphasised by an almost total lack of rearrangements involving chromosome 3. These melanomas appear, at least at the level of cytogenetics, to lose either an entire copy or maintain two normal copies. In a series of over 100 tumors only four cases actually had visible rearrangements of chromosome 3 (unpublished data Sheffield). The breakpoints involved were diverse, 3p24–25, 3p13–14, 3q13, and 3q21, with both arms of chromosome 3 affected. Other reports in the literature exist of such changes, again evidence suggests both arms are involved, with the smallest regions of involvement shown to be at 3p25, 3p13, 3q13–21 and 3q24–26.[15–17] Structural rearrangements can highlight chromosomal regional hotspots and indicate specific gene involvement. The scarcity of chromosome 3 structural alterations in uveal melanomas, would suggest the presence of a highly specific mechanism, in which the loss of an entire chromosome 3 plays a fundamental role, probably because such a loss would be the most efficacious way to target multiple genes resident on a single chromosome. Chromosome 3 is the location of numerous genes linked in some manner with the development and progression of cancer.[18] The relevant genes on chromosome 3, involved in uveal melanoma, however await identification, although recent evidence implicates one potential candidate gene, the TGF-β R2 gene. The gene is located at 3p21–22, and breakpoints and loss of heterozygosity (LOH) of this region have been reported in uveal melanoma,[19] whilst TGF-β itself has been shown to regulate negatively uveal melanoma proliferation.[19] Additional studies have however effectively eliminated other potential candidate genes, such as the Von Hippel Lindau (*VHL*) and Thyroid hormone receptor β (*THRB*) genes.[15,20]

The high frequency of chromosome 3 loss suggests that it is essentially for the malignant transformation of the uvea. There is also little heterogeneity for monosomy 3, and when loss of chromosome 3 is present, it is so within all abnormal cells of the tumor population analysed. This would imply that the change itself is one of the earlier predisposing changes associated with uveal melanoma initiation, and that other chromosome alterations subsequently follow. Parrella and associates proposed a bifurcated tumor pathway with mutual exclusivity of the loss of chromosome 3 and the gain of 6p,[14] although this theory has not been supported by other studies.[10,20–22] Chromosome 3 loss does however seem to be an important part of a sequence of genetic changes more common to certain forms of uveal melanoma. Monosomy 3 has been found to occur more frequently in those tumors with gain of chromosome 8, and although choroidal melanomas can have monosomy 3, a much higher incidence for abnormalities of both chromosomes 3 and 8 is found in tumors arising from the ciliary body.[10–12,23–27] Whether all tumors have chromosome 3 loss at the molecular level remains to be established, but it is clear that even apparently normal copies of chromosome 3 can harbour small deletions[15] and in extreme cases isodisomy has been reported, in which an entire copy of chromosome 3 is lost, and the remaining homologue, presumably with all its imperfections, is duplicated.[28]

## ISOCHROMOSOME 8

As has been briefly mentioned, loss of chromosome 3 is more frequently found in those melanomas that also have abnormalities of chromosome 8. This relationship seems to be quite specific, and is certainly more often associated with tumors possessing a ciliary body component.[10–12,23–27] The abnormalities of chromosome 8 are themselves highly consistent, representing as they do amplification of the long arm, or 8q. These amplifications are predominantly in the form of an isochromosome, in which both arms of the chromosome are derived from the long arm of chromosome 8, in effect also producing a deletion of the short arm. In some uveal melanomas, the amplification occurs as a straightforward gain of an entire chromosome 8, a change that is also found in melanomas with choroidal involvement.[21,27] There is however an interesting tendency to acquire additional amplifications of 8q. In the simplest form chromosome 8 is gained, followed by the development of an isochromosome 8q (or other form of amplification), finally culminating in the accumulation of multiple copies of i(8)(q10). This process itself is even evident within individual tumors, where sub lines co-exist possessing just a single extra copy of chromosome 8, a single i(8)(q10), or with several additional i(8)(q10); other chromosome abnormalities are maintained within all sub lines.[21,26,28,29] It is however clear that the majority of evidence suggests that loss of chromosome 3 occurs prior to abnormalities of chromosome 8,[13,14,29] and that abnormalities of 8 appear to be secondary chromosome changes associated with clonal evolution.[9,13,29] The study of metastatic lesions is in itself problematic, mainly because of their unavailability as post-mortems are not routinely performed. In the few studies that have looked at metastases, abnormalities of chromosome 8 have been found in all eight cases, but not always abnormalities of 3.[7,22,30] In combination these results imply that genes on 8q are perhaps more important in the progression of the tumor, potentially even providing the driving force for the establishment of metastatic disease.

The regions involved on chromosome 8 are again large, and could effectively target many genes important in cancer development and progression. Cytogenetic studies initially defined the smallest region of amplification as 8q21–qter,[10] whilst later studies, in combination with CGH, refined the region to 8q23–24–qter.[31,32] More recently, studies using a combination of spectral karyotyping (SKY) and CGH, have found that in actuality two distinct regions of 8q may be specifically amplified, at 8q21.1–21.2 and again at 8q23–24.[17] At present we can only speculate as to which genes in uveal melanoma may be the targets of such amplifications, but an obvious candidate is the *MYC* oncogene, which is located at 8q24, and therefore falls within the second region identified by Naus and associates.[17] Whether *MYC* is specifically amplified as the preferred target, or is co-amplified because of its proximity to an otherwise unknown gene, remains to be established. What is known is that *MYC* amplification, as determined by FISH (Fluorescence *in situ* Hybridization), occurs at a higher frequency than would be expected from cytogenetic observations.[33] It is estimated that at least 30% of uveal melanomas have specific amplification of *MYC*, and that this gain itself also occurs later in the genetic progression of uveal melanoma.[33] If *MYC* is the potential target, its ultimate effect appears to be contradictory in uveal melanoma, as conflicting evidence has suggested both an association with poor prognosis,[34] and latterly, increased expression is consistently associated with a good outcome.[35–37] Until the location and extent of amplification on 8q is additionally refined, the candidate genes will remain unidentified.

## CHROMOSOME 6

From the first cytogenetic reports of uveal melanoma, chromosome 6 abnormalities were implicated.[7,8] These changes are now some of the most consistent non-randomly associated with these melanomas (Table 7.1). The rearrangements however affect both arms of the chromosome, resulting in deletions of 6q and gains of 6p. Although these changes can occur independently, they are often present in the form of an i(6)(p10), and therefore, assuming the change is not additional, encompass both the deletion of the long arm, and the gain of the short arm in a single alteration.[10,21,25] The breakpoints on chromosome 6q can be quite diverse, whereas those on the short arm are consistently located towards the centromeric region.[21] The smallest regional gain on 6p has been established as 6pter–p21,[31] but for the long arm the regional involvement is less defined, and often the whole arm is deleted through the formation of an isochromosome.[10,21,25] Evidence has suggested that isochromosome formation, whether of chromosome 1, 6 or 8 appears to be more often associated with the presence of monosomy 3.[22] Certainly cytogenetic studies confirm that chromosome 3 loss and i(6)(p10) alterations are found together.[10,21,25] The situation is however confused, and, as mentioned previously, a distinct pathway has been suggested in which monosomy 3 is considered to be mutually exclusive to abnormalities of 6p.[14] This observation has been partly confirmed by Tschentscher and associates, who found through a review of the literature, that only 14% of tumors with monosomy 3 also had 6p gains.[15] In addition, in their own microsatellite analysis (MSA) they found at least one of 13 tumors had monosomy 3 and abnormalities of 6p. It would therefore appear that 6p alterations, although far less frequent, are not excluded from tumors with monosomy 3. A possible explanation has been provided by Tschentscher and co-workers, who highlighted the limitations of MSA in the study of chromosome gains, such as i(6)(p10) and i(8)(q10).[15] It is therefore worth bearing in mind that cytogenetic studies will miss a substantial amount of genetic change at a molecular level, but that purely MSA studies can equally distort the picture. When more studies have used a combination of techniques on individual tumors, we will gain a truer picture.

Alterations of chromosome 6 appear to be a common feature of most melanocytic tissues as comparable changes have also been reported in the few iris melanomas so far detailed.[38] More importantly they are also one of the most frequently found aberrations in cutaneous melanomas,[39] where more in-depth study has been undertaken of their role, and specifically the regions that are affected.[40,41] It is possible that the same genes implicated in cutaneous melanoma are also integral to the development of uveal melanoma. Because of the nature of chromosome 6 rearrangements in uveal melanoma, again affecting both arms, it seems likely that numerous genes are important. Potential targets located in the region 6pter–p21, thought to be involved in uveal melanoma, include genes that could affect cell cycle and angiogenesis, such as *CDKN1A*, or *VEGF*.[31,42,43] Abnormalities of 6p could also substantially affect the immunological behaviour of the tumor, as the genes encoding MHC class I molecules and *TNFα* are also localized to this region.[18] Some comparison of 6p abnormalities with altered HLA expression in uveal melanoma has been undertaken, but as the effects could be wide ranging, no clear relationship has as yet been established.[44] The regions involved on the long arm are less obvious, often the whole arm is affected, but cytogenetic studies also appear to imply that potentially at least two regions may be selectively deleted. The first seems to be a reasonably clear-cut distal deletion affecting 6q24–q27. The other breakpoints would suggest targeting of a region first around 6q13–q15, and potentially a third region at 6q21–q22.[10,21,25–27,32,45] The delineation of smallest regions is complicated by the manner of 6q rearrangements in uveal melanoma, which tend to produce loss from the breakpoint onwards, rather than small interstitial deletions.[10,21,25–27,32,45] It is however likely that some of these rearrangements are complex and 6q material may be dispersed amongst other abnormalities. With the use of additional techniques such as SKY, it is likely that the regions typically involved on 6q will be refined.

## CHROMOSOME 1

In common with cutaneous melanomas, uveal melanomas also have consistent changes of chromosome 1. Rearrangements of the distal part of the short arm of chromosome 1 are one of the most frequent abnormalities of skin melanomas, occurring in about 80% of all cases.[39,46] In uveal melanoma the abnormalities of chromosome 1 are again quite specific, and comparable with those of cutaneous melanoma as they mainly give rise to deletions of 1p. They are however less frequent, being found in approximately 30% of all uveal melanomas.[10,14,21,25,32] Cytogenetic studies suggest that chromosome 1 changes are perhaps more common amongst melanomas with a ciliary body component, although this observation has not been confirmed by FISH[10,21,25,32] (Naus et al. unpublished results). The frequency for chromosome 1 deletion is certainly less than that observed for chromosomes 3 and 8 (Naus et al. unpublished results), suggesting that the abnormality may be subsequent to the other changes. In addition, cytogenetic studies have found a higher incidence of 1p rearrangements in larger melanomas,[21] implying the changes may relate to progression, as has been proposed for cutaneous melanoma.[10,47] Furthermore, recent data has found that loss of chromosome 1p is only present in primary uveal melanoma that had metastasized, and in metastases themselves.[22] It would seem likely that rearrangements of chromosome 1 are indicative of more advanced melanomas, suggesting that chromosome 1 is the location of a uveal melanoma metastatic suppressor gene, or genes.[22]

The rearrangements of chromosome 1 are in themselves interesting, as they appear to fall into two categories, the net result of both being deletions of 1p. In some uveal melanomas deletions of defined regions have been identified, whilst in others the entire short arm is lost, mainly as the result of unbalanced translocations.[10,21,25] There is also an increased specificity in the selection of these translocation partners, with a preponderance for D group involvement.[10,21,25] In addition the breakpoints themselves are also highly consistent, often affecting heterochromatic regions, possibly highlighting the inherent weakness of highly repetitive DNA.[21] In their recent study using CGH, Aalto and associates were able to define a minimal overlapping region around 1p31.[22] Cytogenetic studies however found breakpoints over a larger region spanning 1p12–p36, but interestingly also identified a smallest regional involvement distinct from that suggesting by Aalto and associates, at 1p32–p36.[10,21,25,32] This more distal region has been confirmed to be involved in approximately 30% of uveal melanomas, using FISH for 1p36.[48] The evidence would again suggest that more than one gene located on chromosome 1 is important in the development of uveal melanoma. Certainly genes postulated to be involved in the cutaneous form could also be involved in uveal melanoma, for example deletions of *CDC2L*, a gene encoding a protein kinase isoform located to 1p36, are found in cutaneous melanoma.[49]

## OTHER CHROMOSOME CHANGES

Although uveal melanomas do not characteristically have high levels of chromosome aberrations, in common with other malignancies, they show a correlation between the acquisition of additional chromosome losses and gains and increasing tumors size, suggesting that such numerical alterations are coincidental.[21] Other chromosomes abnormalities, including those of chromosomes 2, 9, 10, 11, 21 and the sex chromosomes appear however to have a more tangible association.[10,21,24–27,32,50,51] Of these other chromosome changes the commonest by far affecting the majority of male patients, is loss of the Y chromosome. Although this change may be artifactual, related to patient age or cultural conditions, its occurrence is mainly associated with the presence of other abnormalities, and is infrequently found in samples of patients blood[20,26,52] (Sheffield unpublished data), suggesting an as yet undetermined role, but has been proposed to relate to tumor progression.[10,25] Trisomy 21 is also speculated to be associated with tumor progression, as the gain of 21 appears to be secondary to those of other chromosomes including 3, 6 and 8. In addition the gain appears to be more frequent in melanomas with involvement of chromosomes 3 and 8 and consequently seems to associate with tumors of the ciliary body.[10,21,24–27,32]

Certain chromosome abnormalities appear common to both uveal and cutaneous melanoma, principally those affecting chromosomes 1 and 6. Cutaneous melanomas also have non-random loss and deletions of other chromosomes including 9p, 10q, and 11.[53,54] Alterations of these chromosomes are less frequent in uveal melanoma, but seemingly target comparable regions to those affected in cutaneous melanoma.[10,21,24–27,32] Deletions of chromosome 9 are considered to be an early event in cutaneous melanoma pathogenesis, and target a familial melanoma susceptibility gene, p16, or *CDKN2/MTS-1/INK4A*, which is located at 9p21.[53,55,56] In uveal melanoma cytogenetic studies have identified tumors which have rearrangements or deletions of 9p, and also of 9q, but they are an infrequent alteration occurring in less than 10% of uveal melanomas.[21,25–27,32,51] CGH studies, although suggesting a higher incidence of 9p alteration in uveal melanomas, are also contradictory, identifying both increased loss and gain for the region,[31,45] whilst MSA implies imbalances of approximately 20% for 9p.[13] The p16 gene may not be the target of these deletions, as studies suggest that its deletion is rare in uveal melanoma,[57] and it is thought that inactivation of p16 is achieved by other methods, including altered methylation status and mutations, which have been identified in about 30% of uveal melanomas.[58–60]. At present it is unclear at what point p16 may be implicated in uveal melanoma pathogenesis, but its inactivation appears to be more important that cytogenetic studies alone would suggest, and it is possible that as in cutaneous melanoma it is a relative early event.

Another clear comparison between the two forms of melanoma involves chromosome 11 abnormalities, which are found in approximately 20% of uveal melanomas.[10,21,24–27,32] In the majority of cases these rearrangements are highly specific targeting the regions 11p15, or 11q23–q25.[21,24] The 11q region also appears to be affected in cutaneous melanoma, and has been related to poor outcome.[61,62] It is unclear how such alterations of chromosome 11 may relate to uveal melanoma development, but deletions or rearrangements of the 11q23–q25 region appear to be more often observed in melanomas with choriodal involvement, and or tumors of a spindle morphology.[21,25,27,31] The role of other chromosome changes shared by both forms of melanoma is unclear. Deletion of 10q is relatively frequent in cutaneous melanoma, with the *PTEN* gene at 10q23 identified as the potential target.[63] In uveal melanoma however, 10q deletions or rearrangements are rare, seen in less than 10% of tumors[21,25,27] and mutations of *PTEN* have not been identified in uveal melanoma cell lines.[64] Other chromosomes were originally thought to be of potential importance to uveal melanoma, but later investigations have failed to support their involvement. For example, deletions of chromosome 2 were initially identified and associated with these melanomas,[50] but subsequent cytogenetic and MSA studies have shown minimal abnormalities of chromosome 2.[10,14,21,24–27,31,32]

Abnormalities of all chromosomes have been reported for uveal melanoma, but until additional information is gained, it is not possible to identify if these other abnormalities are of relevance or occur as a result of increasing instability associated with tumor progression.

## CLINICAL RELEVANCE OF CHROMOSOME CHANGES

For the majority of solid malignancies chromosome changes have little or no direct clinical value. Analysis of posterior uveal melanomas established early the potential that chromosome changes could have in clinical assessment. From the outset, monosomy 3 and 8q were mainly associated with ciliary body melanomas,[11,23–25] and have been latterly related to an epithelioid cell type,[65,66] both factors are considered to be poor prognostic indicators.[67] Such associations suggested that chromosome changes themselves may be of use in determining the prognosis of these melanomas.

Most of the commonest changes found in uveal melanoma, those of 1, 3, 6, and 8, have now been correlated with patient survival. Prescher and co-workers were the first to report on a direct association, finding a strong correlation between loss of chromosome 3 and a poor prognosis of the patient. They observed that all patients with normal copies of chromosome 3 ($n = 24$) survived 3 years after diagnosis, whereas only 57% of those patients with monosomy 3 ($n = 30$) survived the same interval.[12] In a later study, Sisley and associates confirmed the prognostic value of monosomy 3, and they also demonstrated a strong inverse correlation between the presence of extra copies of 8q and survival.[13] In addition a dosage effect was identified, in which increased amplification of 8q correlated with a reduced disease free interval.[13] A link between chromosome changes and prognosis was also established by White and associates, demonstrating a correlation between chromosome 3 loss and 8q and poor prognosis, but the changes were however only predictive when found together.[20] In addition the study also identified a protective effect provided by chromosome 6 abnormalities, even in the presence of monosomy 3 and additional copies of 8q.[20] This observation is interesting but as the effect relates to an overrepresentation of 6p and a loss of 6q, it remains unclear how this biological relationship has developed,[20] and whether one or both arms are important in this protection. The potential value of FISH in determining prognostically relevant chromosome changes was demonstrated by a recent study, in which the relative imbalance in copy numbers of chromosomes 3 and 8 was determined, and correlated to long-term patient survival.[68] An imbalance in chromosome 3 and 8 copy number was shown to significantly correlate with patient survival over a minimum follow up of nine years.[68] Only those patients with a genetic imbalance for chromosomes 3 and 8 died from metastatic disease, with the median survival being 37 months, whilst for the group with no abnormalities median survival was 114 months.[68] In combination it is clear from these studies that assessment of monosomy 3 and gains of chromosome 8 is a significant prognostic indicator. The variations attributed to the significance of other chromosomes, whether individually or combined, may relate to the different techniques used, and with additional studies such anomalies are likely to be resolved.

Genetic studies appear to have clearly identified evidence of the relationship between certain chromosome changes and prognosis, and, as more information is made available, the potential exists to further define the involvement of not only the commonest changes, but also those of the less frequently observed abnormalities. Cytogenetic analysis still has an important part to play and will assist in establishing which chromosome abnormalities are essential to uveal melanoma development. With the introduction of techniques such as FISH, CGH and SKY we also have the potential to more fully characterize the abnormalities associated with these melanomas. The use of procedures such as FISH and MSA can also provide an alternative to cytogenetic analysis for patient prognosis, and because these techniques require smaller amounts of tumor material, the potential exists to adapt the procedure to the assessment of small *in situ* lesions, using fine needle aspiration biopsies (FNAB). These biopsies have already been determined to be suitable for chromosome and FISH analysis, and despite only sampling a small portion of the lesion appear to provide a good approximation of the lesion in its entirety.[48,69] FISH analysis on FNAB was found to provide results in 100% of cases, as, unlike cytogenetic analysis, the specimen need not be cultured.[48] The way is open to the routine use of chromosome changes in the prognostic assessment of uveal melanomas, but depending on the techniques employed variations in the prognostic relevance of individual chromosomes may be introduced. In addition, with continued study of these tumors other, more relevant genetic alterations may be identified, some of which like those of chromosome 6 may identify moderating effects. Crucially, until we know which genes are important in these transactions, and how we can effectively combat their influence we will have little extra to offer patients.

## SUMMARY

In cutaneous melanoma a reasonably well defined model of tumor progression has been developed, in which certain chromosome abnormalities are assigned to phases of progression. The changes in uveal melanoma are less well established, but a preliminary model can be proposed in which changes of chromosomes 3 and 6 are earlier in the scheme, and those of chromosomes 1, 8 and 21 subsequent and potentially related to the transition to metastatic disease.[21] Which chromosome abnormalities are actually the initiating changes essential for uveal melanoma pathogenesis has yet to be determined, and prior to the obvious alterations of chromosomes 3 and 6, there could be a subtle sequence of genetic alteration.

Our knowledge of the chromosome changes of uveal melanoma has increased exponentially in the last decade, but despite this dramatic rise, in total only about 250 cases have been studied with cytogenetics or FISH, and a further 40 cases with CGH, since most of the studies have referred to repeatedly used cohorts. It is clear from MSA studies that more genetic changes potentially exist than suggested by cytogenetic studies alone, but analysis of the chromosomes of posterior uveal melanoma has provided valuable insights into the necessary genetic requirements for its development and progression. In addition, the clinical relevance of chromosomes 1, 3, 6 and 8 abnormalities has been established, and continued cytogenetic investigation has much to add, refining regional involvement and more fully characterizing abnormalities.


## ACKNOWLEDGMENTS

We would like to express our gratitude to Yorkshire Cancer Research, NHS Executive Trent, and the Medical Research Council for support. Our thanks to the contributions made to studies by Mr Kirtikbhai A Patel, Mr Neil Cross, Ms Nicola Tattersall and Ms Fleur Talbot. Also thank you to Arran and Bethany for their patience.

This work was also supported by the Revolving Fund of the University Hospital Rotterdam, The Dutch Foundation Fighting against Blindness and the Rotterdam Blindness Foundation. We would like to thank Dr Annelies de Klein, Dr Gre Luyten, Dr Cornelia Mooy and Dr Dion Paridaens for their enthusiasm and contributions to the studies.


## REFERENCES


1. Nowell PC, Hungerford DA. A minute chromosome in human chronic granulocytic leukaemia. *Science.* 1960;132:1497.
2. Sandberg AA, Chen Z. Cancer cytogenetics and molecular genetics—Clinical implications (review). *Int J Oncology.* 1995;7:1241–1251.
3. Mitelman F, Johansson B, Merten F, eds. *Mitelman database of Chromosome Abberrations in Cancer. The Cancer Genome Anatomy Project*. 2001. Available from: http://cgap.nci.nih.gov/Chromosomes/Mitelman.
4. Nowell PC. The clonal evolution of tumor cell populations. *Science.* 1976;194:23–28.
5. Nowell PC. Mechanisms of tumor progression. *Cancer Res.* 1986;46:2203–2207.
6. Sandberg AA, Turc-Carel C, Gemmill RM. Chromosomes in solid tumors and beyond. *Cancer Res.* 1988;48:1049–1059.
7. Rey JA, Bello MJ, DeCompos JM, Ramos MC, Benitez J. Cytogenetic findings in a human malignant melanoma metastatic to the brain. *Cancer Genet Cytogenet.* 1985;16:179–183.
8. Griffin CA, Long PP, Schachat AP. Trisomy 6p in an ocular melanoma. *Cancer Genet Cytogenet.* 1988;32:129–132.
9. Horsman DE, Sroka H, Rootman J, White VA. Monosomy 3 and isochromosome 8q in a uveal melanoma. *Cancer Genet Cytogenet.* 1990;45:249–253.
10. Prescher G, Bornfeld N, Becher R. Non-random chromosomal abnormalities in primary uveal melanoma. *J Natl Cancer Inst.* 1990;82,1765–1769.
11. Sisley K, Rennie IG, Cottam DW, Potter AM, Potter CW, Rees RC. Cytogenetic findings in six posterior uveal melanomas: involvement of chromosomes 3, 6 and 8. *Genes Chromosomes Cancer.* 1990;2:205–209.
12. Prescher G, Bornfeld N, Hirche H, Horsthemke B, Karl-Heinz Jokel, Becher R. Prognostic implications of monosmy 3 in uveal melanoma. *Lancet.* 1996;347:1222–1225.
13. Sisley K, Rennie IG, Parsons MA, Jacques R, Hammond DW, Bell SM, Potter AM, Rees RC. Abnormalities of chromosomes 3 and 8, in posterior uveal melanoma, correlate with prognosis. *Genes Chromosomes Cancer.* 1997;19:22–28.

14. Parrella P, Sidransky D, Merbs SL (1999). Allelotype of posterior uveal melanoma: implications for a bifurcated tumor progression pathway. *Cancer Res.* 1999;59: 3032–3037.
15. Tschentscher F, Prescher G, Horsman DE, White VA, Rieder H, Anastassiou G, Schilling H, Bornfeld N, Bartz-Schmidt KU, Horsthemke B, Lohmann DR, Zeschnigk M. Partial deletions of the long and short arm of chromosome 3 point to two tumor suppressor genes in uveal melanoma. *Cancer Res.* 2001;61:3439–3442.
15a. McNamara M, Felix C, Davison EV, Fenton M, Kennedy SM. Assessment of chromosome 3 copy number in ocular melanoma using fluorescence *in situ* hybridisation. *Cancer Genet Cytogenet.* 1998;98:4–8.
16. Blasi MA, Roccella E, Balestrazzi E, Del Porto G, De Felice N, Roccella M, Rota R, Grammatico. 3p13 region: A possible location of a tumor suppressor gene involved in uveal melanoma. *Cancer Genet Cytogenet.* 1999;108:81–83.
17. Naus NC, Van Drunen E, De Klein A, Luyten GPM, Paridaens DA, Alers JC, Ksander B, Beverloo HB, Slater RM. Characterization of complex chromosomal abnormalities in uveal melanoma by fluorescent in situ hybridization, spectral karyotyping and comparative geneomic hybridization. *Genes Chromosomes Cancer.* 2001;30:267–273.
18. Online Mendelian Inheritance in Man (OMIM), Johns Hopkins University, 1966–2001. Available from: http://www3.ncbi.nlm.nih.gov/Omim/.
19. Myatt N, Aristodemou P, Neale MH, Foss AJE, Hungerford JL, Bhattacharya S, Cree IA. Abnormalities of the transforming growth factor-beta pathway in ocular melanoma. *J Pathol.* 2000;192:511–518.
20. White VA, Chambers JD, Courtright PD, Chang WY, Horsman DE. Correlation of cytogenetic abnormalities with the outcome of patients with uveal melanoma. *Cancer.* 1998;83:354–359.
21. Sisley K, Parsons MA, Garnham J, Potter AM, Curtis DI, Rees RC, Rennie IG. Association of specific chromosome alterations with tumor phenotype in posterior uveal melanoma. *Br J Cancer.* 2000;82:330–338.
22. AaltoY, Eriksson L, Seregard S, Larsson O, Knuutila S. Concomitant loss of chromosome 3 and whole arm losses and gains of chromosomes 1,6, or 8 in metastasizing primary uveal melanoma. *Invest Ophthalmol Vis Sci.* 2001;42:313–317.
23. Sisley K, Cottam DW, Rennie IG, Parsons MA, Potter AM, Potter CW, Rees RC. Non-random abnormalities of chromosomes 3, 6, and 8 associated with posterior uveal melanoma. *Genes Chromosomes Cancer.* 1992;5:197–200.
24. Dahlenfors R, Tornqvist G, Wettrell K, Mark J. Cytogenetical observations in nine ocular malignant melanomas. *Anticancer Res.* 1993;3:1415–1420.
25. Horsman DE, White VA. Cytogenetic analysis of uveal melanoma. Consistent occurrence of monosomy 3 and trisomy 8q. *Cancer.* 1993;71:811-819.
26. Wiltshire RN, Elner VM, Dennis T, Vine AK, Trent JM. Cytogenetic analysis of posterior uveal melanoma. *Cancer Genet Cytogenet.* 1993;66:47–53.
27. Singh AR, Boghosian-Sell L, Wary KK, Shields CL, De Potter P, Donoso LA, Shields JA, Cannizzaro LA. Cytogenetic findings in primary uveal melanoma. *Cancer Genet Cytogenet.* 1994;72:109–115.
28. White VA, McNeil K, Thiberville L, Horsman DE. Acquired homozygosity (isodisomy) of chromosome 3 during clonal evolution of a uveal melanoma: association with morphologic heterogeneity. *Genes Chromosomes Cancer.* 1996;15:138–143.
29. Prescher G, Bornfeld N, Becher R. Two subclones in a case of uveal melanoma: Relevance of monosmy 3 and multiplication of chromosome 8q. *Cancer Genet Cytogenet.* 1994;77:144–146.

30. Parada LA, Maranon A, Hallen M, Tranberg KG, Stenram U, Bardi G, Johansson B. Cytogenetic analysis of secondary liver tumors reveal significant differences in genomic imbalances between primary and metastatic colon carcinomas. *Clin Exp Metastasis.* 1999;17:471–479.
31. Speicher MR, Prescher G, du Manoir S, Jauch A, Horsthemke B, Bornfeld N, Becher R, Cremer T. Chromosomal gains and losses in uveal melanoma detected by comparative genomic hybridization. *Cancer Res.* 1994;54:3817–3823.
32. Prescher G, Bornfeld N, Friedrichs W, Seeber S, Becher R. Cytogenetics of twelve cases of uveal melanoma and patterns of nonrandom anomalies and isochromosome formation. *Cancer Genet Cytogenet.* 1995;80:40–46.
33. Parrella P, Caballero OT, Sidransky D, Merbs SL. Detection of c-myc amplification in uveal melanoma by fluorescent in situ hybridization. *Invest Ophthalmol Vis Sci.* 2001; 42: 1679–1684.
34. Royds JA, Sharrard RM, Parsons MA, Lwary J, Rees RC, Cottam DW, Wagner B, Rennie IG. c-myc oncogene expression in uveal melanoma. *Graefes Arch Clin Exp Ophthalmol.* 1992;230:366–371.
35. Mooy CM, Luyten GPM, De Jong PTVM, Luider TM, Stijnen T, Van de Ham F, Van Vroonhoven CC, Bosmam FT. Immunohistochemical and prognostic analysis of apoptosis and proliferation in uveal melanoma. *Am J Pathol.* 1995;147:1097–1104.
36. Chana JS, Cree IA, Foss AJE, Hungerford JL, Wilson GD. The prognostic significance of c-myc oncogene expression in uveal melanoma. *Melanoma Res.* 1998;8:139–144.
37. Chana JS, Wilson GD, Cree IA, Alexander RA, Myatt N, Neale M, Foss AJE, Hungerford JL. c-myc, p53, and Bcl-2 expression and clinical outcome in uveal melanoma. *Br J Ophthalmol.* 1999;83:110–114.
38. Sisley K, Brand C, Parsons MA, Maltby E, Rees RC, Rennie IG. Cytogenetics of iris melanomas disparity with other uveal melanomas. *Cancer Genet Cytogenet.* 1998;101:128–133.
39. Fountain JW, Bale SJ, Housman DE, Dracoploi NC. Genetics of melanoma *Cancer Surv.* 1990;9:645–671.
40. Lee JH, Miele ME, Hicks DJ, Phillips KK, Trent JM, Weissman BE, Welch DR. KiSS-1, a novel human malignant melanoma metastasis-suppressor gene. *J Natl Cancer Inst.* 1996;88:1731–1737.
41. Miele ME, Jewett MD, Goldberg SF, Hyatt DL, Morelli C, Gualandi F, Rimessi P, Hicks DJ, Weissman BE, Barbanti-Brodano G, Welch DR. A human melanoma metastasis-suppressor locus maps to 6q16.3–q23. *Int J Cancer.* 2000;86:524–528.
42. Demetrick DJ, Matsumoto S, Hannon GJ, Okamoto K, Xiong Y, Zhang H, Beach DH. Chromosomal mapping of the genes for the human cell cycle proteins cyclin C (CCNC), cyclin E (CCNE), p21 (CDKN1) and KAP (CDKN3). *Cytogenet Cell Genet.* 1995;69: 190–192.
43. Vincenti V, Cassano C, Rocchi M, Persico G. Assignment of the vascular endothelial growth factor gene to human chromosome 6p21.3. *Circulation.* 1996;93:1493–1495.
44. Metzelaar-Blok JA, Jager MJ, Moghaddam PH, Van der Slik AR, Giphart MJ. Frequent loss of heterozygosity on chromosome 6p in uveal melanoma. *Hum Immunol.* 1999;60:962–969.
45. Gordon KB, Thompson CT, Char DH, O'Brien JM, Kroll S, Ghazvini S, Gray JW. Comparative genomic hybridization in the detection of DNA copy number abnormalities in uveal melanoma. *Cancer Res.* 1994;54:4764–4768.
46. Zhang J, Glatfelter AA, Taetle R, Trent JM. Frequent alterations of evolutionary conserved regions of chromosome 1 in human malignant melanoma. *Cancer Genet Cytogenet.* 1999;111:119–123.

47. Dracopoli NC, Bale SJ. Genetic aspects of cutaneous malignant melanoma. *Semin Oncol.* 1988;15:541–548.
48. Naus NC, Verhoeven ACA, Van Drunen E, Slater R, Mooy CM, Paridaens DA, De Klein A. Detection of genetic prognostic markers in uveal melanoma biopsies using fluorescent in situ hybridisation. *Clin Cancer Res.* 2002;8:534–539.
49. Nelson MA, Ariza ME, Yang JM, Thompson FH, Taetle R, Trent JM, Wymer J, Massey-Brown K, Broome-Powell M, Easton J, Lahti JM, Kidd VJ. Abnormalities in the p34cdc2-related PITSLRE protein kinase gene complex (CDC2L) on chromosome band 1p36 in melanoma. *Cancer Genet Cytogenet.* 1999;108:91–99.
50. Mukai S, Dryja TP. Loss of alleles at polymorphic loci on chromsomes 2 in uveal melanoma. *Cancer Genet Cytogenet.* 1986;22:45–53.
51. Magauran RG, Gray B, Small KW. Chromosome 9 abnormality in choroidal melanoma. *Am J Ophthalmol.* 1994;117:109–111.
52. Singh AD, Donoso LA, Jackson L, Shields CL, De Potter P, Shields JA. Familial uveal melanoma absence of constitutional cytogenetic abnormalities in 14 cases. *Arch Ophthalmol.* 1996;114:502–503.
53. Healy E, Rehman I, Angus B, Rees JL. Loss of heterozygosity in sporadic primary cutaneous melanoma. *Genes Chromosom Cancer.* 1995;12:152–156.
54. Nelson MA, Radmacher MD, Simon R, Aickin M, Yang JM, Panda L, Emerson J, Roe D, Adair L, Thompson F, Bangert J, Leong SPL, Taetle R, Salmon S, Trent J. Chromosome abnormalities in malignant melanoma: clinical significance of non-random chromosome abnormalities in 206 cases. *Cancer Genet Cytogenet.* 2000;122:101–109.
55. Gruis NA, Van der Velden PA, Sandkuijl LA, Prins DE, Weaver-Feldhaus J, Kamb A, Bergman W, Frants RR. Homozygotes for CDKN2 (p16) germline mutation in dutch familial melanoma kindreds. *Nat Genet.* 1995;10:351–353.
56. Piepkorn M. Melanoma genetics: an update with focus on the CDKN2A (p16)/ARF tumor suppressors. *J Am Acad Dermatol.* 2000;42:705–722.
57. Ohta M, Berd D, Shimizu M, Nagai H, Cotticelli MG, Mastrangelo M, Shields JA, Shields CL, Croce CM, Huebner K. Deletion mapping of chromosome region 9p21–p22 surrounding the CDKN2 locus inmelanoma. *Int J Cancer.* 1996;65:762–767.
58. Merbs SL, Sidransky D. Analysis of p16 (CDKN2/MTS-1/INK4A) alterations in primary sporadic uveal melanoma. *Invest Ophthamol Vis Sci.* 1999;40:779–783.
59. Van der Velden PA, Metzelaar-Blok JA, Bergman W, Monique H, Hurks H, Frants RR, Gruis NA, Jager MJ. Promoter hypermethylation: a common cause of reduced p16 (INK4a) expression in uveal melanoma. *Cancer Res.* 2001;13:5303–5306.
60. Edmunds SC, Kelsell DP, Hungerford JL, Cree IA. Mutational analysis of selected genes in the TGFbeta, Wnt, pRb, and p53 pathways in primary uveal melanoma. *Invest Ophthalmol Vis Sci.* 2002;43:2845–2851.
61. Herbst RA, Larson A, Weiss J, Cavanee WK, Hampton GM, Arden KC. A defined region of loss of heterozygosity at 11q23 in cutaneous malignant melanoma. *Cancer Res.* 1995;55:2494–2496.
62. Robertson GP, Goldberg EK, Lugo TG, Fountain JW. Functional localization of a melanoma suppressor gene to a small (≤2 Mb) region on 11q23. *Oncogene.* 1999;18:3173–3180.
63. Guldberg P, Straten P, Birck A, Ahrenkiel V, Kirkin AF, Zeuthen J. Disruption of the MMAC!/PTEN gene by deletion or mutation is a frequent event in malignant melanoma. *Cancer Res.* 1997;57:3660–3663.
64. Naus NC, Zuidervaart W, Rayman N, Slater RM, Van Drunen E, Ksander B, Luyten GPM, De Klein A. Mutation analysis of the PTEN gene in uveal melanoma cell lines. *Int J Cancer.* 2000;87:151–153.

65. Scholes AG, Liloglou T, Maloney P, Hagan S, Nunnj, Hiscott P, Damato BE, Grierson I, Field JK. Loss of heterozygosity on chromosomes 3, 9, 13, and 17 including the retinoblastoma locus, in uveal melanoma. *Invest Ophthalmol Vis Sci.* 2001;11:2472–2477.
66. Scholes AGM, Damato BE, Nunn J, Hiscott P, Grierson I, Field JK. Monosomy 3 in uveal melanoma: Correlation with clinical and histologic predictors of survival. *Invest Ophthalmol Vis Sci.* 2003;44:1008–1011.
67. Mooy CM, De Jong PT. Prognostic parameters in uveal melanoma: a review. *Surv Ophthalmol.* 1996;41:215–228.
68. Patel KA, Edmondson ND, Talbot F, Parsons MA, Rennie IG, Sisley K. Prediction of prognosis in patients with uveal melanoma using fluorescence in situ hybridization. *Br J Ophthalmol.* 2001;85:1440–1444.
69. Sisley K, Nichols C, Parsons MA, Farr R, Rees RC, Rennie IG. Clinical applications of chromosome analysis, from fine needle aspiration biopsies, of posterior uveal melanoma. *Eye.* 1998;12:203–207.

A.E. DIRECTOR-MYSKA, J.S. WHITE AND I.W. McLEAN

# 8. Molecular Cytogenetic Characterization of Ten Uveal Melanoma Cell Lines

## INTRODUCTION

Uveal melanoma is the most common malignant intraocular tumor observed in adults, and often results in blindness and/or death. Epidemiological studies show an incidence of approximately six per million per year in the Caucasian population, and within this population it is more common in lightly pigmented eyes.[1] Tumors are generally classified using a modified version of the Callender classification system.[1–3] In this system, uveal melanomas containing epithelioid cells are designated 'mixed-cell type,' melanomas without epithelioid cells are termed 'spindle-cell type,' and tumors with too much necrosis to be classified by cytology are designated 'necrotic type.' The clinical course of the cancer is typically dependent upon the age of the patient, the size of the tumor, the precise location, the cell type, and the size of the nucleoli.[4,5] At the time of treatment, approximately 50% of patients have hematogenous metastasis.[1] Because of the slow evolution of the metastatic process with the time to death being as long as 50 years, some of the patients with metastasis die of other diseases.

Previous studies have shown that oculo(dermal) melanocytosis, neurofibromatosis type 1, Li–Fraumeni syndrome, and familial atypical multiple mole and melanoma (FAMMM) syndrome are predisposing factors.[6] Due to the strong link between sunlight and cutaneous melanoma, researchers have also considered sunlight as a potential cause for uveal melanoma; the results have been ambiguous.[7–10] There have been rare cases of familial uveal melanoma, thought to be inherited in an autosomal dominant fashion and as yet unlinked to any genetic locus or cytogenetic anomaly.[11,12]

There is mounting cytogenetic evidence that copy number abnormalities are prevalent within uveal melanoma.[4,13,14] Classical cytogenetic analysis suggests that the most frequent abnormalities occur in chromosomes 3, 6, 8 and that monosomy 3 is associated with a poor prognosis.[5,13,15,16] Other recurrent anomalies have been noted on 7q, 9p, and 13q.[4] Abnormalities of chromosome 6 are also seen in cutaneous melanoma, which suggests the cancers may share some common genetic alterations.[17] However, classical cytogenetic studies, while useful in elucidating structural abnormalities, are time consuming and require fresh tissue. Furthermore, classical cytogenetics has proven difficult and ambiguous when analyzing solid tumors and their associated cell lines. Techniques such as comparative genomic hybridization (CGH) and spectral karyotyping (SKY) may yield more information.

CGH and SKY are both fluorescence *in situ* hybridization (FISH) techniques. The key to such methodologies lies in the structure and properties of DNA. The double helical structure of DNA is held in place by hydrogen bonds that pair purine with pyrimidine, and can be disrupted by heat or changes in pH. Disruption of purine-pyrimidine hydrogen bonds results in the dissociation of the paired strands and thus the denaturation of the DNA molecule. Marmur et al.,[18] demonstrated that the denaturation process was reversible and complementary strands would readily combine to reform an intact DNA molecule. The characteristic ability of DNA to denature and subsequently renature is the underpinning of any nucleic acid hybridization experiment.

FISH has been applied to many types of samples and there are many different protocols for probe labeling and visualization using directly or indirectly labeled probes. Direct labels allow visualization of the fluorescent signal almost immediately after hybridization. Indirect labels require multi-step amplification before the fluorescent signal is bright enough to be viewed. In either case, direct or indirect label, multiple fluorochromes with different excitation and emission properties can be used to detect more than one target on the same sample.[19] Multiple fluorochrome detection is the basis of both CGH and SKY.[20,21]

CGH is an *in situ* hybridization technique useful in detecting relative copy number changes throughout an entire genome.[20,22] It is essentially the dual application of fluorescence *in situ* hybridization (FISH), wherein total genomic tumor DNA as well as total genomic DNA from normal diploid tissue are differentially labeled and then simultaneously hybridized to normal metaphase chromosomes. Whereas classical cytogenetics identifies structural and numerical alterations of the chromosomes, CGH elucidates amplification (gain) and deletion (loss) of DNA sequences within tumor genome as compared to the normal, diploid genome. Alterations detected by CGH may not be detectable via classical cytogenetic techniques. CGH is not limited to fresh tissue, which increases its applicability to the study of cancer and other diseases.[20]

SKY, another *in situ* hybridization technique, is applicable to fresh material only. This particular technique allows for the simultaneous visualization and karyotyping of all human chromosomes using twenty-four distinct colors.[21] The colors are created by varying combinations of five fluorochromes (rhodamine, Texas-Red, C-Cy5, D-FITC, and E-Cy5.5) used to create twenty-four separate whole chromosome paints. These twenty-four differentially labeled whole chromosome paints are simultaneously hybridized to metaphase chromosome spreads from the tissue of interest, visualized with antibodies, and analyzed by a specialized imaging system. Once imaged, a SKY hybridization reveals structural (exchanges between chromosomes) and numerical (extra chromosomes) chromosome aberrations, similar to classical cytogenetics, but with more resolution.

In this study we have analyzed ten uveal melanoma cell lines (Table 8.1) by CGH and SKY to identify genomic and chromosomal alterations. The cell lines were

Table 8.1. Uveal melanoma cell lines used in this study.

| Cell line | Tumor | Media | Reference |
|---|---|---|---|
| 92-1 | Primary | RPMI 1640 | 27; courtesy of M.J.Jager |
| MEL270 | Primary | RPMI 1640 | 28; courtesy of B.R. Ksander |
| MEL285 | | RPMI 1640 | Courtesy of B.R. Ksander |
| MEL290 | Primary | RPMI 1640 | Courtesy of B.R. Ksander |
| OCM1 | | Ham's F-12 | 29; courtesy of J. Kan-Mitchell |
| OCM3 | | Ham's F-12 | Courtesy of J. Kan-Mitchell |
| OCM8 | | Ham's F-12 | Courtesy of J. Kan-Mitchell |
| OM431 | Primary | Ham's F-12 | 30; courtesy of D.M. Albert |
| OMM1 | | DMEM | 31; courtesy of G.P. Luyten |
| OMM2.3 | Metastatic | RPMI 1640 | Courtesy of B.R. Ksander |

derived from ten uveal melanomas with varying malignant potential and at least two of these cell lines were derived from metastatic tumors.

## TECHNIQUES

### UVEAL MELANOMA CELL LINES

Ten uveal melanoma cell lines were obtained from the Department of Ophthalmology, University of Texas Southwestern Medical Center at Dallas (Dallas, TX), and were maintained in culture using standard techniques (Table 8.1). 'Test DNA' for use in CGH was extracted using standard phenol/chloroform extraction procedures. Metaphase chromosome spreads for use in SKY were prepared on slides via conventional cytogenetic techniques.[23]

### COMPARATIVE GENOMIC HYBRIDIZATION (CGH)

Reference samples for the entire study were collected from a single normal male and a single normal female donor with informed consent. Metaphase chromosome spreads were prepared from normal, cultured human peripheral blood lymphocytes (HPBLs) via conventional techniques.[23] Briefly, the cells were arrested at metaphase, swelled with a hypotonic solution and dropped onto clean glass slides. Phenol/chloroform extraction procedures were used to isolate 'reference DNA' from normal HPBLs.

Whole genomic probes were generated via nick translation of extracted DNA. Reference DNA was labeled with digoxigenin-11-dUTP (Roche Molecular Biochemicals, Indianapolis, IN) while test DNA had biotin-16-dUTP (Roche Molecular Biochemicals, Indianapolis, IN) incorporated into the fragments. Labeled DNA fragments were sized by agarose gel electrophoresis and ethidium bromide staining. Optimal probe size was seen as a smear of DNA between 200- and 800-bp in length. CGH was performed as described by Kallioniemi and colleagues.[20] In brief, reference and test probes were simultaneously hybridized to

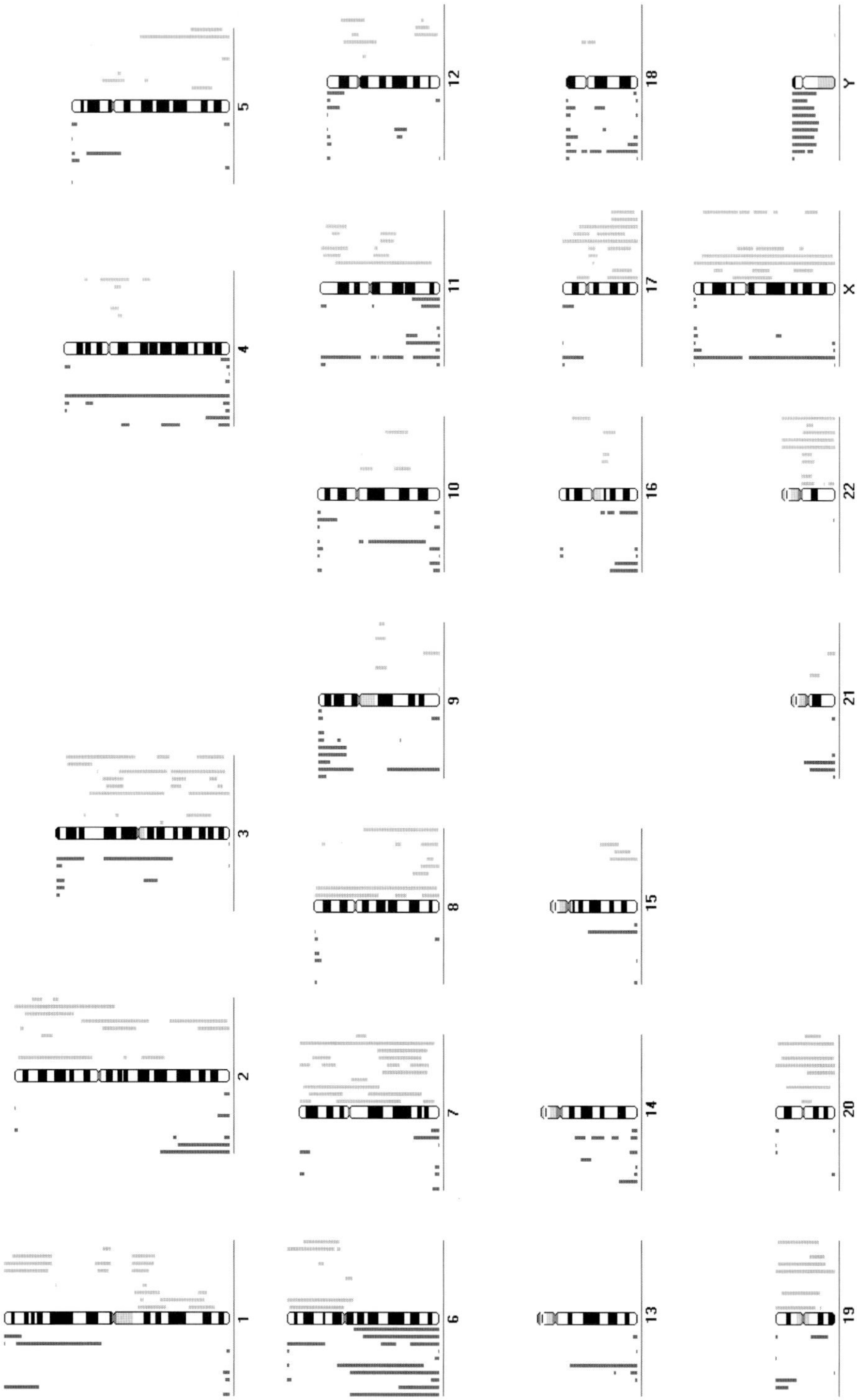
1
2
3
4
5
6
7
8
9
10
11
12
13
14
15
16
17
18
19
20
21
22
X
Y

normal metaphase chromosomes in the presence of 70% formamide/2x SSC, human Cot-1 DNA (Gibco BRL® Life Technologies, Inc., Gaithersburg, MD) and salmon testes DNA (Sigma Co., St. Louis, MO) at 37°C for two nights. Antibody detection was performed on the third day using previously described techniques.[20] Biotinylated-test-DNA signals were detected with avidin-conjugated FITC (Vector Labs, Burlingame, CA), and digoxigenin-11-dUTP-labeled reference DNA was visualized using TRITC-conjugated antibodies (Sigma Co., St. Louis, MO). Following antibody detection procedures, slides were counter-stained with 4′,6-diamidino-2-phenylindole (DAPI) (Sigma Co., St. Louis, MO). Finally, a coverslip was mounted over an antifade solution to complete each of the slides.

Image acquisition and analysis were performed on a Leica Q550CW cytogenetics workstation, which includes a LEICA DM-RXA fluorescent microscope (Leica Inc., Exton, PA), and a SenSys cooled CCD camera (Photometrics Ltd., Tuscon, AZ). The images acquired include individual FITC, TRITC, and DAPI images of each metaphase spread. These images were combined to yield a CGH image suitable for analysis in the Leica QCGH software. An inverse DAPI image was used to approximate G-banding in order to karyotype each metaphase spread. A minimum of ten metaphase spreads were captured and analyzed for each cell line. CGH ratio profiles were compiled for each of the spreads, and used to generate mean ratio profiles for each cell line (Fig. 8.1). The copy number threshold was selected based upon published literature as well as desired sensitivity for detection. The lower threshold was set at 0.8 copies and ratio values less than 0.8 were considered losses (deletions). The upper threshold was set at 1.2 copies, and values exceeding 1.2 were considered gains (amplifications).

Ninety-five percent confidence intervals were applied to each of the collective means (Fig. 8.2). Regions of interest and minimal common regions were determined by comparison of the average profiles for all of the cell lines (Fig. 8.3). Regions of interest include entire chromosome amplifications and deletions as well as high level amplifications or deletions. Sex chromosomes were excluded from the analysis. While significant gains and losses were observed on these

---

Fig. 8.1. Quantitative profile comparison data for ten uveal melanoma cell lines. The mean gains and losses for each cell line are shown. Gains appear as bars to the right of each ideogram; losses appear as bars to the left of each ideogram. This figure is read from the bars immediately flanking the ideogram, on either side, outward. The innermost cell line is 92-1, followed by MEL270, MEL285, MEL290, OCM1, OCM3, OCM8, OM431, OMM1, and OMM2.3. Copy number abnormalities in the heterochromatin of chromosomes 1, 3, 9, 13, 14, 15, 16, 19, 21, and 22 were eliminated. While significant gains and losses were observed on chromosomes X and Y, information on the sex of the parent tumor was not available in all cases. Therefore, only the CGH results for the autosomes were considered (sex chromosome data does not appear). Whole chromosome gains were observed in a non-random fashion for several chromosomes within the cell lines. Chromosome 22 was gained in 30% of the cell lines as well, including OCM3, OCM8, and OMM1. OCM3 also gained an entire chromosome 17. Chromosome 8 was gained in MEL270, while chromosome 7 was gained in its entirety in OMM1. A loss of chromosome 4 was seen in OCM3. Gains and losses seen in at least 50% of the cell lines are shown in Figure 8.3.

chromosomes, information on the sex of the parent tumor was not available for all cell lines. Therefore, only the autosomes were considered in our analysis.

The uveal melanoma cell lines utilized in this study were of an indeterminate number of passages and thus may have contained artifacts. Therefore, the threshold for determination of minimal common regions was gain or loss of a defined region in at least half of all cell lines (Fig. 8.3). The minimal common regions were pinpointed based upon the most recent chromosome ideogram and genome mapping data available.

Previously reported CGH and classical cytogenetic data were compared with the minimal common regions observed in this study (Tables 8.2 and 8.3). Data obtained in this study were compared with the published literature and publicly available genomic databases in order to generate a table correlating regions of amplification and/or deletion with specific genes (Table 8.4). Given our results, these genes may be involved in uveal melanoma and will require further study to confirm such involvement.

## SPECTRAL KARYOTYPING

SKY was performed using the SkyPaint™ hybridization kit (Applied Spectral Imaging, Inc., Carlsbad, CA) and results were visualized using the SkyVision™ spectral imaging system (Applied Spectral Imaging, Inc., Carlsbad, CA). Metaphase spreads were prepared from each of the uveal melanoma cell lines as described previously. Fresh slides were allowed to age at room temperature for a week and then hybridized with SkyPaint™ (Applied Spectral Imaging, Inc., Carlsbad, CA) probes as indicated in the manufacturer's protocol. Selected metaphase slides were treated with a pepsin-HCl solution, washed twice in 1x PBS, once in 1x PBS/$MgCl_2$, and then dehydrated in a series of ethanol dilutions (70%, 85%, and 100%). The SkyPaint™ probe mixture (Applied Spectral Imaging, Inc., Carlsbad, CA) and slides were denatured. Ten microliters of probe was applied to each slide, the slides were coverslipped, sealed with rubber cement (Elmer's Products, Inc., Columbus, OH) and incubated at 37°C for two nights. On the third day the rubber cement seals and coverslips were removed. The slides were washed once in 50% formamide/2x SSC, twice in 1x SSC, and finally in 4x SSC/0.1% Tween 20. A series of antibody layers were then applied according to the manufacturer's protocol (Applied Spectral Imaging, Inc., Carlsbad, CA). Following these layers the slides were washed three times in 4x SSC/0.1% Tween 20 and once in distilled water. The slides were allowed to dry and were then counter-stained with a DAPI/antifade solution (Applied Spectral Imaging, Inc., Carlsbad, CA), and coverslipped. Images were captured and analyzed using the SpectraCube® and a SkyVision™ workstation (Applied Spectral Imaging, Inc., Carlsbad, CA).

All spectral karyotyping results presented in this paper utilize standard cytogenetic nomenclature as defined in ISCN 1995.[24] The following is a brief list of the abbreviations used in this paper and their meanings: t = translocation, der = derivative, dic = dicentric, del = deletion, ins = insertion, i = isochromosome, mr = multiple rearrangements, and R = Roberstsonian translocation.

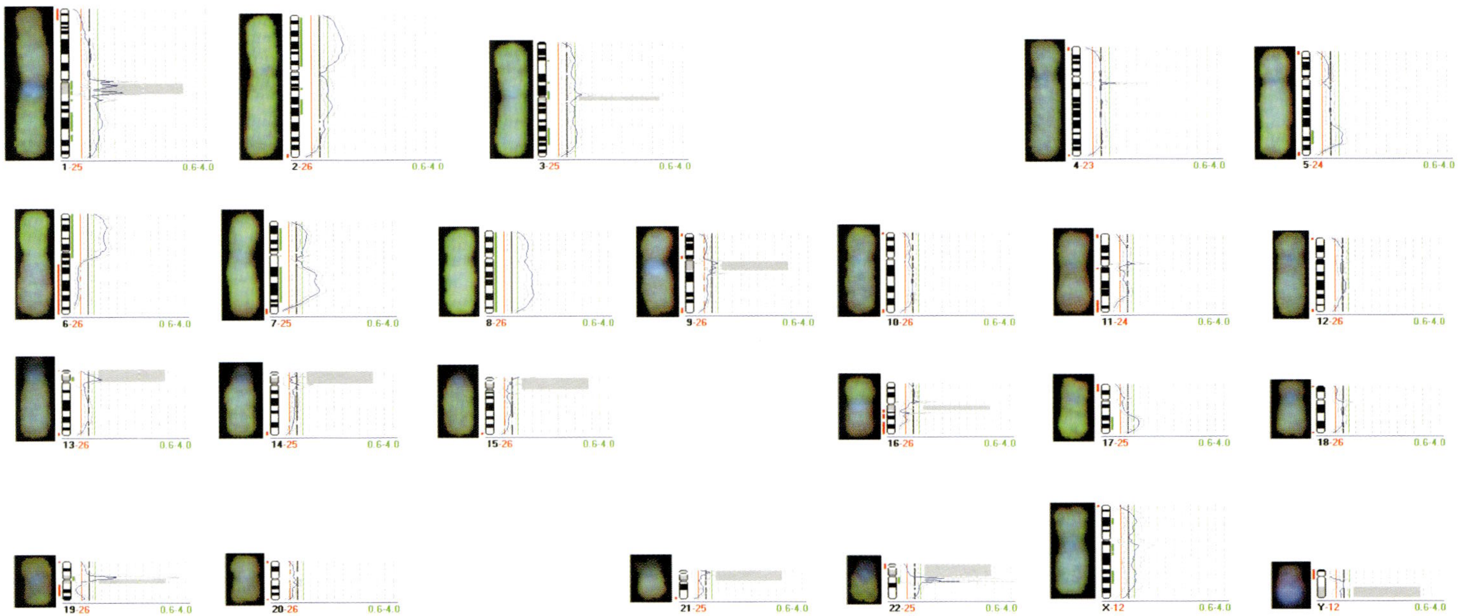


Fig. 8.2. CGH profile data for MEL270 complete with 95% confidence intervals. The Leica QCGH image analysis software (Leica Inc., Exton, PA) generates 95% confidence intervals for mean CGH profile data once all metaphase spreads have been appropriately karyotyped. A minimum of ten metaphase spreads was analyzed to generate the mean for each cell line. The above profile was created from MEL270 data. As the profile deviates from a 1:1 ratio for copy number between tumor and normal (indicated by the black line) and moves toward the right beyond the green line (1.2 copies) or to the left beyond the red line (0.8 copies), an amplification or deletion is indicated. Events can be better visualized by the bars to the right and left of each ideogram. Gains appear as green bars to the right of the ideogram, while losses appear as red bars on the left. The color chromosome images to the left of each ideogram and associated profile are from a single representative MEL270 spread which contributed to the mean data for that cell line. The purpose of these images is to demonstrate the translation of cell line CGH data to mean profile data. Note the relatively narrow confidence intervals for the profiles on chromosomes 6 and 8. The less the variation (width) in the confidence interval, the greater the certainty that can be assigned to the relative copy numbers in the data. These kinds of data are generated for the mean profile data from each cell line during analysis.

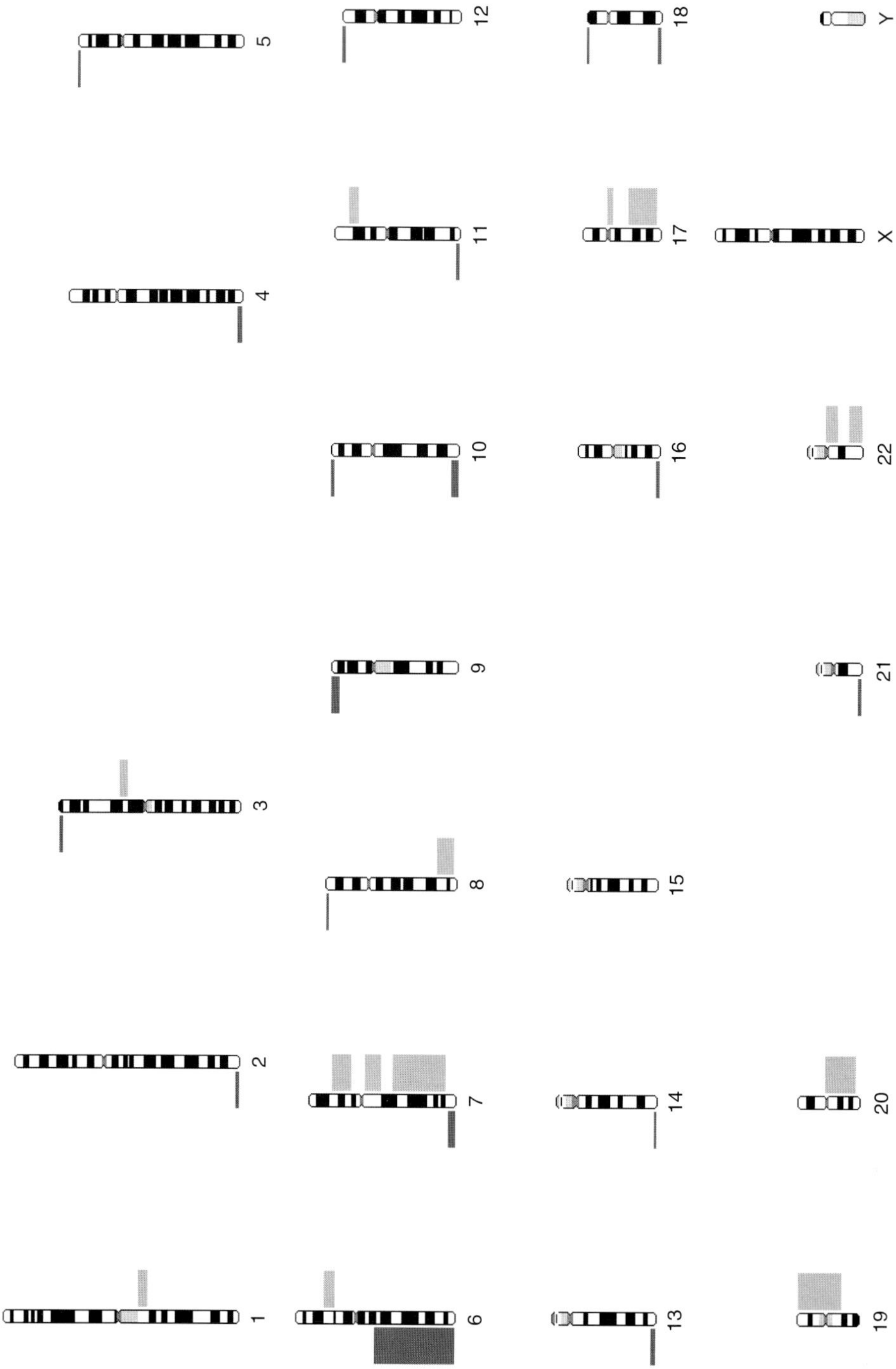

1
2
3
4
5
6
7
8
9
10
11
12
13
14
15
16
17
18
19
20
21
22
X
Y

## RESULTS

### COMPARATIVE GENOMIC HYBRIDIZATION

The frequencies of partial gain on the autosomes (Fig. 8.1) were as follows: 70% of cell lines evidenced gain on 1q, 80% on 2p, 70% on both arms of chromosome 3, 50% on 5p, 60% on 5q, 60% on 7p, 100% on 7q, 70% on 8q, 50% each on 11p and 11q, 60% on 12q, 100% on 17q, 50% on 19p, 60% on 19q, 70% on 20q, and 90% on 22q. Specific regions of amplification are enumerated in Table 8.2, and illustrated in Figure 8.1. Whole chromosome gains observed in separate cell lines include: chromosome 7 (OMM1), chromosome 8 (MEL270), and chromosome 17 (OCM3). Whole chromosome gains were observed in three of the cell lines for chromosomes 20 (OCM3, OCM8, and OMM1) and 22 (OCM3, OCM8, and OMM2.3).

The frequencies of partial loss on the autosomes (Fig. 8.1) were as follows: 50% on 2q, 50% on 3p, 90% on 4q, 50% on 5p, 100% on 6q, 60% on 7q, 50% on 8p, 90% on 9p, 70% on both arms of chromosome 10, 80% on 11q, 80% on 12p, 50% on 13q, 70% on 14q, 50% on 16q, 80% on 18p, 90% on 18q, and 50% on 21q. Specific regions of loss are enumerated in Table 8.3, and illustrated in Figure 8.1. A whole chromosome loss was observed in one cell line on chromosome 4 (OCM3).

Chromosomes 3, 5, 8, 9, 10, 12, and 18 frequently contained p-terminal deletions, while several q-terminal deletions were seen on chromosomes 2, 4, 7, 10, 11, 13, 14, 16, 18, and 21. In distillation of the mean profile data (Fig. 8.1) to the minimal common regions (Fig. 8.3), the relative size of the common terminal losses is illustrated. In some cases, the terminal losses expand beyond the distal portion of the chromosome; in other cases, the loss is strictly terminal.

The gain of 6p, and the loss of 6q, were apparent in each line to varying degrees. A focal gain near 8q24 was also seen in six of the ten cell lines. Monosomy 3 was approached in MEL285, but the mean for distal 3q traced the normal 1:1 ratio line of the profile. Chromosome 3 gains were found in all cell lines save MEL285 and MEL290.

Gain was not seen for any portion of chromosome 9p, 13, 14, 15p and 21p. There was no loss of any portion of 13p, 14p, 15p, 17q, 21p, and 22p. It should be noted that these regions are largely, if not completely, heterochromatic in origin (except 17q).

---

Fig. 8.3. Minimal common regions of gain and loss in ten uveal melanoma cell lines. Minimal common regions were designated as copy number abnormalities manifest in at least half of all cell lines. The uveal melanoma cell lines utilized in this study were of an indeterminate number of passages. Since it was suspected that the cell lines contained artifacts, no copy number aberrations seen in fewer than half of the cell lines were analyzed. The minimal common regions were pinpointed based upon the most recent chromosome ideogram and publicly available genome mapping data. Gains, or amplifications, are represented as bars to the right of each ideogram; losses, or deletions, are represented as bars to the left of each ideogram. It is evident that chromosomes 1, 3, 6, 7, 8, 9, 11, 17, 19, 20, and 22 were involved in significant amplifications and deletions. These involve gains and losses that either encompass, expand beyond, or are entirely distinct from the telomeres, centromeres, and heterochromatic regions. Copy number abnormalities in the heterochromatin of chromosomes 1, 3, 9, 13, 14, 15, 16, 19, 21, and 22 were eliminated. Only autosomes were considered in analyzing gains and losses, thus the X and Y chromosomes show no data.

Table 8.2. A comparison of gains seen in ten uveal melanoma cell lines compared with previously reported chromosomal abnormalities in uveal melanoma.

| Gains observed[a] | | Cell lines[b] | Gains reported by CGH[a] | | Reference | Gains reported by classical cytogenetics[a] | | Reference |
|---|---|---|---|---|---|---|---|---|
| 1q21.1–q21.2 | (60%) | 1,2,3,6,7,8 | 1q | (9.1%) | 13 | | | |
| 1q21.2 | (60%) | 1,3,4,6,7,8 | | | | | | |
| 3p13–p14.1 | (50%) | 2,5,6,7,10 | | | | | | |
| 6p21.2–p21.3 | (50%) | 1,2,7,9,10 | 6p | (45.5%) | 13 | 6p | (46.3%) | 16 |
| | | | 6p | (57%) | 14 | 6p | (25%) | 32 |
| | | | 6p | (42%) | 14 | 6p12–6pter | (25%) | 32 |
| | | | 6p | (40%) | 4 | | | |
| | | | 6p21-pter | (54.5%) | 13 | | | |
| 7p13–p15.2 | (50%) | 2,3,6,7,9 | | | | | | |
| 7q11.21–q11.23 | (50%) | 1,3,4,9,10 | 7q | (70%) | 4 | | | |
| 7q21.2–q21.3 | (60%) | 1,2,3,7,8,9 | | | | | | |
| 7q21.3–q22.1 | (60%) | 1,2,5,7,8,9 | | | | | | |
| 7q22.1–q31.1 | (70%) | 1,2,5,6,7,8,9 | | | | | | |
| 7q31.1–q31.3 | (50%) | 2,5,7,8,9 | | | | | | |
| 7q31.3–q33 | (60%) | 2,5,6,7,8,9 | | | | | | |
| 7q34–q35 | (50%) | 1,5,6,8,9 | | | | | | |
| 8q24.1–q24.2 | (60%) | 1,2,4,5,8,10 | 8q | (54.5%) | 13 | 8q | (48.1%) | 16 |
| 8q24.2–q24.3 | (60%) | 1,2,5,6,8,10 | 8q | (100%, fresh) | 14 | 8 | (25%) | 32 |
| 8q24.3 | (60%) | 1,2,5,8,10 | 8q | (57%, fixed) | 14 | 8q | (50%) | 32 |
| | | | 8q | (100%) | 4 | 8q13.1–8qter | (25%) | 32 |
| | | | 8q24–qter | (63.6%) | 13 | | | |

| | | | | | |
|---|---|---|---|---|---|
| 11p14–p15.1 | (50%) | 3,4,5,7,8 | 11p | (9.1%) | 13 |
| 17q11.1–q11.2 | (50%) | 3,4,5,6,8 | 17 | (18.2%) | 13 |
| 17q21.3–q22 | (50%) | 1,5,6,7,8 | | | |
| 17q22–q24 | (80%) | 1,2,5,6,7,8,9,10 | | | |
| 17q24 | (70%) | 1,2,5,6,8,9,10 | | | |
| 17q24–q25 | (60%) | 1,2,6,8,9,10 | | | |
| 19p13.3–q12 | (50%) | 1,3,6,7,10 | | | |
| 19q12–q13.1 | (60%) | 1,3,6,7,8,10 | | | |
| 19q13.1–q13.2 | (50%) | 3,6,7,8,10 | | | |
| 20p11.1–q11.1 | (50%) | 1,3,6,7,9 | 20 | (14%) | 14 |
| 20q11.1–q11.2 | (70%) | 1,3,5,6,7,9,10 | | | |
| 20q11.2–q13.1 | (60%) | 3,5,6,7,9,10 | | | |
| 20q13.1–q13.3 | (50%) | 3,5,6,7,9 | | | |
| 22q11.1–q11.2 | (80%) | 1,2,4,5,6,7,8,10 | 22 | (9.1%) | 13 |
| 22q11.2–q12.1 | (90%) | 1,2,4,5,6,7,8,9,10 | 22q | (9.1%, fresh) | 14 |
| 22q13.2 | (50%) | 1,6,7,8,10 | 22q | (42%, fixed) | 14 |
| 22q13.3–qter | (50%) | 1,6,7,8,10 | | | |

[a] The percentage in parentheses is the frequency of occurrence for a given gain.

Table 8.3. A comparison of losses seen in ten uveal melanoma cell lines compared with previously reported chromosomal abnormalities in uveal melanoma.

| Losses observed[a] | | Cell lines[b] | Losses reported by CGH[a] | | Reference | Losses reported by classical, cytogenetics[a] | | Reference |
|---|---|---|---|---|---|---|---|---|
| 2q37.3–qter | (50%) | 2,5,8,9,10 | | | | | | |
| 3p26–pter | (50%) | 3,4,6,7,8 | 3 | (45.5%) | 13 | 3 | (80%) | 15 |
| | | | 3 | (57%, fresh) | 14 | 3 | (50%) | 16 |
| | | | 3 | (85%, fixed) | 14 | 3 | (100%) | 32 |
| | | | 3 | (70%) | 4 | | | |
| | | | 3 | (57%) | 5 | | | |
| 4q35–4qter | (90%) | 1,2,3,4,6,7,8,9,10 | 4q | (14%) | 14 | | | |
| 5p15.3–pter | (50%) | 2,4,6,7,10 | | | | | | |
| 6q14–q21 | (50%) | 1,2,6,7,10 | 6q | (45.5%) | 13 | 6q | (46.3%) | 16 |
| 6q21–q22.2 | (60%) | 1,2,3,6,7,10 | 6q | (42%, fresh) | 14 | 6q | (25%) | 32 |
| 6q22.2–q23.3 | (60%) | 1,2,6,7,9,10 | 6q | (28%, fixed) | 14 | 6q12–6qter | (25%) | 32 |
| 6q23.3–q25.2 | (70%) | 1,2,3,6,7,9,10 | | | | | | |
| 6q25.2–q26 | (60%) | 1,2,3,7,9,10 | | | | | | |
| 6q26–q27 | (70%) | 1,2,3,7,8,9,10 | | | | | | |
| 6q27–qter | (90%) | 1,2,3,4,5,7,8,9,10 | | | | | | |

| | | | | | | | | |
|---|---|---|---|---|---|---|---|---|
| 7q36–qter | (60%) | 2,3,4,7,8,10 | | | | | | |
| 8p23.3–pter | (50%) | 3,4,6,7,10 | 8p | (28%) | 14 | 8p | (25%) | 32 |
| 9p23–p24 | (50%) | 6,7,8,9,10 | 9p21–pter | (27.3%) | 13 | 9p | (25%) | 32 |
| 9p24–pter | (90%) | 1,2,4,5,6,7,8,9,10 | 9p21–pter | (27.3%) | 13 | 9p23–9pter | (25%) | 32 |
| 10p15.1–pter | (70%) | 2,3,4,6,7,8,10 | | | | | | |
| 10q26.2–qter | (60%) | 2,4,7,8,9,10 | | | | | | |
| 11q25–qter | (80%) | 1,2,5,6,7,8,9,10 | 11q23–qter, | (18.2%) | 13 | | | |
| | | | 11q | (42%) | 14 | | | |
| 12p13.3–pter | (80%) | 1,2,3,4,6,7,8,10 | 12p | (9.1%) | 13 | | | |
| 13q34–qter | (50%) | 2,4,6,7,8 | | | | | | |
| 14q32.3–qter | (60%) | 2,3,5,7,8,9 | | | | | | |
| 16q24–qter | (50%) | 2,7,8,9,10 | 16q | (18.2%) | 13 | | | |
| 18p11.31–pter | (80%) | 2,3,4,6,7,8,9,10 | | | | | | |
| 18q23–qter | (70%) | 1,2,4,7,8,9,10 | | | | | | |
| 21q22.3–qter | (50%) | 2,7,8,9,10 | | | | | | |

[a] The percentage in parentheses is the frequency of occurrence for a given loss.
[b] See Table 1.

Table 8.4. A correlation of copy number abnormalities in ten uveal melanoma cell lines and genes associated with uveal melanoma or its predisposing factors.

| Gain/Loss observed[a] | | Cell lines[b] | Gene | Locus[c] | Function | Source[c,d] |
|---|---|---|---|---|---|---|
| + 1q21.1–1q21.2 | (60%) | 1,2,3,6,7,8 | TNFSF6 | 1q23 | tumor necrosis factor ligand | OMIM #134638 |
| + 1q21.2 | (60%) | 1,3,4,6,7,8 | | | | |
| – 2q31–q32 | (20%) | 9,10 | alpha4 integrin subunit gene | 2q31–q32 | transcriptional regulator of alpha4 integrin subunit gene in metastasis | 33 |
| + 6p21.2–p21.3 | (50%) | 1,2,7,9,10 | HLA-G | 6p21.3 | histocompatability antigen | OMIM #142871 |
| – 6q14–q21 | (50%) | 1,2,6,7,10 | ? | 6q12–q21 | putative tumor suppressor gene | 34 |
| – 6q21–q22.2 | (60%) | 1,2,3,6,7,10 | AIM1 | 6q21 | absent in melanoma | OMIM #601797 |
| + 7q21.2–q21.3 | (60%) | 1,2,3,7,8,9 | MDR1 | 7q21.1–q21.2 | produces P-gp pump protein, causes drug resistance in cancer cells | 35 |
| + 8q24.1–q24.2 | (60%) | 1,2,4,5,8,10 | c-myc | 8q24 | oncogene | 36 |
| – 9p23–p24 | (50%) | 6,7,8,9,10 | CDKN2 (p16) | 9p21 | tumor suppressor, involved in FAMMM and Li–Fraumeni | 6 |
| – 9p24–pter | (90%) | 1,2,4,5,6,7,8,9,10 | FCM critical region | 9p13–p22 | familial cutaneous melanoma critical region | 12 |
| | | | CMM2 | 9p21 | cutaneous malignant melanoma | OMIM #155601 |
| | | | TYRP1 | 9p23 | tyrosinase-related protein 1 | OMIM #115501 |
| – 10q26.2 qter | (60%) | 2,4,7,8,9,10 | DMBT1 | 10q25.3–q26.1 | deleted in malignant brain tumors | OMIM #601969 |

| | | | | | | |
|---|---|---|---|---|---|---|
| + 11p14–p15.1 | (50%) | 3,4,5,7,8 | HRAS | 11p15.5 | v-Ha-Ras oncogene | 6 |
| – 11q25–qter | (80%) | 1,2,5,6,7,8,9,10 | Tyrosinase | 11q13.5–q14.1 | melanoma associated antigen | 37 |
| – 12p13.3–pter | (80%) | 1,2,3,4,6,7,8,10 | KRAS | 12p12.1 | v-Ki-Ras 2 oncogene | 6 |
| – 13q34–qter | (50%) | 2,4,6,7,8 | BRCA2 | 13q12.2–q12.3 | breast cancer susceptibility locus | 38 |
| – 16q24–qter | (50%) | 2,7,8,9,10 | MC1R | 16q24.3 | melanocortin 1 receptor | OMIM #155555 |
| – 17p13–pter | (30%) | 2,9,10 | p53 | 17p13.1 | tumor suppressor, involved in Li–Fraumeni | 6 |
| + 17q11.1–q11.2 | (50%) | 3,4,5,6,8 | NF1 | 17q11.2 | neurofibromatosis | OMIM #162200 |
| + 17q21.3–q22 | (50%) | 1,5,6,7,8 | BRCA1 | 17q21 | breast cancer | OMIM #113705 |
| + 17q22–q24 | (80%) | 1,2,5,6,7,8,9,10 | PRKCA | 17q22–q23.2 | protein kinase C | OMIM #176960 |
| + 19p13.3–q12 | (50%) | 1,3,6,7,10 | STK11 | 19p13.3 | serine/threonine protein kinase II | OMIM #602216 |
| + 19q12–q13.1 | (60%) | 1,3,6,7,8,10 | MEL | 19p13.2–cen | oncogene MEL, Ras-associated protein | OMIM #165040 |
| + 19q13.1–q13.2 | (50%) | 3,6,7,8,10 | MIA | 19q13.32–q13.33 | melanoma inhibitory activity | OMIM #601340 |
| + 22q11.2–q12.1 | (90%) | 1,2,4,5,6,7,8,9,10 | EWSR1 | 22q12 | Ewing sarcoma breakpoint | OMIM #133450 |
| | | | LFS | 22q12.1 | Li–Fraumeni | OMIM #151623 |
| | | | NF2 | 22q12.2 | neurofibromatosis | OMIM #101000 |

[a] The percentage in parentheses is the frequency of occurrence for a given gain.
[b] See Table 8.1.
[c] Loci without an OMIM reference were pinpointed using The International RH Mapping Consortium—GeneMap '99 at http://www.ncbi.nlm.nih.gov/genemap99/.
[d] All references to OMIM refer to http://www.ncbi.nlm.nih.gov/Omim/ and were collected by doing a general keyword search of 'melanoma.'

These commonalities serve in narrowing the list of possible genes involved in this cancer. Data were not analyzed for either of the sex chromosomes.

Our results incorporate the genes putatively involved with uveal melanoma onset and progression. Copy number gains (Table 8.2) and losses (Table 8.3) correlate with the minimal common regions (Fig. 8.3). Data from Tables 8.2 and 8.3 were used to identify genes likely to be involved in uveal melanoma (Table 8.4). These genes are known to be linked to uveal melanoma or its predisposing factors and/or are related to cell cycle control.

### SPECTRAL KARYOTYPING

SKY revealed many structural and numerical chromosome aberrations. Among the most striking observations was the near triploid to near tetraploid nature of several cell lines and the presence of unusually complex chromosomal rearrangements (Fig. 8.4 and 8.5B).

A minimum of three metaphase spreads were analyzed per cell line. A total of 2,663 chromosome structures were analyzed. The percent of aberrations ranged from 0% for the Y chromosome to 62% for chromosome 17 (Table 8.5). Chromosomes 1, 7, 12, and 17 were involved in structural aberrations in greater than 50% of the metaphases and cell lines. The high frequency of these aberrations suggests that chromosomes 1, 7, 12, and 17 may contain genes of significance in the establishment and/or progression of uveal malignant melanoma. Structural aberrations involving chromosomes 2, 3, 4, 5, 6, 8, 9, 10, 11, 13, 16, 19, 20, and X were seen in five or more cell lines, but occurred less than 50% of the time in the chromosomes in which they were observed. The fact that these aberrations occurred in five or more cell lines suggests that they may also contain genes of significance in uveal malignant melanoma. Chromosomes 1, 3, 8, 17, 19, 20, and 22 were often involved in numerical aberrations. Complex aberrations involving more than two chromosomes were seen frequently in MEL290, OCM1, OCM3, and OCM8 (Fig. 8.4).

## DISCUSSION

Certain anomalies seen in uveal melanoma fresh and fixed tissues have been reported with great consistency, and a cross-section of available data is provided on Tables 8.2 and 8.3. There remains a critical need for large-scale profiling of the genomic changes in uveal melanoma, in particular because the majority of studies have been relatively small and have employed techniques with lower resolution. Monosomy 3, gain of 6p, loss of 6q, and gain of 8q are the most prevalent cytogenetic aberrations to date in the literature.[5,13,15,16] Our data also demonstrate gain of 6p, loss of 6q, and gain of 8q, but do not show monosomy 3. In fact, gains on chromosome 3 were seen in 8 of the 10 cell lines. This is in contrast to the majority of the literature, but is a finding corroborated by a recent study of two cell lines and five fresh tumors.[25] In addition, gains and losses not previously identified in uveal melanoma were found in this study. This suggests the question: are cell lines vastly different than the tumor from which they originated, or has cell culture produced artifacts?

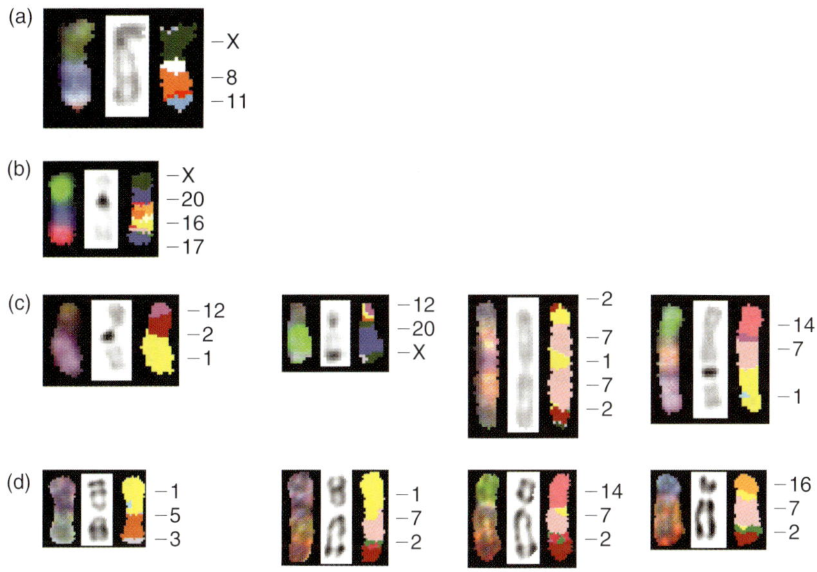


Fig. 8.4. Complex aberrations detected by Spectral Karyotyping. Spectral karyotyping (SKY) employs 24 distinctly labeled chromosome-specific probes, thus allowing for the identification of all the chromosomes involved in complex rearrangements. SKY was performed on 10 uveal melanoma cell lines and revealed complex chromosomal rearrangements in 4 of the lines. (A) MEL290. (B) OCM1. (C) OCM3. (D) OCM8.

In addition to the cytogenetic aberrations of chromosomes 3, 6 and 8, other recurrent anomalies have been noted on 7q, 9p, and 13q.[4] Our results show that copy number alteration events occurred on each of these chromosomes, similar to those in the literature (Tables 8.2 and 8.3). We also observed a 7q deletion and a 13q deletion that were unsubstantiated in the literature (Table 8.3).

To ensure appropriate determination of novel gains and losses, the heterochromatic regions near the centromere and telomeric regions had to be assessed for reliability. The telomeric ends of each of the chromosomes are highly repetitive, as are the heterochromatic regions near the centromeres of chromosomes 1, 3, 9, 13, 14, 15, 16, 19, 21, 22, and Y. The thresholds were set at 0.8 and 1.2 copy numbers, and profile data exceeding those thresholds were considered regions of deletion or amplification, respectively. Although Cot-1 DNA is used to suppress the binding of probe to the heterochromatic regions near the centromere, these areas and the telomeric repeats tend to bind inconsistently, producing artifacts in the data that may or may not be present in the cell lines. These regions of copy number alteration were evaluated individually. Unless the copy number abnormalities spanned the heterochromatic region, the abnormalities in the heterochromatin near the centromeres of chromosomes 1, 3, 9, 13, 14, 15, 16, 19, 21, and 22 were not considered to be accurate data (chromosome Y was not involved in the analysis due to study design). For any modifications of the data, judgements were made based upon profile-by-profile analysis as well as analysis of those means generated from the individual

(a)

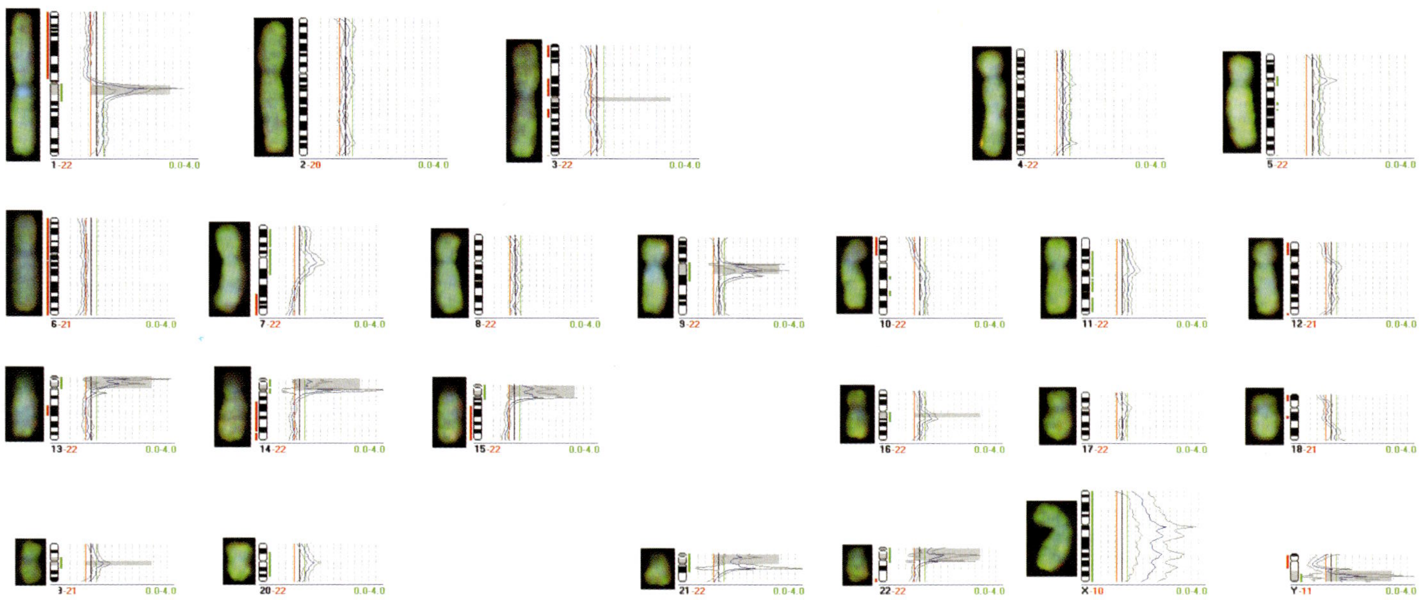

Fig. 8.5 (a). Comparison of a CGH mean profile with a SKY karyotype from a single cell line. (A) The Leica QCGH image analysis software (Leica Inc., Exton, PA) generates 95% confidence intervals for mean CGH profile data once all metaphase spreads have been appropriately karyotyped. A minimum of ten metaphase spreads was analyzed to generate the mean for each cell line. The above profile was created from MEL285 data. Note the relatively narrow confidence intervals. The color chromosome images to the left of each ideogram and associated profile are from a single representative MEL285 spread which contributed to the mean data for that cell line. CGH revealed the following gains and losses: a loss of 1p; a normal chromosome 2; a tendency toward loss of chromosome 3; a normal chromosome 4; tendency toward gain of chromosome 5; loss of chromosome 6; gain of 7p to proximal 7q and loss of distal 7q; a normal chromosomes 8 and 9; loss of 10 p and tendency toward gain 10q; gain of chromosome 11; loss chromosome 12p; tendency toward loss 13; loss of chromosomes 14 and 15; normal chromosomes 16 and 17; loss 18p and tendency toward gain 18q; a normal chromosome 19; gain of chromosome 20, normal chromosomes 21 and 22; gain of the X chromosome; and a very discordant signal for the Y chromosome.

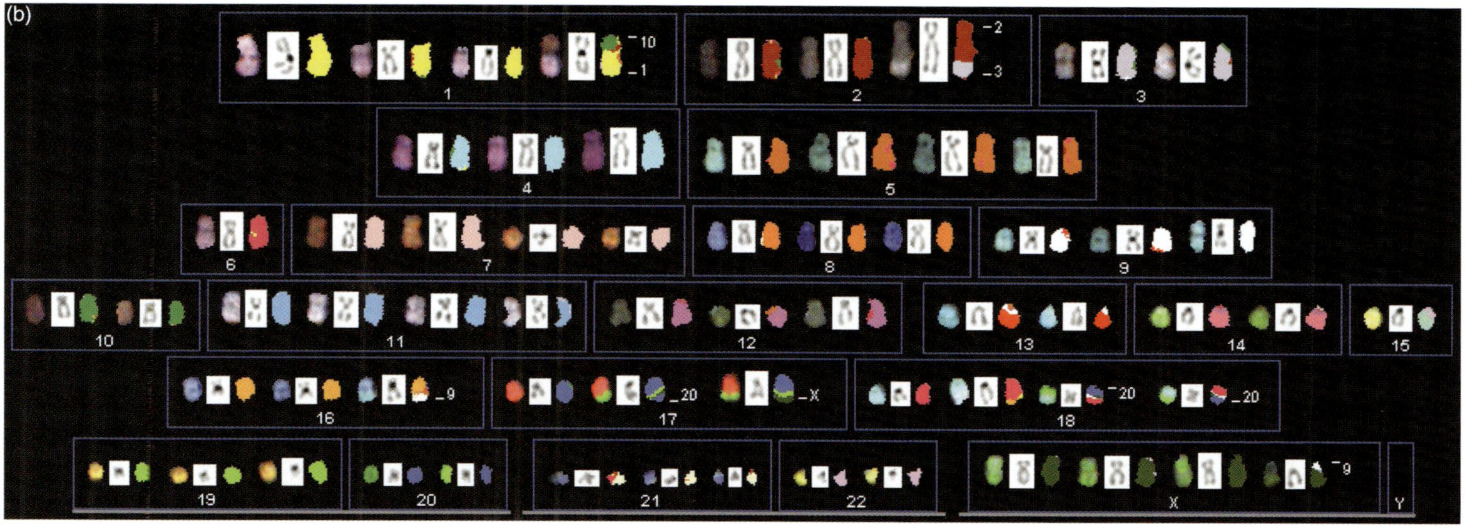


Fig. 8.5 (b). Comparison of a CGH mean profile with a SKY karyotype from a single cell line. (B) A SKY karyotype of a single metaphase spread from the cell line MEL285. Unlike CGH data which represents the gains and losses seen throughout the genome of an entire population of cells, a SKY karyotype is a snapshot of the chromosomal aberrations (and thereby the entire genome) of a single cell. A chromosome-by-chromosome comparison of the CGH profile and the SKY karyotype reveals that the majority of gains and losses identified by CGH can be explained by both structural and numerical chromosome aberrations in the cell line as evidenced by the SKY karyotype. The SKY karyotype revealed a single normal chromosome 1, two chromosomes del(1)(p?), and one der(1)t(1;10); two normal chromosomes 2 and one der(2)t(2;3); two normal chromosomes 3; three normal chromosomes 4; four normal chromosomes 5; one normal chromosome 6; two normal chromosomes 7 and two chromosomes der(7)(p); three normal chromosomes 8; three normal chromosomes 9; two chromosomes del(10)(p?); four normal chromosomes 11; three chromosomes del(12)(p?); two normal chromosomes 13; two normal chromosomes 14; one normal chromosome 15; two normal chromosomes 16 and one der(16)t(9;16); one normal chromosome 17, one der(17)t(17;20), and one der(17)t(17;X); two normal chromosomes 18 and two der(18)t (18;20); three normal chromosomes 19; two normal chromosomes 20; three normal chromosomes 21; two normal chromosomes 22; three normal chromosomes X and one der(X)t(9;X); and no chromosome Y.

profiles for each case. Following assessment of these regions, it remained clear that chromosomes 1, 3, 6, 7, 8, 9, 11, 17, 19, 20, and 22 were involved in significant amplifications and/or deletions. These involve gains and losses that encompass, expand beyond, or are entirely distinct from the telomeres and/or the heterochromatic regions near the centromeres.

Terminal deletions on chromosomes 2q, 3p, 4q, 5p, 7q, 8p, 9p, 10p, 10q, 11q, 12p, 13q, 14q, 16q, 18p, 18q, and 21q extended beyond the telomeric regions (Figs 8.1 and 8.3). By comparing the regions of gain and loss for each line (Fig. 8.2) with the minimal common regions (Fig. 8.3), it is evident that in some cell lines the losses are strictly terminal, while in others losses encompass much larger regions of the chromosomes. In fact, many of the terminal losses expand beyond the distal portion of the chromosome, and thereby are considered significant and warrant further study. The losses that are strictly terminal are of decreased significance since they may be an artifact of hybridization. Therefore, all chromosomes save chromosome 15 were involved in amplification or deletion events that remained significant after consideration of the heterochromatin and distal terminal portions. In some cases our findings were well supported by the published literature, and in others our findings were unique to the characterization of uveal melanoma thus far.

We chose to define minimal common regions as either gains or losses shared between at least half of the cell lines. The use of minimal common regions was predicated upon the voluminous data set compiled when all ten of the cell line means are simultaneously compared. The desired level of sensitivity dictated the use of 50% as a cutpoint for similarities in the data; any cutpoint below 50% would incur far too many commonalties to be of value. Determining minimal common regions allows for the assessment of the similarities associated with uveal melanoma cell lines, and more importantly, allows for localization of probable genes involved in areas of over- or under-expression.

In contrast, there are regions of interest expressing copy number alterations that are unique to a single or a few cell lines. While a great deal of commonalties were expected within the data, each of the ten cell lines is different, and was cultured either from a primary tumor or a metastasis. These regions of interest were also noted; this includes entire chromosome gains and losses as well as high level amplifications or deletions. These regions may only involve a single cell line, or may encompass all ten cell lines; this helps to differentiate between cell lines and may help to account for growth patterns, mechanisms of metastasis, etc. seen in the parent tumor. In other words, regions of interest may help explain commonalties among some of the tumors as well as the differences between the tumors. It should be noted that information regarding the parent tumors is available in some, but not all, cases (Table 8.1).

Table 8.4 does not represent an exhaustive or definitive list of genes involved in uveal melanoma, rather it is an attempt to determine genes putatively involved with this cancer. For the most part, these genes were chosen because they were contained within the minimal common regions (Fig. 8.3). Many of these genes were identified in the literature and also on publicly available databases such as Online Mendelian Inheritance in Man (OMIM). The proposed mechanism or involvement of the gene is stated where possible (Table 8.4). It was found that the regions of amplification and deletion determined in this study correlate with genes known to be involved in the development or progression of uveal melanoma or its predisposing factors. Comparisons of this study with the literature strongly suggest that these ten uveal melanoma cell lines have minimally drifted from the genome of the parent tumor, and are appropriate models for gene dosage alterations within uveal malignant melanoma. If these cell lines are representative of uveal melanoma as a whole, then acceptance of them as models for gene dosage alteration lends validity to our characterization of uveal melanoma and it would follow that our novel amplifications and deletions are worthy of further study.

This is of course assuming the parent tumors of these cell lines were similar to previously characterized tumors. This determination lends validity to our contribution toward characterization of uveal melanoma, particularly with regard to our novel amplifications and deletions.

CGH cannot account for all chromosomal rearrangements and ploidy aberrations seen in SKY. Similarly, SKY cannot account for all of the specific copy number abnormalities seen in CGH. It is important to bear in mind that SKY results are determined on a per cell basis, whereas CGH results are based on the DNA content of a population of cells and is therefore a genomic average. SKY results provide information regarding structural anomalies in addition to copy number abnormalities. SKY is able to resolve the majority of inter-chromosomal exchanges, but not intra-chromosomal rearrangements. SKY results commonly coincided with the observed gains and losses of CGH (Fig. 8.5; Table 8.6). SKY demonstrates that the amplifications and deletions seen in CGH are the result of either numerical or structural abnormalities.[25] The merging of these two data sets thus adds credence to the individual results of each.

While CGH demonstrated significant gene dosage abnormalities within these ten uveal melanoma cell lines, it is inherently incapable of identifying the underlying chromosomal aberrations that cause them. Such unidentifiable aberrations are primarily structural in nature, including translocations and isochromosomes, but also numerical aberrations such as changes in ploidy and instances of mosaicism are not resolved in CGH. SKY results revealed unexpected chromosomal aberrations of many types, including several complex aberrations (Fig. 8.4) and many recurrent aberrations (Fig. 8.5; Table 8.5). The combination of structural and numerical chromosome aberrations identified by SKY corroborates the gains and losses identified in these cell lines by CGH (Fig. 8.5; Table 8.6). Numerical aberrations seen in SKY include the whole chromosome gains found in CGH for three of the cell lines for chromosomes 20 (OCM3, OCM8, and OMM1) and 22 (OCM3, OCM8, and OMM2.3). Additionally, structural rearrangements elucidated by SKY contribute to the copy number gain of chromosome 20 in the case of OCM3 (der (20)t(20;3) and der(20)(12;20;X) and OCM8 (der(20)t(20;3) and der(20)(3;20;12)). Whole chromosome gains were observed singly for chromosome 7 (cell line OMM1), chromosome 8 (cell line MEL270), and chromosome 17 (cell line OCM3) via CGH. Again, SKY revealed whole chromosome gains or rearrangements that contribute to gains as exemplified by t(8;12) in MEL270. SKY results did not coincide with the gain of chromosome 17 in OCM3, but rather a loss was indicated. A whole chromosome loss of chromosome 4 in OCM3 was not corroborated by SKY,

Table 8.5. Structural chromosome aberrations identified by SKY.

| Chromosome | % Aberrations[a] | Lines with aberrations | Frequent aberrations[b] |
|---|---|---|---|
| 1 | 60.3 (141) | 7/10 | deletion [7]<br>(1;10) [5]<br>(1;16) [3] |
| 2 | 43.4 (131) | 7/10 | (2;1) [3]<br>(2;12) [3] |
| 3 | 47.6 (168) | 10/10 | deletion [4]<br>(3;7) [4]<br>(3;10) [4] |
| 4 | 22.7 (110) | 7/10 | |
| 5 | 38.7 (124) | 7/10 | marker [3]<br>duplication 5p [3] |
| 6 | 34.9 (106) | 8/10 | |
| 7 | 57.2 (180) | 9/10 | (7;3) [4]<br>(7;17) [3] |
| 8 | 44.8 (154) | 9/10 | (8;11) [3] |
| 9 | 19.1 (94) | 5/10 | |
| 10 | 37.9 (103) | 8/10 | (10;1) [4]<br>(10;3) [3] |
| 11 | 42.7 (124) | 7/10 | deletion or marker [4]<br>(11;8) [3] |
| 12 | 57.4 (129) | 6/10 | deletion or marker [3]<br>(12;2) [3] |
| 13 | 20.9 (86) | 6/10 | |
| 14 | 12.9 (85) | 4/10 | |
| 15 | 25.0 (96) | 3/10 | |
| 16 | 47.9 (119) | 7/10 | (16;17) [3] |
| 17 | 62.0 (142) | 8/10 | (17;7) [3]<br>(17;16) [3] |
| 18 | 14 (86) | 2/10 | |
| 19 | 25.2 (103) | 5/10 | |
| 20 | 50.0 (120) | 6/10 | |
| 21 | 9.5 (63) | 1/10 | |
| 22 | 14.3 (112) | 2/10 | |
| X | 42.5 (80) | 9/10 | 20 [3] |
| Y | 0.0 (7) | 0/10 | |

[a] The number in parentheses is the total number of chromosomes analyzed.
[b] The number in brackets is the number of cell lines in which the particular aberration was identified.

but there was an instance where only two copies of chromosome 4 and a der(4)t(4;5) were present. The SKY results strongly demonstrate that the gains and losses identified by CGH are by no means due to numerical chromosome aberrations alone. Instead, structural rearrangement of the genome significantly contributes to the amplification or deletion of DNA sequences and thus has a strong effect on the results found by CGH. As an example, the existence of an isochromosome 6p with two normal copies of chromosome 6, as revealed by SKY in MEL270, yields four copies of 6p and only two copies of the 6q arm which explains the CGH results for that cell line (Fig. 8.2). This occurred in MEL270, and was mirrored in the CGH

Table 8.6. A comparison of chromosome aberrations identified by SKY with gains and losses identified by CGH.

| Chromosome | Structural aberrations[a] | Numerical aberrations | Gains by CGH[b] | Losses by CGH[b] |
|---|---|---|---|---|
| 1 | t, dic, del, ins, mr | | 1q21.1–q21.2 | |
| 2 | t, dic, del, ins, mr | | | 2qter |
| 3 | t, dic, del, ins | Aneusomy | 3p | 3pter |
| 4 | t, del | | | 4qter |
| 5 | t, del, i | | | 5p |
| 6 | t, del, i | | 6p | 6q |
| 7 | t, dic, del, mr | Aneusomy | 7p<br>7q | 7qter |
| 8 | t, del, i, mr | Aneusomy | 8q24.1–q24.3 | 8pter |
| 9 | t | Aneusomy | | 9p |
| 10 | t, ins, del | | | 10p and 10qter |
| 11 | t, ins, del | Aneusomy | 11p | 11qter |
| 12 | t, ins, del | Aneusomy | | 12pter |
| 13 | tls | | | 13qter |
| 14 | t, mr, R | | | 14qter |
| 16 | t, mr | | | 16qter |
| 17 | t, mr | Aneusomy | 17q | |
| 18 | | | | 18pter and 18qter |
| 19 | t, mr | Aneusomy | 19 | |
| 20 | t, mr | Aneusomy | 20 | |
| 21 | | Aneusomy | | 21 |
| 22 | i | Aneusomy | 22 | |

[a] t = translocation, dic = dicentric, del = deletion, ins = insertion, i = isochromosome, mr = multiple rearrangements, R = Robertsonian translocation.

[b] Gains and losses have been generalized for ease of presentation. For a more accurate delineation see Tables 8.2 and 8.3.

results that show a gain of 6p and loss of 6q for that cell line. Another group of researchers engaged in the application of CGH, SKY and FISH (fluorescence *in situ* hybridization) to characterize uveal melanoma, has recently revealed data very similar to our own for MEL270.[25] This delicate interplay between CGH and SKY was evidenced in the vast majority of the data, and SKY results for individual metaphases were found to support most of the genomic changes resolved in CGH. Together, SKYand CGH are complimentary techniques that reveal a highly developed picture of the cancer genome.

## SUMMARY

We used comparative genomic hybridization (CGH) and spectral karyotyping (SKY) to elucidate genomic alterations within ten uveal malignant melanoma cell lines often used as models for the disease. Extensive copy number abnormalities were identified by CGH; and frequent structural and numerical chromosomal aberrations were revealed by SKY. Comparison of CGH and SKY results revealed that chromosomal rearrangement played a significant role in the generation of

DNA sequence copy number abnormalities identified by CGH. Distillation of our results revealed several chromosomal regions likely to contain genes involved in the development and metastasis of uveal malignant melanoma, and speculations regarding the identity of these genes were made. This cell line analysis is an important step in the developing cytogenetic characterization of this disease.


## ACKNOWLEDGEMENTS

We would like to thank the originators of the cell lines for sharing their data and preliminary characterizations of each derived cell line. A debt of gratitude is owed to Dr. Jerry Y. Niederkorn and Ms. Elizabeth Mayhew, both at the Department of Ophthalmology at the University of Texas Southwestern Medical Center at Dallas, in Dallas, TX, for their assistance in obtaining the uveal melanoma cell lines. Drs. Timothy J. O'Leary and Robert L. Becker, Armed Forces Institute of Pathology, Washington, DC, were of great help in modifying both our experimental methods and data analysis.


## REFERENCES


1. McLean W, Gamel JW. Uveal (intraocular) melanoma. *Cancer J.* 1996;9:20–25.
2. Callender GR. Malignant melanotic tumors of the eye: a study of histologic types in 111 cases. *Trans Am Acad Ophthalmol Otolaryngol.* 1931;36:131–142.
3. Char DH. *Ocular Oncology.* New York: Churchill-Livingstone, 1989.
4. Gordon KB, Thompson CT, Char DH, O'Brien JM, Kroll S, Ghazvini S, Gray JW. Comparative genomic hybridization in the detection of DNA copy number abnormalities in uveal melanoma. *Cancer Res.* 1994;54:4764–4768.
5. Prescher G, Bornfeld N, Hirche H, Horsthemke B, Jockel K, Becher R. Prognostic implications of monosomy 3 in uveal melanoma. *Lancet.* 1996;347:1222–1225.
6. Singh AD, Wang MX, Donoso LA, Shields CL, De Potter P, Shields JA. Genetic aspects of uveal melanoma: a brief review. *Semin Oncol.* 1996;23:768–772.
7. Tucker MA, Shields JA, Hartge P, Augsburger J, Hoover RN, Fraumeni JF Jr. Sunlight exposure as risk factor for intraocular malignant melanoma. *N Engl J Med.* 1985;313: 789–792.
8. Egan KM, Seddon JM, Glynn RJ, Gragoudas ES, Albert DM. Epidemiologic aspects of uveal melanoma. *Surv Ophthalmol.* 1988;32:239–251.
9. Holly EA, Aston DA, Char DH, Kristiansen JJ, Ahn DK. Uveal melanoma in relation to ultraviolet light exposure and host factors. *Cancer Res.* 1990;50:5773–5777.
10. Dolin PJ, Foss AJ, Hungerford JL. Uveal melanoma: is solar ultraviolet radiation a risk factor? *Ophthalmic Epidemiol.* 1994;1:27–30.
11. Lynch HT, Anderson DE, Krush AJ. Heredity and intraocular malignant melanoma. Study of two families and review of forty-five cases. *Cancer.* 1968;21:119–125.
12. Singh AD, Donoso LA, Jackson L, Shields CL, De Potter P, Shields JA. Familial uveal melanoma: absence of constitutional cytogenic abnormalities in 14 cases. *Arch Ophthalmol.* 1996;114:502–503.
13. Speicher MR, Prescher G, Du Manoir S, Jauch A, Horsthemke B, Bornfeld N, Becher R, Cremer T. Chromosomal gains and losses in uveal melanomas detected by comparative genomic hybridization. *Cancer Res.* 1994;54:3817–3823.
14. Ghazvini S, Char DH, Kroll S, Waldman FM, Pinkel D. Comparative genomic hybridization analysis of archival formalin-fixed paraffin-embedded uveal melanomas. *Cancer Genet Cytogenet.* 1996;90:95–101.

15. White VA, McNeil BK, Horsman DE. Acquired homozygosity (isodisomy) of chromosome 3 in uveal melanoma. *Cancer Genet Cytogenet*. 1998;102:40–45.
16. White VA, Chambers JD, Courtright PD, Chang WY, Horsman DE. Correlation of cytogenetic abnormalities with the outcome of patients with uveal melanoma. *Cancer*. 1998;83:354–359.
17. Griffin CA, Long PP, Schachat AP. Trisomy 6p in an ocular melanoma. *Cancer Genet Cytogenet*. 1988;32:129–132.
18. Marmur J, Rownd R, Schildkraudt. Denaturation and renaturation of deoxyribonucleic acid. *Prog Nucleic Acid Res*. 1963;1:231–300.
19. Reid T, Baldini A, Rand TC, Ward DC. Simultaneous visualization of seven different DNA probes by *in situ* hybridization using combinatorial fluorescence and digital imaging microscopy. *Proc Natl Acad Sci USA*. 1992;89:1388–1392.
20. Kallioniemi A, Kallioniemi OP, Sudar D, Rutovit D, Gray J, Waldman F, Pinkel D. Comparative genomic hybridization for molecular cytogenetic analysis of solid tumors. *Science*. 1992;258:818–821.
21. Schrock E, Du Manoir S, Veldman T, Schoell B, Wienberg J, Ferguson-Smith MA, Ning Y, Ledbetter DH, Bar-Am I, Soenksen D, Garini Y, Ried T. Multicolor spectral karyotyping of human chromosomes. *Science*. 1996;273:494–497.
22. Thompson CT, Gray JW. Cytogenetic profiling using fluorescence *in situ* hybridization (FISH) and comparative genomic hybridization (CGH). *J Cell Biochem Suppl*. 1993;17G:139–143.
23. Tucker JD, Lee DA, Ramsey MJ, Briner J, Olsen L, Moore DH 2nd. On the frequency of chromosome exchanges in a control population measured by chromosome painting. *Mutat Res*. 1994;313:193–202.
24. Mitelman F, ed. *ISCN 1995. An International System for Human Cytogenetic Nomenclature* (1995). Basel, 1995.
25. Naus NC, Van Drunen E, De Klein A, Luyten GP, Paridaens DA, Alers JC, Ksander BR, Beverloo HB, Slater RM. Characterization of complex chromosomal abnormalities in uveal melanoma by fluorescence *in situ* hybridization, spectral karyotyping, and comparative genomic hybridization. *Genes Chromosomes Cancer*. 2001;30:267–273.
26. Online Mendelian Inheritance in Man, OMIM (TM). McKusick-Nathans Institute for Genetic Medicine, Johns Hopkins University (Baltimore, MD) and National Center for Biotechnology Information, National Library of Medicine (Bethesda, MD), 2000. Available from: URL: http://www.ncbi.nlm.nih.gov/omim/
27. De Waard-Siebinga I, Blom DJ, Griffioen M, Schrier PI, Hoogendoorn E, Beverstock G, Danen EH, Jager MJ. Establishment and characterization of an uveal-melanoma cell line. *Int J Cancer*. 1995;62:155–161.
28. Chen PW, Murray TG, Uno T, Salgaller ML, Reddy R, Ksander BR. Expression of MAGE genes in ocular melanoma during progression from primary to metastatic disease. *Clin Exp Metastasis*. 1997;15:509–518.
29. Kan-Mitchell J, Mitchell MS, Rao N, Liggett PE. Characterization of uveal melanoma cell lines that grow as xenografts in rabbit eyes. *Invest Ophthalmol Vis Sci*. 1989;30:829–834.
30. Albert DM, Ruzzo MA, McLaughlin MA, Robinson NL, Craft JL, Epstein J. Establishment of cell lines of uveal melanoma. Methodology and characteristics. *Invest Ophthalmol Vis Sci*. 1984;25:1284–1299.
31. Luyten GP, Naus NC, Mooy CM, Hagemeijer A, Kan-Mitchell J, Van Drunen E, Vuzevski V, De Jong PT, Luider TM. Establishment and characterization of primary and metastatic uveal melanoma cell lines. *Int J Cancer*. 1996;66:380–387.
32. Wiltshire RN, Elner VM, Dennis T, Vine AK, Trent JM. Cytogenetic analysis of posterior uveal melanoma. *Cancer Genet Cytogenet*. 1993;66:47–53.

33. Larouche N, Larouche K, Beliveau A, Leclere S, Salesse C, Pelletier G, Guerin SL. Transcriptional regulation of the alpha 4 integrin subunit gene in the metastatic spread of uveal melanoma. *Anticancer Res.* 1998;18:3539–3547.
34. Copeman MC. The putative melanoma tumor-suppressor gene on human chromosome 6q. *Pathology.* 1992;24:307–309.
35. Dunne BM, McNamara M, Clynes M, Shering SG, Larkin AM, Moran E, Barnes C, Kennedy SM. MDR1 expression is associated with adverse survival in melanoma of the uveal tract. *Hum Pathol.* 1998;29:594–598.
36. Blom DJ, Mooy CM, Luyten GP, Kerkvliet S, Ouwerkerk I, Zwinderman AH, Schrier PI, Jager MJ. Inverse correlation between expression of HLA-B and c-myc in uveal melanoma. *J Pathol.* 1997;181:75–79.
37. Luyten GP, Van der Spek CW, Brand I, Sintnicolaas K, De Waard-Siebinga I, Jager MJ, De Jong PT, Schrier PI, Luider TM. Expression of MAGE, gp100, and tyrosinase genes in uveal melanoma cell lines. *Melanoma Res.* 1998;8:11–16.
38. Houlston RS, Damato BE. Genetic predisposition to ocular melanoma. *Eye.* 1999; 13:43–46.

GABRI VAN DER PLUIJM*, CLEMENS LÖWIK AND MARTINE DECKERS

# 9. Developing Mouse Bone as an *in vitro* Model to Study Angiogenesis

## INTRODUCTION

In order to study the process of angiogenesis and to test the (anti)-angiogenic potential of newly developed agents, suitable assays are essential. Fetal mouse long bones are well-known models to study cartilage differentiation and osteoclastic resorption. We show here the outgrowth of PECAM-1 positive tube-like structures from such bone rudiments. This feature can be used to study angiogenesis *in vitro*. The area of outgrowth significantly increased with culture time as shown by computerized image analysis of PECAM-1 positive tube-like structures. Treatment with rhVEGF stimulated the formation of tube-like structures. Outgrowth of tube-like structures was partly dependent on endogenous VEGF-A since treatment with anti-mVEGF-A and sFLT1 both strongly inhibited the formation of the tube-like structures.

Treatment of explants with the angiogenesis inhibitor endostatin resulted in inhibition of the formation of the PECAM-1 positive tube-like structures. Tube formation required activation of matrix metalloproteinases since treatment of the bones with an inhibitor of matrix metalloproteinases completely inhibited migration and tube formation.

In conclusion, we describe a new *in vitro* model to study angiogenesis that can be used to test the angiogenic or anti-angiogenic potential of novel test compounds and which combines the multi-cellularity of *in vivo* assays with the accessibility and flexibility of *in vitro* assays.

## MODELS OF ANGIOGENESIS

Angiogenesis, the development of vessels from pre-existing vessels, is essential for a variety of physiologic processes including organ development,[1,2] wound healing and reproduction.[3,4] In adults it is usually related to pathological conditions such as rheumatoid arthritis, diabetic retinopathy, tumor progression and metastasis.[5,6] Highly vascularized tumors are often associated with poor prognosis.[7] The identification of circulating anti-angiogenic factors in tumor-bearing animals and

* To whom correspondence should be addressed.

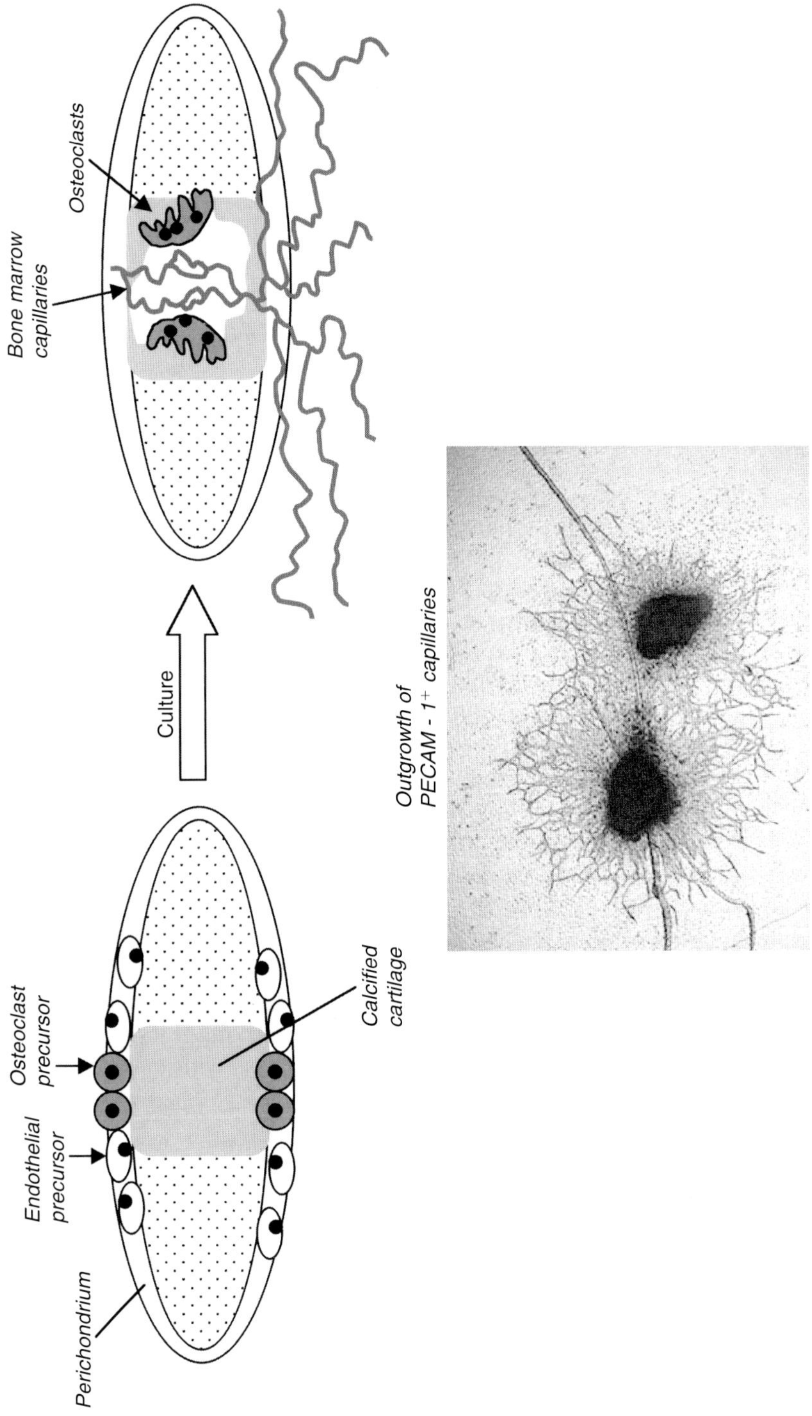
Perichondrium
Endothelial precursor
Osteoclast precursor
Calcified cartilage
Culture
Bone marrow capillaries
Osteoclasts
Outgrowth of PECAM - 1+ capillaries

humans[8–10] led to the postulation that the activation state of endothelial cells is determined by the balance between endogenous angiogenic and anti-angiogenic factors. This implies that if levels of inhibitors are sufficiently high, the angiogenic response will be switched off. This might enable interventions of tumor progression by using anti-angiogenic compounds,[11] e.g., directed against endothelial growth factors, growth factor receptors, proteolytic enzymes or extra-cellular matrix molecules.[12–14] On the other hand, pro-angiogenic therapy may provide a promising strategy for patients suffering from vascular insufficiency.[15]

To study the process of angiogenesis and to test the (anti)-angiogenic potential of newly developed agents, suitable assays are essential. The most commonly used *in vivo* assays are the corneal micropocket assay, the chorioallantoic membrane (CAM) assay and dorsal skin-fold assay.[16–18] To study the efficacy of angiogenic compounds the corneal micropocket is often used since it comprises an avascular environment. The efficacy of anti-angiogenic compounds in inhibiting growth factor induced-vascularization or spontaneous vascularization is usually studied in a vascular environment, such as the CAM assay or in the dorsal skin-fold assay. Although these assays have proven their use they have their limitations (for a review see ref. 19): (i) complicated surgical techniques are required; (ii) the number of test compounds that can be assayed, e.g., in the micropocket assay, is limited; (iii) simultaneous assessment of both angiogenic and anti-angiogenic compounds in the same assay without the addition of exogenous growth factors is not feasible. Most *in vitro* assays used are based on the assessment of proliferation[20] or migration of endothelial cells,[21–23] but lack non-endothelial cells such as macrophages which are known to contribute markedly to the angiogenic response *in vivo*.[24] Furthermore, primary endothelial cells or endothelial cell lines often require a coating of extracellular matrix components to study tube formation.[25,26]

## FETAL MOUSE LONG BONES: A NEW *IN VITRO* ANGIOGENESIS ASSAY

Fetal mouse long bones (metatarsals) are well-known models to study cartilage differentiation and osteoclastic resorption.[27,28] At day 17 during fetal development mouse metatarsals consist of hypertrophic cartilage which is mineralized at the center (Fig. 9.1). At this stage during embryonic development osteoclast-precursors are still confined to the surrounding perichondrium and will differentiate and fuse to form multinucleated osteoclasts that will invade and resorb the calcified cartilagenous matrix.[28] At this developmental stage CD31/PECAM-1 positive endothelial cells are still located in the perichondrium (Fig. 9.1). When 17-day-old

Fig. 9.1. The principle of the *in vitro* angiogenesis assay using fetal mouse bone rudiments (17-day-old fetal mouse metatarsals). At time of explantation (day 17 after gestation) endothelial precursors (and osteoclast-precursors) are still confined to the perichondrium (left hand panel). During culture PECAM-1 positive capillaries (right hand panels) will grow out from the bone rudiments (and osteoclasts will form and resorb the calcified cartilage). The area of outgrowth is significantly increased with culture time and can be analyzed by computerized image analysis of PECAM-1 positive tube-like structures (see Fig. 9.2)

metatarsals were dissected and cultured, fibroblast-like cells started to migrate away from the bone explant.[29] After five to six days of culture a resorption cavity was formed, due to osteoclastic activity, which expanded during culture, leaving eventually only the cartilage ends (Figs 9.1 and 9.2). After seven days of culture, formation of tube-like structures over the fibroblast-like cells was observed.[29] These tube-like structures stained positively for PECAM-1. After 10 to 14 days of culture, this area was further increased resulting in a densely branched network of PECAM-1 positive tube-like structures (Figs 9.1 and 9.2). The area of outgrowth significantly increased with culture time[29] and can be measured using image analysis (Fig. 9.2) expressed as pixels per area.

This method has several advantages. The *in vitro* angiogenesis assay combines the multicellularity of *in vivo* assays with the flexibility of *in vitro* systems, without

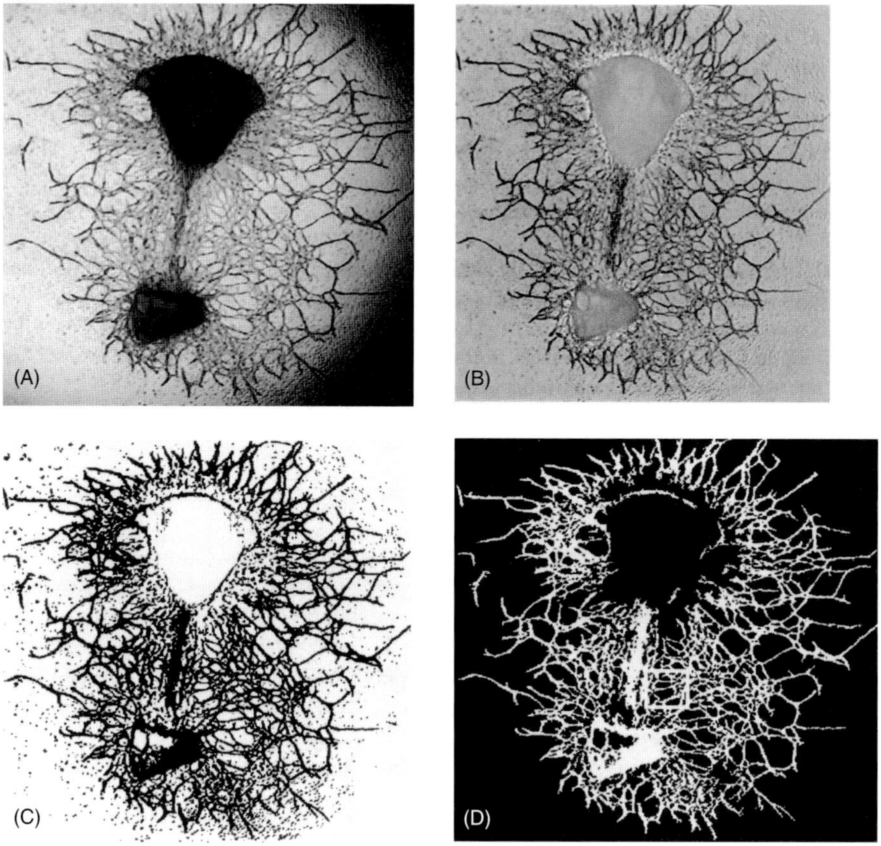


Fig. 9.2. Image processing. Quantification of the formation of PECAM-1 positive tube-like structures was performed in sequential steps.[29] (A) Image captured by CCD camera. (B) Image from which background is subtracted and reverted into a grayscale image. (C) Binary image after manual adjustment on a scale of 1 : 255. (D) Masked image devoid of cell debris and PECAM-1 negative stromal cells in which areas >50 pixels are shown. (Reproduced with permission.[29])

the requirement of complicated surgical techniques.[29] Furthermore, the formation of tube-like structures can be assessed without the need of exogenous growth factors or a coating of extracellular matrix molecules and the response to inhibitors or stimulators of angiogenesis can be quantified by image analysis.[29]

## EFFECT OF EXOGENOUS rhVEGF-A

Treatment of metacarpals with two doses of exogenous rhVEGF-A (10 or 100 ng/ml) resulted in a significant stimulation of the total area of outgrowth as depicted in Figure 9.3. Representative images of PECAM-1 stained control and VEGF-A treated bones are shown in Figure 9.3.

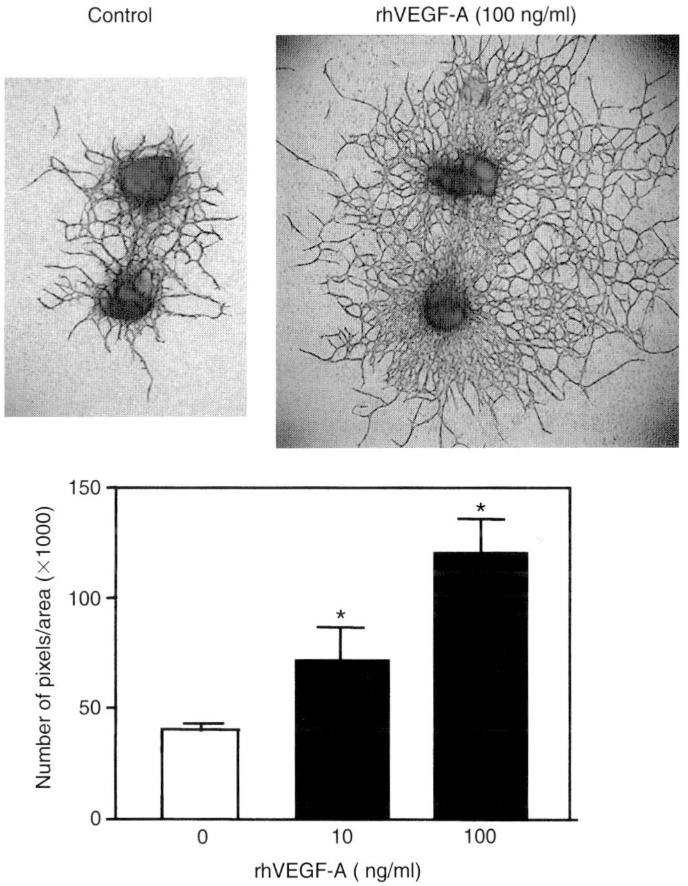


Fig. 9.3. Effect of rhVEGF-A on the formation of PECAM-1 positive tube-like structures. Fetal mouse metacarpals were treated with 10 or 100 ng/ml rhVEGF-A. After 14 days of culture the number of PECAM-1 positive pixels per area was quantified (see Fig. 9.2). rhVEGF-A dose dependently and significantly stimulated the formation of tube-like structures. * $= p \leq 0.05$ as compared to controls, $n = 6$. Representative images of PECAM-1 staining of control and VEGF-treated (100 ng/ml) cultures after 14 days of culture. (Reproduced with permission.[29])

## THE ROLE OF ENDOGENOUS VEGF-A

To determine whether endogenous mouse VEGF-A was required for the formation of PECAM-1 positive tube-like structures, cultures were treated with a functional blocking antibody directed against mouse VEGF-A (anti-mVEGF-A) or with truncated VEGF receptor-1 (sFlt1).[30] Treatment with anti-mVEGF-A from day 7 to day

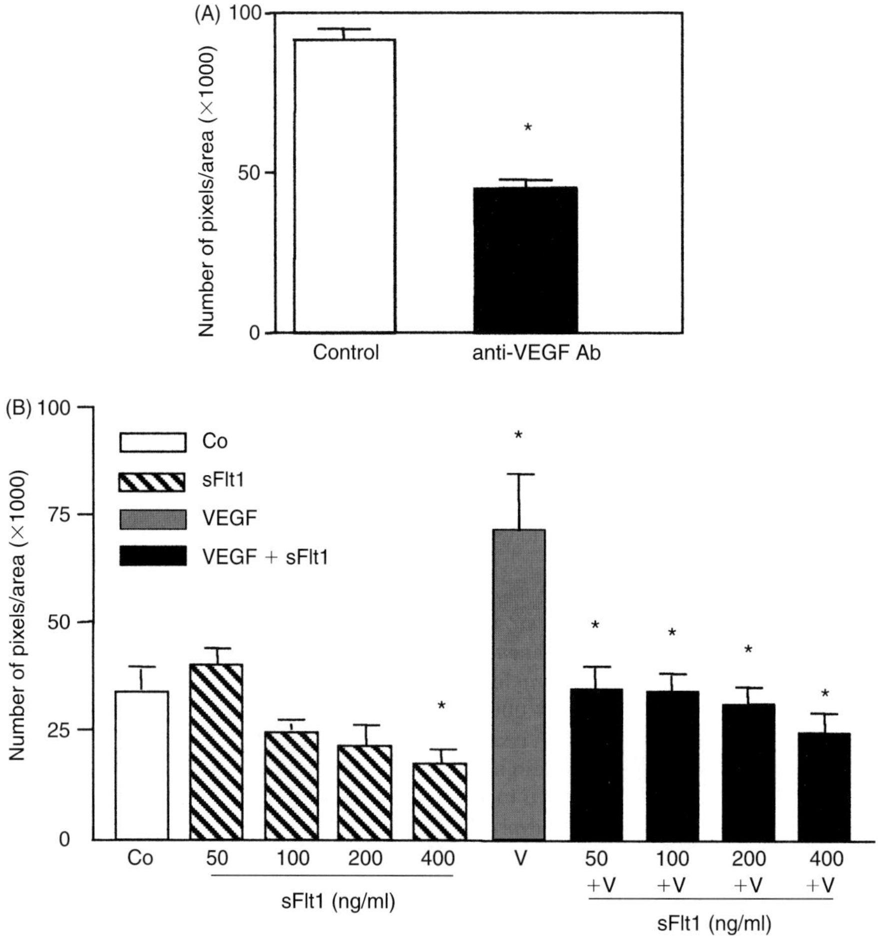


Fig. 9.4. Effect of a functional blocking antibody against mVEGF-A (Fig. 9.4A) and soluble Flt1/sFlt1 (Fig. 9.4B) on the formation of PECAM-1 positive tube-like structures. Fetal mouse metatarsals were treated with anti-mouse VEGF-A antibody (1 μg/ml) from day 7 to day 14 of culture. Fetal mouse metatarsals were treated with various doses of sFlt1 for 14 days in presence or absence of 10 ng/ml rhVEGF-A. sFlt1 dose-dependently inhibited the formation of tube-like structures both in the presence and absence of rhVEGF-A. * $= p \leq 0.05$ as compared to controls, # $= p \leq 0.05$ as compared to VEGF-A treated cultures, $n = 6$. The number of PECAM-1 positive pixels per area was quantified after 14 days of culture as described earlier.[29] (Co) control; (V) rhVEGF-A. (Reproduced with permission.[29])

14 resulted in 40% (± 5%) inhibition of the formation of PECAM-1 positive tube-like structures as shown in Figure 9.4A. Treatment with sFlt1 from day 3 onwards dose-dependently inhibited the formation of PECAM-1 positive tube-like structures (Fig. 9.4B). Similarly, treatment of metatarsals with a combination of rhVEGF-A and various doses sFlt1 completely reversed the formation of PECAM-1 positive tube-like structures to control levels (Fig. 9.4B). This suggests that sFlt1 inhibits both human and mouse VEGF-A-induced formation of tube-like structures.

### EFFECT OF ENDOSTATIN

To test the angiostatic properties of soluble recombinant human endostatin derived from an embryonic kidney cell line (EBNA 293 cells[22]) metatarsals were treated with rhEndostatin (Fig. 9.5A). Treatment with rhEndostatin at a concentration of 1 and 5 μg/ml significantly inhibited the formation of PECAM-1 positive tube-like structures after 14 days of treatment (Fig. 9.5A). Outgrowth of fibroblast-like cells, however, was not blocked by treatment with rhEndostatin, indicating that this agent exerts an endothelial-specific effect.

## EFFECT OF MATRIX METALLOPROTEINASE INHIBITORS

To test whether matrix metalloproteinases are involved in tube formation, metatarsals were cultured in the presence of marimastat ($10^{-6}$ M), a broad spectrum matrix metalloproteinase inhibitor. Treatment with marimastat strongly inhibited the outgrowth of PECAM-1 positive capillaries. Histological section reveal that PECAM-1 endothelial cells remained in close proximity of the fetal bone explant after culture. Most likely the migration of the PECAM-1 positive cells (and subsequent formation of tube-like structures) was directly inhibited by marimastat (Fig. 9.5B). In contrast, treatment with aprotinin, an inhibitor of plasmin activity, had no effect.[29] This suggests that the formation of PECAM-1 positive tube-like structures in our assay acts via a MMP-dependent process rather than a plasmin-dependent process.

## CONCLUSION

Fetal long bones of specific developmental stages, representing different stages of endochondral bone formation, are well-known models to study chondrocyte differentiation (E15)[31,32] or osteoclastic resorption (E17).[28,33] Here we describe the use of E17 mouse metatarsals as a simple and quantitative assay to study the formation of capillary-like structures in response to angiogenic (VEGF) and anti-angiogenic factors (endostatin, marimastat). These tube-like structures exhibited an endothelial-like morphology and expressed the endothelial markers PECAM-1 (CD31) and collagen type IV.[29]

In conclusion, we have developed a novel *in vitro* angiogenesis assay in which the angiogenic as well as angiostatic potential of various classes of compounds can be tested.[29] Spontaneous tube formation occurred even in the absence of a coating of extra-cellular matrix proteins and exogenous growth factors. This model combines both the flexibility and accessibility of *in vitro* models with the complexity of *in vivo*

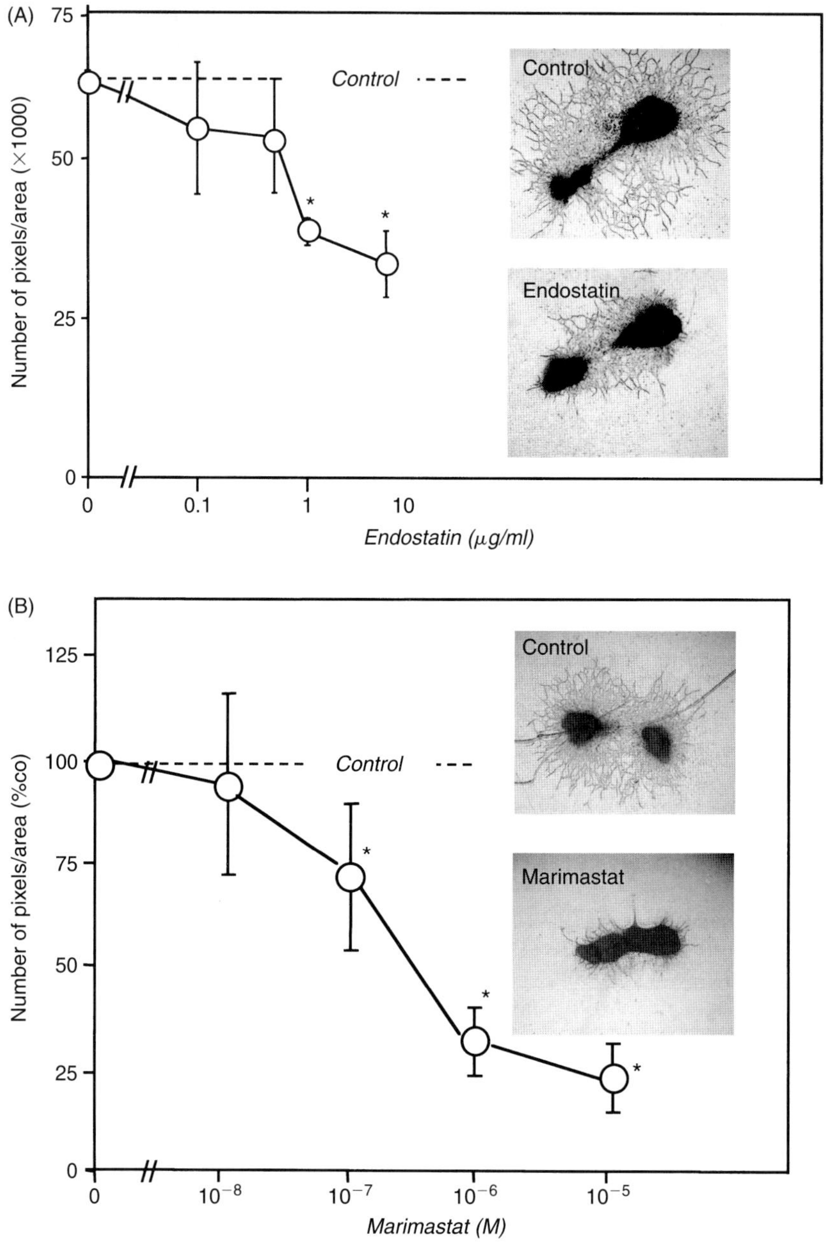


Fig. 9.5. Effect of rhEndostatin and marimastat on the formation of PECAM-1 positive tube-like structures. Fetal mouse metatarsals were treated with various concentrations soluble rhEndostatin (A) and marimastat (B) for 14 days. Both rhEndostatin and marimastat significantly inhibited formation of tube-like structures. * $= p \leq 0.05$ as compared to controls, $n = 6$. (Fig. 9.5A, adapted from ref. 29. Reproduced with permission.)

assays, in particular the contribution of inflammatory cells and stromal cells that interact with endothelial cells. With the growing demand for easy and reproducible *in vitro* angiogenesis assays and the growing interest in the specific properties of endothelial cells this assay provides a new tool for screening agents for potential clinical use and further research in the field of angiogenesis.

## REFERENCES


1. Adams RH, Wilkinson GA, Weiss C, Diella F, Gale NW, Deutsch U, Risau W, Klein R. Roles of ephrinB ligands and EphB receptors in cardiovascular development: demarcation of arterial/venous domains, vascular morphogenesis, and sprouting angiogenesis. *Genes Dev.* 1999;3:295–306.
2. Erlebacher A, Filvaroff E, Gitelman SE, Derynck R. Toward a molecular understanding of skeletal development. *Cell.* 1995;80:371–378.
3. Tamura H, Greenwald GS. Angiogenesis and its hormonal control in the corpeus luteum of the pregnant rat. *Biol Reprod.* 1987;36:1149–1154.
4. Nissen NN, Polverini PJ, Koch AE, Volin MV, Gamelli RL, DiPietro LA. VEGF mediates angiogenic activity during the proliferative phase of wound healing. *Am J Pathol.* 2000;152:1445–1452.
5. Folkman J. Angiogenesis in cancer, vascular, rheumatoid and other disease. *Nat Med.* 1995;1:27–31.
6. Ellis LM, Fidler IJ. Angiogenesis and metastasis. *Eur J Cancer.* 1996;32A:2451–2460.
7. Szabo S, Sandor Z. The diagnostic and prognostic value of tumor angiogenesis. *Eur J Surg Suppl.* 1998;582:99–103.
8. Fidler IJ, Ellis LM. The implications of angiogenesis for the biology and therapy of cancer metastasis. *Cell.* 1998;79:185–189.
9. O'Reilly MS, Boehm T, Shing Y, Fukai N, Vasios G, Lane WS, Flynn E, Birkhead JR, Olsen BR, Folkman J. Endostatin: an endogenous inhibitor of angiogenesis and tumor growth. *Cell.* 1997;88:277–285.
10. Sten-Linder M, Linder C, Strander H, Munck-Wikland E, Wersall P, Linder S, Wiman B. Angiostatin fragments in urine from patients with malignant disease. *Anticancer Res.* 1999; 19:3409–3414.
11. Hanahan D, and Folkman J. Patterns and emerging mechanisms of the angiogenic switch during tumorigenesis. *Cell.* 1996;86:353–364.
12. Millauer B, Shawver LK, Plate KH, Risau W, Ullrich A. Glioblastoma growth inhibited *in vivo* by a dominant-negative Flk-1 mutant. *Nature.* 1994;367:576–579.
13. Fisher C, Gilbertson-Beadling S, Powers EA, Petzold G, Poorman R, Mitchell MA. Interstitial collagenase is required for angiogenesis *in vitro*. *Dev Biol.* 1994;62:499–510.
14. Ingber D. Extracellular matrix as a solid-state regulator in angiogenesis: identification of new targets for anti-cancer therapy. *Semin Cancer Biol.* 1992;3:57–63.
15. Rosengart TK, Lee LY, Patel SR, Sanborn TA, Parikh M, Bergman GM, Hachamovich R, Szulc M, Kligfield PD, Okin PM, Hahn RT, Devereux RM, Post MR, Hackett NR, Foster T, Grasso TM, Lesser ML, Isom OW, Crystal RG. Angiogenesis gene therapy: phase I assessment of direct intramyocardial administration of an adenovirus vector expressing VEGF121 cDNA to individuals with clinically significant severe coronary artery disease. *Circulation.* 1999;100:468–474.
16. Fournier GA, Lutty GA, Watt S, Fenselau A, Patz A. A corneal micropocket assay for angiogenesis in the rat eye. *Invest Ophthalmol Vis Sci.* 1981;21:351–354.
17. Kenyon BM, Voest EE, Chen CC, Flynn E, Folkman J, D'Amato RJ. A model of angiogenesis in the mouse cornea. *Invest Ophthalmol Vis Sci.* 1996;37:1625–1632.

18. Jakob WG, Jentzsch KD, Mauersberger B, Heder G. The chick embryo choriallantoic membrane as a bioassay for angiogenesis factors: reactions induced by carrier materials. *Exp. Pathol. (Jena)* 1978;15:241–249.
19. Jain RK, Schlenger K, Yuan F. Quantitative angiogenesis assays: progress and problems. *Nat Med.* 1997;3:1203–1208.
20. Gospodarowicz D, Greenburg G, Bialecki H, Zetter BR. Factors involved in the modulation of cell proliferation *in vivo* and *in vitro*: the role of fibroblast and epidermal growth factors in the proliferative response of mammalian cells. *In Vitro.* 1978;14:85–118.
21. Zetter BR. Migration of endothelial cells is stimulated by tumour-derived factors. *Nature* 1980;5759:41–43.
22. Yamaguchi N, Anand-Apte B, Lee M, Sasaki T, Fukai N, Shapiro R, Que I, Lowik C, Timpl R, Olsen BR. Endostatin inhibits VEGF-induced endothelial cell migration and tumor growth independently of zinc binding. *EMBO J.* 1999;18:4414–4423.
23. Nicosia RF, Ottinetti A. Growth of microvessels in serum-free matrix culture of rat aorta. A quantitative assay of angiogenesis *in vitro. Lab Invest.* 1990;63:115–122.
24. Salvesen HB, Akslen LA. Significance of tumour-associated macrophages, vascular endothelial growth factor and thrombospondin-1 expression for tumour angiogenesis and prognosis in endometrial carcinomas. *Int J Cancer* 1999;84:538–543.
25. Montesano R, Mouron P, Orci L. Vascular outgrowth from tissue explants embedded in fibrin or collagen gels: a simple *in vitro* model of angiogenesis. *Cell Biol Int Rep.* 1985;9:869–875.
26. Koolwijk P, Van Erck MG, De Vree WJ, Vermeer MA, Weich HA, Hanemaaijer R, Van Hinsbergh VW. Cooperative effect of TNFalpha, bFGF, and VEGF on the formation of tubular structures of human microvascular endothelial cells in a fibrin matrix. Role of urokinase activity. *J Cell Biol.* 1996;132:1177–1188.
27. Van der Pluijm G, Löwik CWGM, De Groot H, Alblas MJ, Van der Wee-Pals LJ, Bijvoet OLM, Papapoulos SE. Modulation of PTH-stimulated osteoclastic resorption by bisphosphonates in fetal mouse bone explants. *J Bone Miner Res.* 1991;6:1203–1210.
28. Van der Pluijm G, Most WW, Van der Wee-Pals LJA, De Groot H, Papapoulos SE, Löwik CWGM. Two distinct effects of recombinant human tumor necrosis factor alpha (TNF-alpha) on osteoclast development and subsequent resorption of mineralized matrix. *Endocrinology.* 1991;129;1596–1604.
29. Deckers M, Van der Pluijm G, Dooijewaard S, Kroon M, Van Hinsbergh V, Papapoulos S, Lowik C. Effect of angiogenic and antiangiogenic compounds on the outgrowth of capillary structures from fetal mouse bone explants. *Lab Invest.* 2001;81:5–15.
30. Roeckl W, Hecht D, Sztajer H, Waltenberger J, Yayon A, Weich HA. Differential binding characteristics and cellular inhibition by soluble VEGF receptors 1 and 2. *Exp Cell Res.* 1998;241:161–170.
31. Dieudonné SC, Semeins CM, Goei SW, Vukicevic S, Nulend JK, Sampath TK, Helder M, Burger EH. Opposite effects of osteogenic protein and transforming growth factor beta on chondrogenesis in cultured long bone rudiments. *J Bone Miner Res.* 1994;9:771–780.
32. Haaijman A, Karperien M, Lanske B, Hendriks J, Löwik CW, Bronckers AL, Burger EH. Inhibition of terminal chondrocyte differentiation by bone morphogenetic protein 7 (OP-1) *in vitro* depends on the periarticular region but is independent of parathyroid hormone-related peptide. Bone 1999;25:397–404.
33. Van Beek E, Van der Wee-Pals L, Van de Ruit M, Nijweide P, Löwik CWGM. Leukemia inhibitory factor inhibits osteoclastic resorption, growth, mineralization, and alkaline phosphatase activity in fetal mouse metacarpal bones in culture. *J Bone Miner Res.* 1993;8:191–198.

SHELLEY BOYD

# 10. Uveal Melanoma and Angiogenesis

## BACKGROUND

Based on the pioneering work of Dr Judah Folkman, countless studies over the last three decades have confirmed the significance of a tumor's blood supply to its growth and dissemination.[1] Uveal melanoma is no exception. Tumor vascularity, both its density and its spatial pattern, is reported to be an independent predictor of survival amongst patients with uveal melanoma.

Blood vessels contribute to the pathogenesis, morbidity, and mortality of uveal melanoma. This is true both locally within the eye, and remotely in the development of metastatic disease. Within the confines of the eye, growth of the primary tumor requires the simultaneous and ongoing growth of its vasculature; the retinal vessels may become hyperpermeable; and neovascularization in the posterior or anterior segments can occur. Local radiation therapy affects both the tumor and the retina, the latter disturbance giving rise to a blinding retinal vasculopathy. Systemic dissemination of uveal melanoma requires the movement of tumor cells through the vascular circulation, while the processes of dormancy and growth of secondary metastatic tumors are also believed to be blood-vessel dependent processes.

In addition to its clinical significance, the vascular pathology associated with uveal melanoma is interesting for several reasons. First, the eye has no lymphatic vessels implying that the metastatic dissemination of uveal melanoma occurs strictly via haematogenous spread. This is unique. In addition, uveal melanoma like breast cancer, is characterized by prolonged periods of dormancy, and, according to at least one theory implies the protracted existence of tumor cells unable to expand until a new vasculature has been established.[1–4] And finally, the majority of clinically-detectable metastatic uveal melanoma spreads to the liver, suggesting heightened affinity for this site or a suitable environment for growth, both of which could be dependent upon the local vasculature.

In the last decade uveal melanoma has become the subject of intense scientific discussion and debate and has set the stage for fruitful analyses of other tumor types. Approximately ten years ago, Dr Folberg and co-workers identified and characterized unique two-dimensional patterns of periodic acid Schiff (PAS)-positive staining on histologic section which, by their presence or absence, were found to be predictive for patient outcome. These vascular patterns are now recognized as an independent prognostic variable for both uveal melanoma and cutaneous melanoma (see Chapters 11–14). More recently, this same group of researchers suggested that fluid- and blood-containing channels can develop between nests of expanding uveal melanoma cells through the development of vessel-like channels which are devoid of endothelial cells.

In the review which follows, the contribution of blood vessel pathology to morbidity and mortality will be presented as it pertains to the growth of the primary tumor, local response of the retinal and iris vasculatures, and the retinovascular response to radiation treatment. The role of the vasculature in dissemination, dormancy and metastases will also be presented.

## INTRODUCTION—A TUMOR AND ITS BLOOD VESSELS

A solid tumor is dependent on its blood supply for its oxygen and nutrients. This is true for both primary and secondary tumors and is one of the tenets of tumor biology. Hypotheses generated upon this tenet include the conversion from benign cancer to invasive cancer, the end of dormancy, and ultimately have led to the rational development of anti-angiogenic therapies. Without a functional vasculature, tumor growth cannot proceed beyond the limits of diffusion.[5]

Within the current body of literature pertaining to tumor vascular biology, one particular concept is worth emphasizing. Intra-tumoral vessels are not conventional vessels—they are not entirely similar to developing vessels nor are they entirely similar to mature, quiescent vessels of the adult. The concept of mature and immature vessels is no doubt too simplistic in tumor biology, and gives way to a multiplicity of vessel descriptions. This diversity of intra-tumoral blood vessels has long been appreciated, and it is likely that the many forms of vessels co-exist and interconvert.[5a] Nonetheless, it is surely true that as a tumor grows so too must its vasculature.

In general, the growth of new blood vessels is described as occurring through two major processes, angiogenesis and vasculogenesis. Vasculogenesis, observed predominantly in the developing embryo is the process by which blood vessel precursor cells spontaneously form spatially-distributed blood islands which mature and coalesce to form a vascular plexus. By contrast, angiogenesis is defined as the sprouting or branching of new vessels from an existing vascular bed. This is also well-described in development and additionally in mature processes such as wound healing or reproductive biology.

In the prevailing theory of tumor growth, blood vessels are believed to arise from the local vascular bed and to grow directly into the tumor. This is angiogenesis. It is known that pre-existent vessels at the site of a growing tumor can become incorporated into a tumor with little change in their structural integrity or character. In this case, the vessels appear simply to have been physically engulfed by the growing tumor; their contribution to tumor growth is not clear. However, evidence from studies of fluorescently-labeled tumor cells shows that single tumor cells can migrate to, and proliferate along pre-existent vessels. These small groups of cells then appear to induce vascular sprouting—a process known as 'incipient angiogenesis'.[6–8] By contrast, some new vessels at the tumor–host interface appear to be under local influence of the tumor and tend to be large and dilated, the so-called 'mother vessels'.[8,9] Adjacent host vessels presumably grow or sprout into a tumor upon appropriate signaling. Another hypothesis suggests an initial incorporation of local host blood vessels with their subsequent collapse once the growing tumor develops its own blood supply.[10–12] Studies in which solid tumors are generated by injecting tumor cells of one species into a different-species host, typically human tumor cells in an immunocompromised mouse, also supports the notion that local, murine vessels grow into the expanding tumor.[13–14]

The process of vasculogenesis has also been described within tumors. In one view, vasculogenesis proceeds by the coalescence of intra-tumoral blood islands, with subsequent separation or subdivision of newly-formed blood conduits into smaller channels by a process known as intusseception.[15–19] In a modified extension of this theory, new blood channels arise spontaneously in spatially-distributed areas within a tumor (similar to vasculogenesis), but not through formation of endothelial-lined vessels, but rather through development of short segments of channels lined by tumor cells.[20,21] This process has been termed 'vasculogenic mimicry.' Another process known as 'vascular mosaicism,' describes the process by which potentially metastatic tumor cells contribute directly to the lumen of the vessel wall;[22,23] such migratory tumor cells may contribute up to four percent of the total lumenal surface.

## PRIMARY UVEAL MELANOMA AND ITS BLOOD VESSELS

Consistent with the foregoing discussion, it is not surprising to find that blood vessels within uveal melanoma are distinct from normal, non-pathological vessels. In particular, the vessels of uveal melanoma do not have the round or elliptical cross-sections which typify most blood vessels. Instead, cross-sections are often irregular, with acute angles and concave walls. They appear, by reasonable interpretation, as though they have been compressed by adjacent nests of growing tumor cells. This is a rather remarkable change in vessel morphology considering that blood vessels within uveal melanoma arise anatomically from the choroidal vasculature, a system of large sinusoidal vessels and fine capillaries. This anatomical connection is confirmed by fluorescein angiography showing the 'dual circulation' of choroidal and tumor filling, distinct from that of the overlying retina. It is also worth noting that cutaneous melanoma, a genetically distinct tumor also derived from the melanocyte, has the same tumor vessel architecture as does uveal melanoma. Like uveal melanoma, cutaneous melanoma is characterized by the development of nests of tumor cells with vessels located in the space between the nests.

## INTRA-TUMORAL VESSELS

### VASCULAR DENSITY

Given the importance of blood vessels to tumor growth, it is not surprising that their density has long been suspected to correlate with prognosis. Nonetheless, controversy exists as to whether vascular density is indeed prognostic in uveal melanoma.[24,25] Similarly, some investigations of cutaneous melanoma have shown greater dependency on the phase of blood vessel growth, whether it be radial or vertical, than on measures of vascular density.[26,27]

Part of the discrepancy in using tumor vessel density as a marker of prognosis may lie in tumor sampling and staining techniques. For instance, as vessel density is often non-homogenous throughout the tumor, 'sampling error' could profoundly impact analysis. To this end, some authors advocate measuring vessel density in so-called 'hot-spots' or regions of highest density.[28] The problem is exacerbated by the choice of endothelial cell marker used for analysis. For example, von Willibrand factor (vWF) is found only within discrete Weibel–Palade bodies—as these vesicles may be absent in short segments of vessels, vessel counts may be falsely low. Vessel quantification may be further complicated if some vessels are not lined in their entirety by endothelial cells, as is suggested to occur with vasculogenic mimicry or vascular mosaicism (see below).

## VASCULAR PATTERNS

Within the last decade a second measure of tumor vascularity, its spatial pattern, has been evaluated as a marker of prognosis in uveal melanoma. Histological examination of uveal melanoma by standard H & E light microscopy shows a homogenous, densely cellular tumor with variable pigmentation, little necrosis and little fibrous tissue. However, when viewed by dark field filter with no nuclear counterstain, PAS-positive strands can be visualize coursing in complex patterns throughout the tumor. When described by the two-dimensional patterns they form, these patterns appear to relate to prognosis.[25,29–38]

Histologically, PAS-patterns are a simple concept, but at the cellular or molecular level, they are not. Though originally called 'vascular patterns' it has become evident that PAS positivity relates to the spatial pattern of extracellular matrix—the vessels lie within some, but not all, of these strands. Reciprocally, it does appear to be true that vessels exist only within these strands. So then, by what means do the spatial patterns of PAS-positive staining correlate with the cellular and molecular mechanisms of disease progression? Put differently, how can the two-dimensional spatial pattern of PAS staining determine long-term prognosis and the likelihood of death due to metastatic disease?

This question has been addressed in at least two ways. The first involves identification of specific molecules within the PAS-positive patterns which may be of biological significance. Such analysis has determined that the two-dimensional pattern of laminin staining correlates strongly with PAS positive pattern,[39–41] and more significantly, that the pattern of laminin positivity, particularly the laminin $\gamma$-2 chain, correlates with patient prognosis.[42] This has been demonstrated for both uveal and cutaneous melanoma.[32,43] Each newly identified, potential molecular target must be assessed by retrospective and prospective analysis of enucleated specimens, correlating the immunohistochemistry with long-term clinical outcome. Ongoing studies of this sort hope to identify many such prognosis-related molecules.

The second method by which PAS-positive patterns have been investigated is through multi-gene analysis using micro-array technology.[21] For this type of investigation, the complete repertoire of messenger RNA (mRNA) from tumors with hi-risk or low-risk patterns was determined. When compared, several groups of genes appeared to be differentially expressed. While yielding vast amounts of data, the results of such functional genomics studies can be summarized as follows: tumors with hi-risk PAS positive patterns and poor prognosis were less differentiated and more 'embryonic' in their gene expression. This is consistent with earlier studies suggesting that less differentiated tumors had a relatively poor prognosis. Again, meaningful interpretation requires the analysis of long-term clinical and molecular data.

To complement these studies, Folberg and co-workers observed that uveal melanoma cells grown *in vitro* do not form a continuous sheet as is commonly seen. Rather, cultured melanoma cells tend to grow in 'rows' or 'clusters' of cells reminiscent of the nests they form *in vivo*.[21,44] These patterns develop in the absence of endothelial or other peri-vascular cell types, and suggest that analysis of the tumor cells themselves is useful and valid in the molecular evaluation of tumor angiogenesis.

As a result of these pioneering studies in uveal melanoma, other tumors are now being investigated for their ability to form vascular patterns *in vivo* and *in vitro*.[45,46] Positive correlation between pattern and prognosis now appears in several tumor types, and it is anticipated that as data are generated from these multiple studies, unique and highly-represented molecules will emerge as new therapeutic targets.

## VASCULOGENIC MIMICRY

Observations of the unique cross-sectional shapes of vessels within uveal melanoma suggest that these vessels are constrained by the tumor nests which abut them. It has been proposed that the 'inter-nest space' of both uveal and cutaneous melanoma could be used as potential conduits for fluid or blood.[20,21,47] Such channels are hypothesized to arise in spatially-distributed pattern, independent of local vascular sprouting (hence the term 'vasculogenic') but, unlike most vessels would not be lined by endothelial cells (hence the term 'mimicry'). In the theory of vasculogenic mimicry, vascular channels have an associated PAS-positive matrix and are lined by tumor cells found at the edge of adjacent septae.[20] This hypothesis is significant as it suggests that at least a portion of a tumor's blood or nutrient supply can be delivered in an endothelium-independent manner. This has implications for both the evaluation of intra-tumoral vessels using endothelial cell markers, and also for the development of therapies which target vascular endothelium exclusively. Vaculogenic mimicry has now been assessed in several tumor types.[48,49]

In a little-cited set of papers evaluating the ability of antibodies to penetrate into the parenchyma of subcutaneous melanoma (a proposed method of immunotherapy), Shockley demonstrated that blood components, particularly antibodies and vital dyes could penetrate throughout much of the tumor, most notably by passage between tumor nests.[50,51] This observation is consistent with the continuous passage of fluids from blood vessels into the inter-septal spaces. Recently, a potential junction between the endothelial-lined and non-endothelial-lined systems has been described.[52]

Nonetheless, significant controversy exists.[53,54] Amongst several arguments presented, some authors suggest that the reported absence of endothelial cells along vascular channels is artifactuous, and likewise that red blood cells noted in the channels are due to dissemination during histological preparation. Nonetheless, authors who originally challenged the concept of vasculogenic mimicry,[22] subsequently demonstrated that fluorescently-tagged tumor cells can contribute directly to the vessel wall,[22] presumably when migrating into the blood stream. They have termed this process 'vascular mosaicism.' Previous authors have also suggested the presence of tumor-cell lined 'vessels.'[55,56]

Similar to the *in vivo* work describing vascular patterns, *in vitro* studies of vasculogenic mimicry demonstrate that fluids can percolate around clusters of melanoma cells grown in culture, being largely excluded from the centre of the nest.[20,44] Micro-array analysis of specimens has suggested that tumor cells capable of forming vascular channels *in vivo* and *in vitro* are considerably de-differentiated and express an embryonic-like phenotype.[57–61]

In addition, 'conventional' angiogenic genes can in some cases be found to be expressed by tumor cells themselves.[22,62] Examples include Tie-2 and VE-cadherin, phosphorylated Eck/EphA2, and again, laminin.[63–67] Similar studies in diverse tumors now support the embryonic-like, and/or angiogenic-like characteristic of tumor cells which may be able to contribute directly to the tumor wall.[45]

## MOLECULAR MEDIATORS OF INTRA-TUMORAL VESSEL GROWTH

Despite the unique properties of some vessels within uveal melanoma, growth of most intra-tumoral vessels is believed to be regulated by a group of genes and proteins common to most forms of angiogenesis. These include the pro-angiogenic cytokines and their receptors, the anti-angiogenic molecules, and other proteins which modify cell–cell and cell–matrix interaction.

The two best described pro-angiogenic molecules are vascular endothelial growth factor (VEGF) and basic fibroblast growth factor (bFGF). Both these molecules lead to endothelial cell proliferation, migration and capillary tube formation both *in vivo* and *in vitro*. VEGF is also a potent vasopermeability factor often found at sites of vascular leakage.[68] bFGF, in addition to being a pro-angiogenic molecule, is a well-described autocrine/paracrine stimulus for proliferation of cutaneous tumor cells.[69–71] bFGF has recently been described in uveal melanoma but its role in autonomous cell proliferation is not described.[72] The effects of VEGF and bFGF are reported to be synergistic in some systems.[73,74]

By comparison with the majority of tumors, VEGF appears to play only a small role in the growth of primary uveal melanoma. In many immunohistochemical and *in situ* hybridization studies it is virtually undetectable,[75,76] and when present, it is found most closely associated with areas of fibrosis or necrosis, both rare findings in uveal melanoma.[72,77] By contrast, VEGF is more frequently described in cultured primary melanoma or melanoma cell lines. This may of course reflect the *in vitro* selection pressures rather than expression patterns found in the tumors *in vivo*.[78–86] Nonetheless, primary uveal melanoma cells derived from enucleated human specimens can support proliferation of primary endothelial cells or endothelial cell lines.[72]

Other angiogenic cytokines/receptors investigated in uveal melanoma include EGF, PDGF and IL-8.[87,88] Expression of these factors is highly variability in tumor lines and primary tumors,[89] however their expression can correlate with metastases or aggressivity in *in vivo* and *in vitro* models.VEGF-C, a marker of the lymphatic system has also been detected in uveal melanoma despite the absence of lymphatic vessels.[90]

Components of the extracellular matrix which may be conducive for vessel formation, and potentially pro-angiogenic cells which move from the circulation into the peri-vascular mesenchyme have also been investigated. These include collagen VI, laminin, fibronection and others.[67,91–95] In addition, macrophages are known to provide pro-angiogenic molecules and can be found in high numbers in uveal melanoma.[96]

Considerable interest has also focused on the role of the integrin molecules in the growth and angiogenesis of cutaneous and uveal melanoma.[97] The integrins are a large family of heterodimeric transmembrane molecules that transmit signals between cells or between a cell and its extra-cellular matrix. Signaling functions include cell adhesion, cell motility, cell survival (particularly during relative anchorage-independent processes such as cell migration),[98,99] and in some cases the provision of unique signals for parallel receptor pathways.[100]

The integrin molecules alphaVbeta3 and alphaVbeta5 were originally described in melanoma, expressed by the tumor cells themselves. These molecules are also found in endothelial cells at the advancing front of newly forming vessels. Numerous studies have determined that the integrin profiles are distinct between uveal and cutaneous melanoma.[91,101,102] Nonetheless, in both cases, numerous endothelial cell and tumor cell functions appear to be mediated through integrin ligation.[13,103,104] Molecules such as fibronectin, vitronection, and laminin serve as ligands for the integrin molecules,[65–67] and as previously discussed, the pattern or distribution of extracellular matrix is significant to melanoma growth and patient prognosis. Hence, the integrin molecules expressed by either tumor or endothelial cells could mediate signaling using laminin or other molecules of the extra-cellular matrix. Overall, the role of specific integrins in determining tumor aggressiveness or vascular growth and patterning is complex.[94,91,105]

Recent studies have focused on the integrin molecules other than avb3 or avb5, particularly $\alpha5\beta1$, $\alpha1\beta1$, $\alpha2\beta1$ and $\alpha6\beta1$, and $\alpha4$.[94,106,107] Changes in $\alpha6\beta1$ and $\alpha4$ may correlate with the aggressive phenotype.[106,108] $\alpha5\beta1$ is also believed to characterize the invasive phenotype.[106]

Metalloproteinases (MMPs) have been described in association with expanding tumors, both in experimental systems and in human samples.[109–113] MMPs are an extensive group of divalent-cation-dependent proteases whose function include, among other things, degradation of the extracellular matrix. These molecules are tightly regulated in terms of their activation, inactivation, and their spatial distribution. The MMPs can be found in association with the advancing edge of newly formed vessels and and so may serve as a 'diamond tip' for extension of growing vessels through the extra-cellular matrix.

Numerous MMPs have been assessed in uveal melanoma. MMP-2 and MMP-9, the most extensively studied, are found in human and experimental melanoma and are correlated with metastatic potential.[85,114–116] Endogenous inhibitors of the MMPs include the tissue inhibitor of metalloproteinase (TIMP) molecules, and these are also found in uveal melanoma.[107,115] Evidence suggests that patients with elevated levels of TIMP-1 and -2 may have a better prognosis than those without.[115] Genetic analysis suggests that abnormalities of TIMP-3 may be characteristic of aggressive uveal melanoma.[116a,b]

Recent studies[14a] using a xenograft model of human cutaneous melanoma grown subcutaneously in a mouse, have shown that MMP-9 is localized to the stroma in advance of the invasive front and also along the intra-tumoral vessels. Species-specific immunohistochemistry demonstrates that the intra-tumor vessels are derived exclusively from the murine host—proteolytic activity may therefore be important not only as the tumor invades the host, but also as the host vessels 'invade' the tumor.

The MMPs also function to cleave and 'unmask' hidden or cryptic molecules contained within larger molecules. Some of these smaller molecules provide regulatory, often negative, signals for cell growth.[117–124] For example, endostatin, is a short segment of collagen XVIII derived through proteolytic cleavage; this molecule is known to down-regulate angiogenesis. Similarly, angiostatin is a proteolytic cleavage product of plasminogen, and also functions as an anti-angiogenic molecule. Angiostatin and endostatin can be produced by a variety of primary and metastatic tumors, and their production by primary tumors is hypothesized in some cases to reduce growth of its metastases.[123,125–127] Inhibition of tumor growth in the cutaneous B16 cell line correlates with gene dosage of exogenously-expressed angiostatin.[128]

Other studies have shown that primary uveal melanoma and cultured melanoma cell lines are capable of producing angiostatin.[88,129,130] It therefore follows that surgical removal of a primary uveal melanoma which is producing angiostatin could lead to accelerated metastatic disease. The relevance of this observation to patient survival is not known as angiostatin may be one of a mix of pro- and anti-angiogenic molecules expressed by the primary tumor, and local production within the eye may be incapable of achieving biological concentrations at remote sites.

Clinical studies, particularly the natural history arm of each of the three major reports of the COMS,[131–133] have failed to indicate any survival advantage of leaving a primary uveal melanoma in place, although significant debate exists.[136,183] This theory was originally suggested by Dr Zimmerman in 1978.[134–136] Based on current investigation, it may be that the local production of angiostatin by primary uveal melanoma could be amongst the factors contributing to the final outcome.

## VASCULAR CHANGES WITHIN EYES HARBOURING UVEAL MELANOMA

Eyes harbouring uveal melanoma, whether treated or untreated, are subject to perturbations of the intrinsic vasculature. In particular the retinal vasculature may become highly permeable, while the retina or iris may undergo frank neovascularization.

## INCREASED VASCULAR PERMEABILITY

Uveal melanoma can be accompanied by retinal detachments with significant subretinal fluid.[137] The presence of retinal detachment is positively correlated with poor outcome in some studies but not all.[137–140] At least one study found that retinal detachment was not predictive of survival after adjusting for tumor size and microvascular patterns.[141]

Even in the absence of retinal detachment, vascular permeability may be increased in the presence of treated or non-treated uveal melanoma. Clinical examination may reveal aqueous flare, while non-invasive measures, including fluorophotometry and tyndallography using the laser-flare meter, can quantify these changes.[142–148] Autoreflectivity of the cornea may also increase in the presence of uveal melanoma, presumably due to accumulation of serum proteins within this structure.[149]

Given that some pro-angiogenic molecules, most notably VEGF, are potent vasopermeability factors,[68] it is not unreasonable to postulate that retinal detachments reflect their local production. VEGF is found elevated in ocular fluids in the presence of uveal melanoma and other tumors.[76,150–153] This is significant because, as described above, very few uveal melanoma actually express VEGF[75]—the source is therefore not fully understood. Theories include the production of VEGF in the outer, hypoxic retina in the presence of retinal detachment. In the absence of detachment, additional explanations include the secondary induction of VEGF in ocular structures such as the retina or iris by basic fibroblast growth factor (bFGF) secreted by the tumor,[72–74,154] the presence of other growth factors,[130,155] and in some cases, by radiation treatment.

Immunohistochemical studies of extravasated albumin show perturbation of the blood-ocular-barrier in the presence of ocular tumors such as retinoblastoma, and significantly have shown that VEGF can be upregulated in the retina at sites remote from the tumor.[156]

The presence of VEGF itself in aqueous fluid of tumor-bearing eye was found to correlate with long-term survival in at least one study,[156a] although the presence of VEGF within the tumor per se, did not.[77]

## INTRA-OCULAR ANGIOGENESIS IN THE PRESENCE OF UVEAL MELANOMA

In 1979, Dr Folkman used aqueous fluid from eyes harbouring ocular tumors to induce blood vessel growth on the chick chorioallantoic membrane. These studies which pre-dated molecular characterization of most of the known pro-angiogenic molecules, clearly demonstrate that ocular fluids from tumor-bearing eyes are pro-angiogenic.

Retinal vessels over the tumor or remote from the tumor may proliferate; rarely choroidal neovascularization has also been reported.[140,157–159] Neovascularization of the iris (NVI) and neovascular glaucoma (NVG) are relatively common and feared complications of both treated and untreated uveal melanoma.[160] Factors which contribute to NVI include large tumor size, presence of retinal detachment, and others.[28,161,162] Many authors note correlation between irradiation and neovascularization (discussed below). VEGF alone is known to induce NVI[163] and threshold levels for NVI in human disease have been determined.[163a]

In addition to the release of pro-angiogenic molecules, some tumors may produce anti-angiogenic agents such as angiostatin as mentioned above. It is also noteworthy that one of the most potent anti-angiogeneic molecules, pigment epithelium derived factor (PEDF), was identified in eyes harbouring retinoblastoma.[164] PEDF concentrations are inversely related to VEGF concentrations in some proliferative vasculopathies[165] but have not yet been reported in uveal melanoma.

## RADIATION-INDUCED VASCULOPATHY

Ophthalmologists have long recognized that local radiation treatment of ocular tumors leads to predictable changes in the retinal vasculature. Visual loss is the ultimate outcome, despite 'successful' local treatment of the tumor. This radiation-induced vasculopathy is characterized by increased vascular permeability, intraretinal haemorrhage, development of microaneurysms, capillary drop-out and frank neovascularization.[28,160,166–169] Pathological analysis of enucleated specimens demonstrates that the endothelial cell is the preferential target of radiation-induced damage.[170]

Radiation therapy of uveal melanoma is usually either by plaque (brachytherapy) or external beam radiation. Early external beam therapies were limited to the proton beam; today the highly focused gamma-knife is also used. Proton beam therapies were frequently complicated by retinal vasculopathy and anterior segment neovascularization.[167–169,171–177] Unfortunately, recent studies of gamma knife radiation treatment also identify a high rate of neovascular glaucoma, in one study as high as 47%.[178–180]

By contrast to external beam irradiation, plaque therapy delivers energy directly to the tumor via the sclera and choroid while minimizing the amount of radiation which must pass through remote ocular structures via multi-beam treatment.[181,182] Many studies using ruthenium, iodine-125 or palladium-103 plaques appear to have lower rates of neovascularization than series using external beam.[28,166,169,183–192] Tumor location, and hence location of the plaque also determines the type and extent of damage.[166,193,194] Several reviews compare tumor and treatment variables against outcome.[28,195] Combination of transpupillary thermotherapy with radiation suggest that lower radiation doses may be given with resultant lower rates of neovascularization.[196,197] Transpupillary thermotherapy has been associated with vascular occlusion but with little neovascularization.[198]

Increased vascular permeability is associated with radiation therapy, and the onset of radiation retinopathy or iris neovacularization correlate with increased intra-ocular protein, as determined by the laser-flare meter.[144] Also, though intraocular VEGF concentrations may be elevated in the presence of uveal melanoma with or without retinal detachment, the highest concentrations detected in enucleated human eyes were those eyes which had received radiation treatment.[153]

Some clinicians will avoid radiation therapy for eyes with clinically-detectable flare due to a perceived high risk of NVI [J Hungerford, personal communication].

## THE VASCULATURE AND METASTATIC UVEAL MELANOMA

### INTRAVASATION/EXTRAVASATION

For metastases to occur it is generally believed that tumor cells must become separated from their neighbouring cells, penetrate through extracellular matrix and basement membrane, enter a nearby vessel, move through the systemic circulation to a new location, and then reverse this process to reside in a peri-vascular location.

The movement of tumor cells out of a primary tumor mass requires a decrease in cohesive signaling[95] and cell migration. It is known that serine/threonine proteases such as plasminogen activator-1, the MMPs, and their inhibitors are present within uveal melanoma, and that these may correlate with metastatic capability, presumably by altering cell adhesion and migration.[106,107,199–202] Integrin expression further determines cell motility and survival.[21,93] It is also known that aggressive uveal melanoma cells with an interconverted phenotype are highly mobile and more likely to metastasize.[60,203]

Numerous investigators have utilized *in vitro* systems to analyse the metastatic potential of uveal melanoma. The Boyden chamber, or modified versions of this chamber, can mimic chemotaxis, cell migration or cell extravasation.[204] Some investigators utilize a synthetic basement membrane such as Matrigel through which tumor cells must migrate, while others additionally add a monolayer of endothelial cells to more closely approximate the barrier presented to a tumor cell by a blood vessel wall.[141,205,206] Though a useful model, it is important to note that *in vitro* findings of this sort are likely to reflect the selective pressures on the cells at the time of assay and may or may not reflect their response *in vivo*.[107]

By contrast, and distinct from intra-lumenal extravasation, it appears that uveal melanoma cells exiting the eye via intra-scleral canals can do so by moving laterally along the external side of the vessels. This abluminal migration of cells is described experimentally[41,207,208] and is observed by clinical pathologists. Systemic dissemination of uveal melanoma may thus arise not only by direct invasion into the lumen, but also after tumor cell movement along the abluminal surface of the scleral vessels and entery into the orbital space. In a rodent model of uveal melanoma it is known that the pattern of distant metastases depends on whether the tumor cells are injected exclusively into the sub-retinal space with no breach of the conjunctiva or whether they are injected through conjunctiva[209,210]—it is therefore presumed that the origin of dissemination, whether intra-ocular or extra-ocular, contributes to the pattern of remote metastases.

### SYSTEMIC CIRCULATION OF TUMOR CELLS

After extravasation, uveal melanoma cells circulate via the systemic blood stream and can be detected using various techniques. Surface markers of the melanocyte lineage can be detected using immunocytochemical techniques, while polymerase chain reaction (PCR) can be used to identify cells expressing mRNA hypothetically unique to these cells. Despite early success,[211] clinicians and investigators have not reliably demonstrated circulating melanoma cells by PCR from patients with known metastatic disease nor in the peri-operative period, a time when tumor cells may be shed from the dissected tumor.[212] Highly sensitive PCR techniques have turned out to be difficult to perform and even more difficult to perform uniformly between laboratories.[213,214] In studies of cutaneous melanoma, the use of two melanoma-associated markers and PCR led to higher frequencies of detection, however, the most sensitive combination of markers was also less specific.[215] In addition, though circulating tumor cells can be detected within peripheral blood, their detection does not necessarily correlate with prognosis.[216] On a strictly theoretical basis, melanoma cells which are found in the blood are not appropriately seated to give rise to secondary tumors in tissue parenchyma. By contrast, a single cell sequestered from the circulation into the appropriate cellular environment, could.

The lymphatic system does not appear to be involved in the dissemination of uveal melanoma. Lymph node involvement is relatively uncommon and is usually associated with extensive conjunctival extension; the eye itself is known to be devoid of lymphatics. The role of the lymphatic system in metastases in tumors other than uveal melanoma is currently an active area of investigation,[217–219] and it is known that unique forms of VEGF and its receptors characterize lymphatic tissue.[220] Perhaps surprisingly, VEGF-C and its receptor, flt-4, markers of the lymphatic system, are found in uveal melanoma in the absence of lymphatic vessels per se.[90]

And finally, in order to generate a metastatic foci, circulating tumor cells must exit the circulation and enter a suitable site. Once detained in the vessels of the target tissue, the intrinsic motility of tumor cells is once again presumably important in the process of tissue invasion

## LIVER METASTASES

Metastatic uveal melanoma demonstrates a strong preference for the liver; up to 80% of patients present with metastases to this organ.[221] Shorter survival times are noted in association with metastatic disease to the liver as apposed to the lung.[222,223]

Although the mechanism by which tumor cells preferentially relocate to a particular organ is not understood, it is generally accepted that the new environment must provide appropriate signals for tumor cell adhesion, survival and proliferation.[224,225] The local environment must not only support growth of the tumor, but also provide its blood supply. It is important to note that subclinical deposition of tumor cells may occur at multiple sites in the body but remain undetected if they cannot enlarge.

It is known that melanoma cell lines expressing epidermal growth factor (EGF) receptors on their surface metastasize to the liver preferentially.[89,226,227] In a retrospective study of archived primary human tumors IGF-1 was also found elevated in more metastatic tumors than in non-metastatic tumors. Kaplan-Meir analysis showed a significant difference in patient survival dependent on IGF-1 expression.[228] Spread to liver can also be blocked through anti-ganglioside antibodies.[229]

Amongst the best-characterized liver-derived growth factors is hepatocyte growth factor (HGF). Its receptor, c-met is found on uveal melanoma cells and their level of expression correlates significantly the metastatic potential of.[60] It appears that HGF can induce the co-expression of both vimentin and keratin intermediate filaments in uveal melanoma cells. These cells with the interconverted phenotype are highly motile and form metastases readily.[60] In studies of vasculogenic mimicry, the interconverted phenotype is highly correlated with *in vivo* and *in vitro* formation of vascular patterns; these in turn relate to death due to metastasis.[58,230,231]

Although little is known regarding angiogenesis within metastatic uveal melanoma, the role of angiogenesis in the growth of the metastases is in general increasing.[232,233] In an experimental model of cutaneous melanoma metastatic to the brain, increased transgene expression of VEGF was associated with increased intra- and peri-tumoral vessel diameter, increased permeability and metastases.[80] These tumors enlarged faster than the equivalent low-VEGF tumors and had an area of central necrosis.[234] In other studies, neither exogenous provision or VEGF, nor anti-sense reduction in VEGF transcripts altered proliferation rates of the tumors.[83]

Once growth is initiated within the liver, life-expectancies are short. Unlike metastatic cutaneous melanoma which often presents with jaundice and other signs of obstructive liver disease, this is generally not observed in uveal melanoma. Rather, cellular dysfunction is biochemically detected. Though the precise mechanism by which metastatic melanoma causes liver dysfunction and death is not known, evidence suggests that melanoma cells can directly induce apoptosis of hepatocytes through the Fas cell-death pathway.[231]

## DORMANCY

Metastatic uveal melanoma can be characterized by protracted periods of dormancy. This is similar to breast carcinoma, and despite efforts in both these and other fields of investigation, little is known regarding the process of dormancy or its cessation. Although the majority of metastatic uveal melanoma are detected within the first three years following detection of the primary tumor, some micrometastases persist for extended periods and are detected decades later.

Two general concepts guide our current understanding of tumor dormancy. The first suggests that tumor growth, limited in size by the peri-vascular diffusion of oxygen and nutrients, reflects a balance between proliferative and apoptotic signaling in the tumor cells per se.[5] An alteration in this balance would determine secondary tumor growth. The second theory suggests that a dormant tumor mass will remain quiescent until angiogenesis is initiated. This latter theory has led to the suggestion of an 'angiogenic switch.'[2–4,235–241] This 'switching' involves simultaneous up- and down-regulation of pro- and anti-angiogenic molecules respectively.

And finally, as introduced earlier, some primary tumors are known to produce anti-angiogenic molecules which may suppress growth at secondary sites.[88,129,242] The extent to which this mechanism plays a role in the regulation of uveal melanoma dormancy is not yet known.

## ANTI-ANGIOGENIC THERAPIES

In the last decade new therapies directed against a tumor's blood supply have been developed. It is hypothesized that loss of a blood supply will destroy a tumor. Numerous anti-angiogenic therapies have been developed, many are in pre-clinical trial, and some are already in clinical use. Some of the targets of anti-angiogenesic therapies include inhibition of the pro-angiogenic growth factors and their receptors, up-regulation of anti-angiogenic molecules, and modulation of related molecules such as the integrins and proteases. Endothelial cell migration, vessel assembly and vessel stability are amongst the targeted cellular processes. New therapies include pharmacological compounds directed against targets of the vasculature, and gene therapies delivered by a variety of means. For reviews of anti-angiogenesis therapies in the treatment of cancer see refs.[109,118,243–264]

It is also apparent that some traditional chemotherapeutic agents also act by reducing angiogenesis. In particular, when some compounds are provided repeatedly at low dose, a technique known as metronomic dosing, some agents take on anti-angiogenic properties.[265–267] Many clinicians and scientists now believe that combinations of anti-angiogenic agents with standard chemotherapeutic drugs will provide much greater cancer control.[258,268–271] At present the choice of which drug combinations will be efficacious is not known.

In a broader context, it must be pointed out that there are currently few clinical measures available to determine whether anti-angiogenesis therapy is effective. The single best measure currently in use is the systemic measurement of plasma levels of circulating VEGF. This is currently in use for highly vascular tumors such as haemangiomas or large bulky tumors secreting high concentrations of cytokines. Large reductions in tumor volume correlate with decreased circulating levels.

It is however now appreciated that some cancers can survive with very low oxygen levels. Clinical studies have confirmed that tumors can adapt to conditions of low oxygen delivery and such resistance to hypoxia can be selected for through anti-angiogenic therapies.[272,273] This potential for anti-angiogenic resistance could be offset by carefully-selected combination therapies.

## SUMMARY AND CONCLUSIONS

Uveal melanoma is a rare tumor with a poor prognosis. Growth of both primary and secondary uveal melanoma requires an imbalance of cellular proliferation over apoptosis and the development of a functional vasculature. The characteristics of this vasculature, both its pattern and possibly its density, are independent prognostic variables with impact on metastases and patient survival.

Abnormal blood vessels play a vital role in primary tumor growth and in the visual morbidity within the eye. Tumor-related vascular changes can occur locally within the eye in the presence of uveal melanoma, and can be exacerbated with radiation treatment. The systemic vasculature permits systemic dissemination of melanoma cells, while new vessels at remote sites permit secondary tumors to grow to clinical significance. Whether the local production of pro- and anti-angiogenic factors by the primary tumor can modify the growth of the secondary tumor remains undetermined.

As with all tumors, the vasculature of uveal melanoma may be a target for anti-angiogenic therapy. Because sustained growth of a tumor requires the simultaneous and sustained growth of its vasculature, combined therapies designed to target both the endothelial and tumor-cell compartments may ultimately provide better control than current regimens.

And finally, it is remarkable that studies of angiogenesis in uveal melanoma, a rare ophthalmic tumor, have had significant impact on the study of highly-prevalent tumors such as cutaneous melanoma and breast carcinoma. The observations of vascular patterns and vascular mimicry, the protracted periods of dormancy and the strict haemotogenous spread, make studies of uveal melanoma relevant for all patients with cancer. Ongoing study will no doubt bring better outcomes for patients with this deadly disease.

## REFERENCES


1. Folkman J. Angiogenesis in cancer, vascular, rheumatoid and other disease. *Nat Med.* 1995;1:27–31.
2. Arbiser JL, Moses MA, Fernandez CA, Ghiso N, Cao Y, Klauber N, Frank D, Brownlee M, Flynn E, Parangi S, Byers HR, Folkman J. Oncogenic H-ras stimulates tumor angiogenesis by two distinct pathways. *Proc Natl Acad Sci USA* 1997;94: 861–866.
3. Hanahan D, Christofori G, Naik P, Arbeit J. Transgenic mouse models of tumor angiogenesis: the angiogenic switch, its molecular controls, and prospects for preclinical therapeutic models. *Eur J Cancer.* 1996;32A:2386–2393.
4. Hanahan D, Folkman J. Patterns and emerging mechanisms of the angiogenic switch during tumorigenesis. *Cell.* 1996;86:353–364.
5. Holmgren L, O'Reilly MS, Folkman J. Dormancy of micrometastases: balanced proliferation and apoptosis in the presence of angiogenesis suppression. *Nat Med.* 1995;1:149–153.

5a. Warren BA. The vascular morphology of tumors. In: Person HI, ed. *Tumor Blood Circulation: Angiogenesis, Vascular Morphology and Blood Flow of Experimental and Human Tumors.* Boca Raton: CRC Press, 1979; 1–48.

6. Folkman J. Incipient angiogenesis. *J Natl Cancer Inst.* 2000;92:94–95.
7. Li CY, Shan S, Cao Y, Dewhirst MW. Role of incipient angiogenesis in cancer metastasis. *Cancer Metastasis Rev.* 2000;19:7–11.
8. Ferrara N. Vascular endothelial growth factor and the regulation of angiogenesis. Recent Prog Horm Res 2000;55:15–35; discussion 35–16.
9. Borgstrom P, Gold DP, Hillan KJ, Ferrara N. Importance of VEGF for breast cancer angiogenesis in vivo: implications from intravital microscopy of combination treatments with an anti-VEGF neutralizing monoclonal antibody and doxorubicin. *Anticancer Res.* 1999;19:4203–4214.
10. Zagzag D, Amirnovin R, Greco MA, Yee H, Holash J, Wiegand SJ, Zabski S, Yançopoulos GD, Grumet M. Vascular apoptosis and involution in gliomas precede neovascularization: a novel concept for glioma growth and angiogenesis. *Lab Invest.* 2000;80:837–849.
11. Zagzag D, Hooper A, Friedlander DR, Chan W, Holash J, Wiegand SJ, Yancopoulos GD, Grumet M. In situ expression of angiopoietins in astrocytomas identifies angiopoietin-2 as an early marker of tumor angiogenesis. *Exp Neurol.* 1999;159:391–400.

12. Holash J, Wiegand SJ, Yancopoulos GD. New model of tumor angiogenesis: dynamic balance between vessel regression and growth mediated by angiopoietins and VEGF. *Oncogene.* 1999;18:5356–5362.
13. Felding-Habermann B, Mueller BM, Romerdahl CA, Cheresh DA. Involvement of integrin alpha V gene expression in human melanoma tumorigenicity. *J Clin Invest.* 1992;89:2018–2022.
14. Gouon V, Tucker GC, Kraus-Berthier L, Atassi G, Kieffer N. Up-regulated expression of the beta3 integrin and the 92-kDa gelatinase in human HT-144 melanoma cell tumors grown in nude mice. *Int J Cancer.* 1996;68:650–662.
14a. Boyd SR, Kinder K, Friedlander M. Melanoma: molecular signalling at the tumour–vessel interface. *Assoc Res Vision Ophthalmol.* 2002; Abstract 1828.
15. Ribatti D, Nico B, Vacca A, Roncali L, Burri PH, Djonov V. Chorioallantoic membrane capillary bed: a useful target for studying angiogenesis and anti-angiogenesis in vivo. *Anat Rec.* 2001;264:317–324.
16. Patan S, Munn LL, Jain RK. Intussusceptive microvascular growth in a human colon adenocarcinoma xenograft: a novel mechanism of tumor angiogenesis. *Microvasc Res.* 1996;51:260–272.
17. Schlatter P, Konig MF, Karlsson LM, Burri PH. Quantitative study of intussusceptive capillary growth in the chorioallantoic membrane (CAM) of the chicken embryo. *Microvasc Res.* 1997;54:65–73.
18. Patan S. TIE1 and TIE2 receptor tyrosine kinases inversely regulate embryonic angiogenesis by the mechanism of intussusceptive microvascular growth. *Microvasc Res.* 1998;56:1–21.
19. Djonov V, Schmid M, Tschanz SA, Burri PH. Intussusceptive angiogenesis: its role in embryonic vascular network formation. *Circ Res.* 2000;86:286–292.
20. Folberg R, Hendrix MJ, Maniotis AJ. Vasculogenic mimicry and tumor angiogenesis. *Am J Pathol.* 2000;156:361–381.
21. Maniotis AJ, Folberg R, Hess A, Seftor EA, Gardner LM, Pe'er J, Trent JM, Meltzer PS, Hendrix MJ. Vascular channel formation by human melanoma cells in vivo and in vitro: vasculogenic mimicry. *Am J Pathol.* 1999;155:739–752.
22. Chang YS, di Tomaso E, McDonald DM, Jones R, Jain RK, Munn LL. Mosaic blood vessels in tumors: frequency of cancer cells in contact with flowing blood. *Proc Natl Acad Sci USA.* 2000;97:14608–14613.
23. Folkman J. Can mosaic tumor vessels facilitate molecular diagnosis of cancer? *Proc Natl Acad Sci USA.* 2001;98:398–400.
24. Foss AJ, Alexander RA, Jefferies LW, Hungerford JL, Harris AL, Lightman S. Microvessel count predicts survival in uveal melanoma. *Cancer Res.* 1996;56: 2900–2903.
25. Lane AM, Egan KM, Yang J, Saornil MA, Alroy J, Albert D, Gragoudas ES. An evaluation of tumor vascularity as a prognostic indicator in uveal melanoma. *Melanoma Res.* 1997;7:237–242.
26. Barnhill RL, Levy MA. Regressing thin cutaneous malignant melanomas ($\leq 1.0$ mm) are associated with angiogenesis. *Am J Pathol.* 1993;143: 99–104.
27. Barnhill RL, Fandrey K, Levy MA, Mihm MC, Jr., Hyman B. Angiogenesis and tumor progression of melanoma. Quantification of vascularity in melanocytic nevi and cutaneous malignant melanoma. *Lab Invest.* 1992;67:331–337.
28. Foss AJ, Alexander RA, Hungerford JL, Harris AL, Cree IA, Lightman S. Reassessment of the PAS patterns in uveal melanoma. *Br J Ophthalmol.* 1997;81:240–246; discussion 247–248.

29. Folberg R, Rummelt V, Parys-Van Ginderdeuren R, Hwang T, Woolson RF, Pe'er J, Gruman LM. The prognostic value of tumor blood vessel morphology in primary uveal melanoma. *Ophthalmology.* 1993;100:1389–1398.
30. MäkitieT, Summanen P, Tarkkanen A, Kivelä T. Microvascular density in predicting survival of patients with choroidal and ciliary body melanoma. *Invest Ophthalmol Vis Sci.* 1999;40:2471–2480.
31. Mäkitie T, Summanen P, Tarkkanen A, Kivelä T. Microvascular loops and networks as prognostic indicators in choroidal and ciliary body melanomas. *J Natl Cancer Inst.* 1999;91:359–367.
32. Warso MA, Maniotis AJ, Chen X, Majumdar D, Patel MK, Shilkaitis A, Gupta TK, Folberg R. Prognostic significance of periodic acid-Schiff-positive patterns in primary cutaneous melanoma. *Clin Cancer Res.* 2001;7:473–477.
33. McLean IW, Keefe KS, Burnier MN. Uveal melanoma. Comparison of the prognostic value of fibrovascular loops, mean of the ten largest nucleoli, cell type, and tumor size. *Ophthalmology.* 1997;104:777–780.
34. Rummelt V, Folberg R, Rummelt C, Gruman LM, Hwang T, Woolson RF, Yi H, Naumann GO. Microcirculation architecture of melanocytic nevi and malignant melanomas of the ciliary body and choroid. A comparative histopathologic and ultrastructural study. *Ophthalmology.* 1994;101:718–727.
35. Rummelt V, Gardner LM, Folberg R, Beck S, Knosp B, Moninger TO, Moore KC. Three-dimensional relationships between tumor cells and microcirculation with double cyanine immunolabeling, laser scanning confocal microscopy, and computer-assisted reconstruction: an alternative to cast corrosion preparations. *J Histochem Cytochem.* 1994;42:681–686.
36. Folberg R, Pe'er J, Gruman LM, Woolson RF, Jeng G, Montague PR, Moninger TO, Yi H, Moore KC. The morphologic characteristics of tumor blood vessels as a marker of tumor progression in primary human uveal melanoma: a matched case-control study. *Hum Pathol.* 1992;23:1298–1305.
37. Sakamoto T, Sakamoto M, Yoshikawa H, Hata Y, Ishibashi T, Ohnishi Y, Inomata H. Histologic findings and prognosis of uveal malignant melanoma in japanese patients. *Am J Ophthalmol.* 1996;121:276–283.
38. Singh AD, Shields CL, Shields JA. Prognostic factors in uveal melanoma. *Melanoma Res.* 2001;11:255–263.
39. Kramer RH, Vu MP, Cheng YF, Ramos DM, Timpl R, Waleh N. Laminin-binding integrin alpha 7 beta 1: functional characterization and expression in normal and malignant melanocytes. *Cell Regul.* 1991;2:805–817.
40. Ramos DM, Cheng YF, Kramer RH. Role of laminin-binding integrin in the invasion of basement membrane matrices by fibrosarcoma cells. *Invasion Metastasis* 1991;11:125–138.
41. Lugassy C, Shahsafaei A, Bonitz P, Busam KJ, Barnhill RL. Tumor microvessels in melanoma express the beta-2 chain of laminin. Implications for melanoma metastasis. *J Cutan Pathol.* 1999;26:222–226.
42. Rummelt V, Mehaffey MG, Campbell RJ, Pe'er J, Bentler SE, Woolson RF, Naumann GO, Folberg R. Microcirculation architecture of metastases from primary ciliary body and choroidal melanomas. *Am J Ophthalmol.* 1998;126:303–305.
43. Thies A, Mangold U, Moll I, Schumacher U. PAS-positive loops and networks as a prognostic indicator in cutaneous malignant melanoma. *J Pathol.* 2001;195:537–542.
44. Chowers I, Folberg R, Livni N, Pe'er J. Comparison of microcirculation patterns and MIB-1 immunoreactivity in iris and posterior uveal melanoma. *Ophthalmology.* 2001;108:367–371.

45. Sood AK, Fletcher MS, Hendrix MJ. The embryonic-like properties of aggressive human tumor cells(1). *J Soc Gynecol Investig*. 2002;9:2–9.
46. Krishnamurthy S, Desai S.Vascular patterns as an aid to cytodiagnosis in fine needle aspiration. *Acta Cytol*. 2001;45:899–901.
47. Folberg R, Chen X, Boldt HC, Pe'er J, Brown CK, Woolson RF, Maniotis AJ. Microcirculation patterns other than loops and networks in choroidal and ciliary body melanomas. *Ophthalmology*. 2001;108:996–1001.
48. Sood AK, Seftor EA, Fletcher MS, Gardner LM, Heidger PM, Buller RE, Seftor RE, Hendrix MJ. Molecular determinants of ovarian cancer plasticity. *Am J Pathol*. 2001;158:1279–1288.
49. Shirakawa K, Tsuda H, Heike Y, Kato K, Asada R, Inomata M, Sasaki H, Kasumi F, Yoshimoto M, Iwanaga T, Konishi F, Terada M, Wakasugi H. Absence of endothelial cells, central necrosis, and fibrosis are associated with aggressive inflammatory breast cancer. *Cancer Res*. 2001;61:445–451.
50. Shockley TR, Lin K, Nagy JA, Tompkins RG, Yarmush ML, Dvorak HF. Spatial distribution of tumor-specific monoclonal antibodies in human melanoma xenografts. *Cancer Res*. 1992;52:367–376.
51. Shockley TR, Lin K, Sung C, Nagy JA, Tompkins RG, Dedrick RL, Dvorak HF, Yarmush ML. A quantitative analysis of tumor specific monoclonal antibody uptake by human melanoma xenografts: effects of antibody immunological properties and tumor antigen expression levels. *Cancer Res*. 1992;52:357–366.
52. Shirakawa K, Kobayashi H, Heike Y, Kawamoto S, Brechbiel MW, Kasumi F, Iwanaga T, Konishi F, Terada M, Wakasugi H. Hemodynamics in vasculogenic mimicry and angiogenesis of inflammatory breast cancer xenograft. *Cancer Res*. 2002;62:560–566.
53. McDonald DM, Munn L, Jain RK.Vasculogenic mimicry: how convincing, how novel, and how significant? *Am J Pathol* 2000;156:383–388.
54. McDonald DM, Foss AJ. Endothelial cells of tumor vessels: abnormal but not absent. *Cancer Metastasis Rev*. 2000;19:109–120.
55. Hammersen F, Endrich B, Messmer K. The fine structure of tumor blood vessels. I. Participation of non-endothelial cells in tumor angiogenesis. *Int J Microcirc Clin Exp*. 1985;4:31–43.
56. Timar J, Toth J. Tumor sinuses- vascular channels. *Pathol Oncol Res*. 2000;6:83–86.
57. Hendrix MJ, Seftor EA, Chu YW, Seftor RE, Nagle RB, McDaniel KM, Leong SP, Yohem KH, Leibovitz AM, Meyskens FL, Jr., et al. Coexpression of vimentin and keratins by human melanoma tumor cells: correlation with invasive and metastatic potential. *J Natl Cancer Inst*. 1992;84:165–174.
58. Chu YW, Seftor EA, Romer LH, Hendrix MJ. Experimental coexpression of vimentin and keratin intermediate filaments in human melanoma cells augments motility. *Am J Pathol*. 1996;148:63–69.
59. Hendrix MJ, Seftor EA, Seftor RE, Kirschmann DA, Gardner LM, Boldt HC, Meyer M, Pe'er J, Folberg R. Regulation of uveal melanoma interconverted phenotype by hepatocyte growth factor/scatter factor (HGF/SF). *Am J Pathol*. 1998;152:855–863.
60. Hendrix MJ, Seftor EA, Seftor RE, Gardner LM, Boldt HC, Meyer M, Pe'er J, Folberg R. Biologic determinants of uveal melanoma metastatic phenotype: role of intermediate filaments as predictive markers. *Lab Invest*. 1998;78:153–163.
61. Bissell MJ. Tumor plasticity allows vasculogenic mimicry, a novel form of angiogenic switch. A rose by any other name? *Am J Pathol*. 1999;155:675–679.
62. Hendrix MJ, Seftor EA, Kirschmann DA, Seftor RE. Molecular biology of breast cancer metastasis. Molecular expression of vascular markers by aggressive breast cancer cells. *Breast Cancer Res*. 2000;2:417–422.

63. Hess AR, Seftor EA, Gardner LM, Carles-Kinch K, Schneider GB, Seftor RE, Kinch MS, Hendrix MJ. Molecular regulation of tumor cell vasculogenic mimicry by tyrosine phosphorylation: role of epithelial cell kinase (Eck/EphA2). *Cancer Res.* 2001;61: 3250–3255.
64. Hendrix MJ, Seftor EA, Meltzer PS, Gardner LM, Hess AR, Kirschmann DA, Schatteman GC, Seftor RE. Expression and functional significance of VE-cadherin in aggressive human melanoma cells: role in vasculogenic mimicry. *Proc Natl Acad Sci USA.* 2001;98:8018–8023.
65. Scott GA, Cassidy L, Tran H, Rao SK, Marinkovich MP. Melanocytes adhere to and synthesize laminin-5 in vitro. *Exp Dermatol.* 1999;8:212–221.
66. Scott GA, Cassidy L. Racl mediates dendrite formation in response to melanocyte stimulating hormone and ultraviolet light in a murine melanoma model. *J Invest Dermatol.* 1998;111:243–250.
67. Seftor RE, Seftor EA, Koshikawa N, Meltzer PS, Gardner LM, Bilban M, Stetler-Stevenson WG, Quaranta V, Hendrix MJ. Cooperative interactions of laminin 5 gamma2 chain, matrix metalloproteinase-2, and membrane type-1-matrix/metalloproteinase are required for mimicry of embryonic vasculogenesis by aggressive melanoma. *Cancer Res.* 2001;61:6322–6327.
68. Connolly DT, Heuvelman DM, Nelson R, Olander JV, Eppley BL, Delfino JJ, Siegel NR, Leimgruber RM, Feder J. Tumor vascular permeability factor stimulates endothelial cell growth and angiogenesis. *J Clin Invest.* 1989;84:1470–1478.
69. Halaban R, Fan B, Ahn J, Funasaka Y, Gitay-Goren H, Neufeld G. Growth factors, receptor kinases, and protein tyrosine phosphatases in normal and malignant melanocytes. *J Immunother.* 1992;12:154–161.
70. Halaban R, Funasaka Y, Lee P, Rubin J, Ron D, Birnbaum D. Fibroblast growth factors in normal and malignant melanocytes. *Ann N Y Acad Sci.* 1991;638:232–243.
71. Szebenyi G, Fallon JF. Fibroblast growth factors as multifunctional signaling factors. *Int Rev Cytol.* 1999;185:45–106.
72. Boyd SR, Tan DS, de Souza L, Neale MH, Myatt NE, Alexander RA, Robb M, Hungerford JL, Cree IA. Uveal melanomas express vascular endothelial growth factor and basic fibroblast growth factor and support endothelial cell growth. *Br J Ophthalmol.* 2002;86:440–447.
73. Stavri GT, Zachary IC, Baskerville PA, Martin JF, Erusalimsky JD. Basic fibroblast growth factor upregulates the expression of vascular endothelial growth factor in vascular smooth muscle cells. Synergistic interaction with hypoxia. *Circulation.* 1995; 92:11–14.
74. Pepper MS, Ferrara N, Orci L, Montesano R. Potent synergism between vascular endothelial growth factor and basic fibroblast growth factor in the induction of angiogenesis in vitro. *Biochem Biophys Res Commun.* 1992;189:824–831.
75. Kvanta A, Steen B, Seregard S. Expression of vascular endothelial growth factor (VEGF) in retinoblastoma but not in posterior uveal melanoma. *Exp Eye Res.* 1996;63:511–518.
76. Stitt AW, Simpson DA, Boocock C, Gardiner TA, Murphy GM, Archer DB. Expression of vascular endothelial growth factor (VEGF) and its receptors is regulated in eyes with intra-ocular tumors. *J Pathol.* 1998;186:306–312.
77. Sheidow TG, Hooper PL, Crukley C, Young J, Heathcote JG. Expression of vascular endothelial growth factor in uveal melanoma and its correlation with metastasis. *Br J Ophthalmol.* 2000;84:750–756.
78. Gitay-Goren H, Halaban R, Neufeld G. Human melanoma cells but not normal melanocytes express vascular endothelial growth factor receptors. *Biochem Biophys Res Commun.* 1993;190:702–708.

79. Liu B, Earl HM, Baban D, Shoaibi M, Fabra A, Kerr DJ, Seymour LW. Melanoma cell lines express VEGF receptor KDR and respond to exogenously added VEGF. *Biochem Biophys Res Commun*. 1995;217:721–727.
80. Claffey KP, Brown LF, del Aguila LF, Tognazzi K, Yeo KT, Manseau EJ, Dvorak HF. Expression of vascular permeability factor/vascular endothelial growth factor by melanoma cells increases tumor growth, angiogenesis, and experimental metastasis. *Cancer Res*. 1996;56:172–181.
81. Fonsatti E, Lamaj E, Coral S, Sigalotti L, Nardi G, Gasparollo A, Colombo MP, Altomonte M, Maio M. In vitro analysis of the melanoma/endothelium interaction increasing the release of soluble intercellular adhesion molecule 1 by endothelial cells. *Cancer Immunol Immunother*. 1999;48:132–138.
82. Bayer-Garner IB, Hough AJ, Jr., Smoller BR. Vascular endothelial growth factor expression in malignant melanoma: prognostic versus diagnostic usefulness. *Mod Pathol*. 1999;12:770–774.
83. Graeven U, Fiedler W, Karpinski S, Ergun S, Kilic N, Rodeck U, Schmiegel W, Hossfeld DK. Melanoma-associated expression of vascular endothelial growth factor and its receptors FLT-1 and KDR. *J Cancer Res Clin Oncol*. 1999;125:621–629.
84. Weber F, Sepp N, Fritsch P. Vascular endothelial growth factor and basic fibroblast growth factor in melanoma. *Br J Dermatol*. 2000;142:392–393.
85. Hofmann UB, Westphal JR, Van Kraats AA, Ruiter DJ, Van Muijen GN. Expression of integrin alpha(v)beta(3) correlates with activation of membrane-type matrix metalloproteinase-1 (MT1-MMP) and matrix metalloproteinase-2 (MMP-2) in human melanoma cells in vitro and in vivo. *Int J Cancer*. 2000;87:12–19.
86. Lacal PM, Failla CM, Pagani E, Odorisio T, Schietroma C, Falcinelli S, Zambruno G, D'Atri S. Human melanoma cells secrete and respond to placenta growth factor and vascular endothelial growth factor. *J Invest Dermatol*. 2000;115:1000–1007.
87. Rofstad EK, Halsor EF. Vascular endothelial growth factor, interleukin 8, platelet-derived endothelial cell growth factor, and basic fibroblast growth factor promote angiogenesis and metastasis in human melanoma xenografts. *Cancer Res*. 2000;60: 4932–4938.
88. Westphal JR, Van't Hullenaar R, Peek R, Willems RW, Crickard K, Crickard U, Askaa J, Clemmensen I, Ruiter DJ, De Waal RM. Angiogenic balance in human melanoma: expression of VEGF, bFGF, IL-8, PDGF and angiostatin in relation to vascular density of xenografts in vivo. *Int J Cancer*. 2000;86:768–776.
89. Danielsen T, Rofstad EK. VEGF, bFGF and EGF in the angiogenesis of human melanoma xenografts. *Int J Cancer*. 1998;76:836–841.
90. Clarijs R, Schalkwijk L, Ruiter DJ, De Waal RM. Lack of lymphangiogenesis despite coexpression of VEGF-C and its receptor Flt-4 in uveal melanoma. *Invest Ophthalmol Vis Sci*. 2001;42:1422–1428.
91. Marshall JF, Rutherford DC, Happerfield L, Hanby A, McCartney AC, Newton-Bishop J, Hart IR. Comparative analysis of integrins *in vitro* and *in vivo* in uveal and cutaneous melanomas. *Br J Cancer* 1998;77:522–529.
92. Daniels KJ, Boldt HC, Martin JA, Gardner LM, Meyer M, Folberg R. Expression of type VI collagen in uveal melanoma: its role in pattern formation and tumor progression. *Lab Invest*. 1996;75:55–66.
93. Elshaw SR, Sisley K, Cross N, Murray AK, MacNeil SM, Wagner M, Nichols CE, Rennie IG. A comparison of ocular melanocyte and uveal melanoma cell invasion and the implication of alpha1beta1, alpha4beta1 and alpha6beta1 integrins. *Br J Ophthalmol* 2001;85:732–738.

94. Anastassiou G, Schilling H, Djakovic S, Bornfeld N. Expression of VLA-2, VLA-3, and alpha(v) integrin receptors in uveal melanoma: association with microvascular architecture of the tumor and prognostic value. *Br J Ophthalmol.* 2000;84:899–902.
95. Rohrbach JM, Wild M, Riedinger C, Kreissig I, Thiel HJ. Premetastatic uveal melanoma cells do not express laminin receptors. *Ger J Ophthalmol.* 1994;3:144–147.
96. Mäkitie T, Summanen P, Tarkkanen A, Kivelä T. Tumor-infiltrating macrophages (CD68(+) cells) and prognosis in malignant uveal melanoma. *Invest Ophthalmol Vis Sci.* 2001;42:1414–1421.
97. Kramer RH, Vu M, Cheng YF, Ramos DM. Integrin expression in malignant melanoma. *Cancer Metastasis Rev.* 1991;10:49–59.
98. Scott G, Cassidy L, Busacco A. Fibronectin suppresses apoptosis in normal human melanocytes through an integrin-dependent mechanism. *J Invest Dermatol.* 1997; 108:147–153.
99. Petitclerc E, Stromblad S, von Schalscha TL, Mitjans F, Piulats J, Montgomery AM, Cheresh DA, Brooks PC. Integrin alpha(v)beta3 promotes M21 melanoma growth in human skin by regulating tumor cell survival. *Cancer Res.* 1999;59:2724–2730.
100. Friedlander M, Brooks PC, Shaffer RW, Kincaid CM, Varner JA, Cheresh DA. Definition of two angiogenic pathways by distinct alpha v integrins. *Science.* 1995;270:1500–1502.
101. Ten Berge PJ, Danen EH, Van Muijen GN, Jager MJ, Ruiter DJ. Integrin expression in uveal melanoma differs from cutaneous melanoma. *Invest Ophthalmol Vis Sci.* 1993; 34:3635–3640.
102. Seftor RE, Seftor EA, Hendrix MJ. Molecular role(s) for integrins in human melanoma invasion. *Cancer Metastasis Rev.* 1999;18:359–375.
103. Cheresh DA. Human endothelial cells synthesize and express an Arg–Gly–Asp-directed adhesion receptor involved in attachment to fibrinogen and von Willebrand factor. *Proc Natl Acad Sci USA.* 1987;84:6471–6475.
104. Cheresh DA, Pytela R, Pierschbacher MD, Klier FG, Ruoslahti E, Reisfeld RA. An Arg–Gly–Asp-directed receptor on the surface of human melanoma cells exists in an divalent cation-dependent functional complex with the disialoganglioside GD2. *J Cell Biol.* 1987;105:1163–1173.
105. Natali PG, Hamby CV, Felding-Habermann B, Liang B, Nicotra MR, Di Filippo F, Giannarelli D, Temponi M, Ferrone S. Clinical significance of alpha(v)beta3 integrin and intercellular adhesion molecule-1 expression in cutaneous malignant melanoma lesions. *Cancer Res.* 1997;57:1554–1560.
106. Beliveau A, Berube M, Rousseau A, Pelletier G, Guerin SL. Expression of integrin alpha5beta1 and MMPs associated with epithelioid morphology and malignancy of uveal melanoma. *Invest Ophthalmol Vis Sci.* 2000;41:2363–2372.
107. Baker JK, Elshaw SR, Mathewman GE, Nichols CE, Murray AK, Parsons MA, Rennie IG, Sisley K. Expression of integrins, degradative enzymes and their inhibitors in uveal melanoma: differences between in vitro and in vivo expression. *Melanoma Res.* 2001;11:265–273.
108. Beliveau A, Berube M, Carrier P, Mercier C, Guerin SL. Tumorigenicity of the mixed spindle-epithelioid SP6.5 and epithelioid TP17 uveal melanoma cell lines is differentially related to alpha5beta1 integrin expression. *Invest Ophthalmol Vis Sci.* 2001; 42:3058–3065.
109. Vihinen P, Kahari VM. Matrix metalloproteinases in cancer: prognostic markers and therapeutic targets. *Int J Cancer.* 2002;99:157–166.
110. Jiang Y, Goldberg ID, Shi YE. Complex roles of tissue inhibitors of metalloproteinases in cancer. *Oncogene.* 2002;21:2245–2252.

111. Giannelli G, Antonaci S. Gelatinases and their inhibitors in tumor metastasis: from biological research to medical applications. *Histol Histopathol.* 2002;17: 339–345.
112. Egeblad M, Werb Z. New functions for the matrix metalloproteinases in cancer progression. *Nature Rev Cancer.* 2002;2:161–174.
113. Coussens LM, Fingleton B, Matrisian LM. Matrix metalloproteinase inhibitors and cancer: trials and tribulations. *Science.* 2002;295:2387–2392.
114. Hofmann UB, Westphal JR, Waas ET, Zendman AJ, Cornelissen IM, Ruiter DJ, Van Muijen GN. Matrix metalloproteinases in human melanoma cell lines and xenografts: increased expression of activated matrix metalloproteinase-2 (MMP-2) correlates with melanoma progression. *Br J Cancer.* 1999;81:774–782.
115. El-Shabrawi Y, Ardjomand N, Radner H. MMP-9 is predominantly expressed in epithelioid and not spindle cell uveal melanoma. *J Pathol.* 2001;194:201–206.
116. Hofmann UB, Westphal JR, Zendman AJ, Becker JC, Ruiter DJ, van Muijen GN. Expression and activation of matrix metalloproteinase-2 (MMP-2) and its co-localization with membrane-type 1 matrix metalloproteinase (MT1-MMP) correlate with melanoma progression. *J Pathol.* 2000;191:245–256.
116a. Zuidervaart W, Van der Velden PA, Nieuwpoort AF, Krose CJM, Ksander BR, Gruis NA, Jager MJ. Gene expression profiling of eleven different uveal melanoma cell lines compared to normal choroidal melanocytes. *Assoc Res Vision Ophthalmol.* 2002:1117.
116b. Van der Velden, P. Zuidervaart W, Hurks MH, Pavey S, Ksander BR, Krijgsman E, Frants RR, Tensen CP, Willemze R, Jager MJ, Gruis NA. Expression profiling reveals that methylation of TIMP3 is involved in uveal melanoma development. *Int J Cancer.* 2003;106:472–479.
117. Cao Y. Endogenous angiogenesis inhibitors: angiostatin, endostatin, and other proteolytic fragments. *Prog Mol Subcell Biol.* 1998;20:161–176.
118. Sledge GW, Jr., Miller KD. Angiogenesis and antiangiogenic therapy. *Curr Probl Cancer.* 2002;26:1–60.
119. Marneros AG, Olsen BR. The role of collagen-derived proteolytic fragments in angiogenesis. *Matrix Biol.* 2001;20:337–345.
120. Pepper MS. Extracellular proteolysis and angiogenesis. *Thromb Haemost.* 2001;86: 346–355.
121. Cao Y. Endogenous angiogenesis inhibitors and their therapeutic implications. *Int J Biochem Cell Biol.* 2001;33:357–369.
122. O'Reilly MS, Holmgren L, Shing Y, Chen C, Rosenthal RA, Cao Y, Moses M, Lane WS, Sage EH, Folkman J. Angiostatin: a circulating endothelial cell inhibitor that suppresses angiogenesis and tumor growth. *Cold Spring Harb Symp Quant Biol.* 1994;59:471–482.
123. Cao Y, Ji RW, Davidson D, Schaller J, Marti D, Sohndel S, McCance SG, O'Reilly MS, Llinas M, Folkman J. Kringle domains of human angiostatin. Characterization of the anti-proliferative activity on endothelial cells. *J Biol Chem.* 1996;271:29461–29467.
124. Folkman J. Angiogenesis inhibitors generated by tumors. *Mol Med.* 1995;1:120–122.
125. O'Reilly MS, Holmgren L, Shing Y, Chen C, Rosenthal RA, Moses M, Lane WS, Cao Y, Sage EH, Folkman J. Angiostatin: a novel angiogenesis inhibitor that mediates the suppression of metastases by a Lewis lung carcinoma. *Cell.* 1994;79:315–328.
126. Kuroi K, Toi M. Circulating angiogenesis regulators in cancer patients. *Int J Biol Markers.* 2001;16:5–26.
127. Kirsch M, Schackert G, Black PM. Angiogenesis, metastasis, and endogenous inhibition. *J Neurooncol.* 2000;50:173–180.

128. Ambs S, Dennis S, Fairman J,Wright M, Papkoff J. Inhibition of tumor growth correlates with the expression level of a human angiostatin transgene in transfected B16F10 melanoma cells. *Cancer Res.* 1999;59:5773–5777.
129. Apte RS, Niederkorn JY, Mayhew E, Alizadeh H. Angiostatin produced by certain primary uveal melanoma cell lines impedes the development of liver metastases. *Arch Ophthalmol.* 2001;119:1805–1809.
130. Ijland SA, Jager MJ, Heijdra BM, Westphal JR, Peek R. Expression of angiogenic and immunosuppressive factors by uveal melanoma cell lines. *Melanoma Res.* 1999;9:445–450.
131. Sieving PA. Fifteen years of work: the COMS outcomes for medium-sized choroidal melanoma. *Arch Ophthalmol.* 2001;119:1067–1068.
132. Earle JD. Results from the Collaborative Ocular Melanoma Study (COMS) of enucleation versus preoperative radiation therapy in the management of large ocular melanomas. *Int J Radiat Oncol Biol Phys.* 1999;43:1168–1169.
133. Mortality in patients with small choroidal melanoma. COMS report no. 4. The Collaborative Ocular Melanoma Study Group. *Arch Ophthalmol.* 1997;115:886–893.
134. Zimmerman LE, McLean IW, Foster WD. Does enucleation of the eye containing a malignant melanoma prevent or accelerate the dissemination of tumor cells. *Br J Ophthalmol.* 1978;62:420–425.
135. Zimmerman LE, McLean IW. An evaluation of enucleation in the management of uveal melanomas. *Int Ophthalmol Clin.* 1980;20:1–31.
136. McLean IW, Zimmerman LE, Foster WD. Survival rates after enucleation of eyes with malignant melanoma. *Am J Ophthalmol.* 1979;88:794–797.
137. Haimovici R, Mukai S, Schachat AP, Haynie GD, Thomas MA, Meredith TA, Gragoudas ES. Rhegmatogenous retinal detachment in eyes with uveal melanoma. *Retina.* 1996;16:488–496.
138. Augsburger JJ, Schroeder RP, Territo C, Gamel JW, Shields JA. Clinical parameters predictive of enlargement of melanocytic choroidal lesions. *Br J Ophthalmol.* 1989; 73:911–917.
139. Brieden SR, Schmidt J, Kroll P. Exudative retinal detachment: a parameter for the effectiveness of irradiation for malignant melanoma? *Ophthalmologe.* 1999;96:1–5.
140. Lee J, Logani S, Lakosha H, Schroeder RP, Simpson R, Jampol LM. Preretinal neovascularisation associated with choroidal melanoma. *Br J Ophthalmol.* 2001;85:1309–1312.
141. Kivelä T, Eskelin S, Mäkitie T, Summanen P. Exudative retinal detachment from malignant uveal melanoma: predictors and prognostic significance. *Invest Ophthalmol Vis Sci.* 2001;42:2085–2093.
142. Frau E, Gregoire-Cassoux N, Offret M, Labetoulle M, Nodarian M, Lautier-Frau M, Offret H. [Rupture of the hemato-ocular barrier, studied by fluorophotometry, in uveal melanoma patients. Preliminary results]. *J Fr Ophtalmol.* 1998;21:409–413.
143. Brooks AM. Experiences with fluorophotometry. *Aust J Ophthalmol.* 1982;10:41–51.
144. Nguyen NX, Kuchle M, Naumann GO. Tumor growth of a choroidal malignant melanoma and aqueous flare. Report of a case. *Ophthalmologica.* 1999;213:194–196.
145. Nguyen NX, Kuchle M, Strunk W. [Tyndallometry for follow-up of iodine-125 brachytherapy of uveal malignant melanomas. Report of 2 patients]. *Klin Monatsbl Augenheilkd.* 1996;209:25–30.
146. Castella AP, Bercher L, Zografos L, Egger E, Herbort CP. Study of the blood-aqueous barrier in choroidal melanoma. *Br J Ophthalmol.* 1995;79:354–357.
147. Küchle M, Nguyen NX, Naumann GO. Quantitative assessment of the blood-aqueous barrier in human eyes with malignant or benign uveal tumors. *Am J Ophthalmol.* 1994;117:521–528.

148. Küchle M, Nguyen NX, Naumann GO. Aqueous flare in eyes with choroidal malignant melanoma. *Am J Ophthalmol*. 1992;113:207–208.
149. Muskens RP, Van Best JA, Bleeker JC, Keunen JE. Corneal autofluorescence in choroidal melanoma or in choroidal naevus. *Br J Ophthalmol*. 2001;85:662–665.
150. Pe'er J, Shweiki D, Itin A, Hemo I, Gnessin H, Keshet E. Hypoxia-induced expression of vascular endothelial growth factor by retinal cells is a common factor in neovascularizing ocular diseases. *Lab Invest*. 1995;72:638–645.
151. Los M, Aarsman CJ, Terpstra L, Wittebol-Post D, Lips CJ, Blijham GH, Voest EE. Elevated ocular levels of vascular endothelial growth factor in patients with von Hippel–Lindau disease. *Ann Oncol*. 1997;8:1015–1022.
152. Aiello LP, Avery RL, Arrigg PG, Keyt BA, Jampel HD, Shah ST, Pasquale LR, Thieme H, Iwamoto MA, Park JE, et al. Vascular endothelial growth factor in ocular fluid of patients with diabetic retinopathy and other retinal disorders. *N Engl J Med*. 1994;331: 1480–1487.
153. Boyd SR, Tan D, Bunce C, Gittos A, Neale MH, Hungerford JL, Charnock-Jones S, Cree IA. Vascular endothelial growth factor is elevated in ocular fluids of eyes harbouring uveal melanoma: identification of a potential therapeutic window. *Br J Ophthalmol*. 2002;86:448–452.
154. Hata Y, Rook SL, Aiello LP. Basic fibroblast growth factor induces expression of VEGF receptor KDR through a protein kinase C and p44/p42 mitogen-activated protein kinase-dependent pathway. *Diabetes*. 1999;48:1145–1155.
155. Graff BA, Bjornaes I, Rofstad EK. Microvascular permeability of human melanoma xenografts to macromolecules: relationships to tumor volumetric growth rate, tumor angiogenesis, and VEGF expression. *Microvasc Res*. 2001;61:187–198.
156. Pe'er J, Neufeld M, Baras M, Gnessin H, Itin A, Keshet E. Rubeosis iridis in retinoblastoma. Histologic findings and the possible role of vascular endothelial growth factor in its induction. *Ophthalmology*. 1997;104:1251–1258.
156a. Jager MJ, Krose CJM, Zuidervaart W, Eilers P, Boyd SR, Van der Pluijm G, Keunen JEE, De Wolff-Rouendaal D, Hurks HMH. Vascular endothelial growth factor (VEGF) in aqueous humor: prognostic factor in uveal melanoma. *Assoc Res Vision Ophthalmol*. 2002; Abstract 1829.
157. Keunen JE, Hooymans JM, Ulbig MW, Shields CL. Retinal neovascularization in choroidal melanoma without retinal ischemia. *Retina*. 2002;22:371–374.
158. Lubin JR, Gragoudas ES, Albert DM. Choroidal neovascularization associated with malignant melanoma: a case report. *Acta Ophthalmol (Copenh)*. 1982;60:412–418.
159. Vine AK. Choroidal melanoma with disc and retinal neovascularization. *Retina*. 1983;3:118–120.
160. Finger PT. Radiation therapy for choroidal melanoma. *Surv Ophthalmol*. 1997;42: 215–232.
161. Foss AJ, Whelehan I, Hungerford JL, Anderson DF, Errington RD, Kacperek A, Restori M, Kongerud J, Sheen M. Predictive factors for the development of rubeosis following proton beam radiotherapy for uveal melanoma. *Br J Ophthalmol*. 1997;81:748–754.
162. Hungerford JL, Foss AJ, Whelahan I, Errington RD, Kacperek A, Kongerud J. Side effects of photon and proton radiotherapy for ocular melanoma. *Front Radiat Ther Oncol*. 1997;30:287–293.
163. Tolentino MJ, Miller JW, Gragoudas ES, Chatzistefanou K, Ferrara N, Adamis AP. Vascular endothelial growth factor is sufficient to produce iris neovascularization and neovascular glaucoma in a nonhuman primate. *Arch Ophthalmol*. 1996;114: 964–970.

163a. Boyd SK, Zachery I, Chakracarthy U, Allen GJ, Wisdom GB, Cree IA, Martin JF, Hykin PG. Correlation of increased vascular endothelial growth factor with neovascularisation and permeability in ischemic central vein occlusion. *Arch Ophthalmol.* 2002;120:1644–1650.
164. Dawson DW, Volpert OV, Gillis P, Crawford SE, Xu H, Benedict W, Bouck NP. Pigment epithelium-derived factor: a potent inhibitor of angiogenesis. *Science.* 1999;285:245–248.
165. Ogata N, Nishikawa M, Nishimura T, Mitsuma Y, Matsumura M. Inverse levels of pigment epithelium-derived factor and vascular endothelial growth factor in the vitreous of eyes with rhegmatogenous retinal detachment and proliferative vitreoretinopathy. *Am J Ophthalmol.* 2002;133:851–852.
166. Gunduz K, Shields CL, Shields JA, Cater J, Freire JE, Brady LW. Plaque radiotherapy of uveal melanoma with predominant ciliary body involvement. *Arch Ophthalmol.* 1999;117:170–177.
167. Gragoudas ES, Li W, Lane AM, Munzenrider J, Egan KM. Risk factors for radiation maculopathy and papillopathy after intraocular irradiation. *Ophthalmology.* 1999;106: 1571–1577; discussion 1577–1578.
168. Gunduz K, Shields CL, Shields JA, Cater J, Freire JE, Brady LW. Radiation retinopathy following plaque radiotherapy for posterior uveal melanoma. *Arch Ophthalmol.* 1999;117:609–614.
169. Finger PT, Berson A, Szechter A. Palladium-103 plaque radiotherapy for choroidal melanoma: results of a 7-year study. *Ophthalmology.* 1999;106:606–613.
170. Saornil MA, Fisher MR, Campbell RJ, Robertson DM, Earle JD, Eagle RC, Jr., Shields JA, Shields CL, Chandra SR, Albert DM. Histopathologic study of eyes after iodine I 125 episcleral plaque irradiation for uveal melanoma. *Arch Ophthalmol.* 1997;115:1395–1400.
171. Egger E, Zografos L, Munkel G, Bohringer T, Bercher L, Chamot L. Results of proton radiotherapy for uveal melanomas. *Front Radiat Ther Oncol.* 1997;30:111–122.
172. Castro JR, Char DH, Petti PL, Daftari IK, Quivey JM, Singh RP, Blakely EA, Phillips TL. 15 years experience with helium ion radiotherapy for uveal melanoma. *Int J Radiat Oncol Biol Phys.* 1997;39:989–996.
173. Guyer DR, Mukai S, Egan KM, Seddon JM, Walsh SM, Gragoudas ES. Radiation maculopathy after proton beam irradiation for choroidal melanoma. *Ophthalmology.* 1992;99:1278–1285.
174. Kim MK, Char DH, Castro JL, Saunders WM, Chen GT, Stone RD. Neovascular glaucoma after helium ion irradiation for uveal melanoma. *Ophthalmology.* 1986;93:189–193.
175. Kincaid MC, Folberg R, Torczynski E, Zakov ZN, Shore JW, Liu SJ, Planchard TA, Weingeist TA. Complications after proton beam therapy for uveal malignant melanoma. A clinical and histopathologic study of five cases. *Ophthalmology.* 1988;95: 982–991.
176. Egan KM, Gragoudas ES, Seddon JM, Glynn RJ, Munzenreider JE, Goitein M, Verhey L, Urie M, Koehler A. The risk of enucleation after proton beam irradiation of uveal melanoma. *Ophthalmology.* 1989;96:1377–1382; discussion 1382–1373.
177. Char DH, Castro JR, Kroll SM, Irvine AR, Quivey JM, Stone RD. Five-year follow-up of helium ion therapy for uveal melanoma. *Arch Ophthalmol.* 1990;108:209–214.
178. Haas A, Pinter O, Papaefthymiou G, Weger M, Berghold A, Schrottner O, Mullner K, Pendl G, Langmann G. Incidence of radiation retinopathy after high-dosage single-fraction gamma knife radiosurgery for choroidal melanoma. *Ophthalmology.* 2002; 109:909–913.

179. Langmann G, Pendl G, Klaus M, Papaefthymiou G, Guss H. Gamma knife radiosurgery for uveal melanomas: an 8-year experience. *J Neurosurg*. 2000;93 Suppl 3:184–188.
180. Marchini G, Gerosa M, Piovan E, Pasoli A, Babighian S, Rigotti M, Rossato M, Bonomi L. Gamma Knife stereotactic radiosurgery for uveal melanoma: clinical results after 2 years. *Stereotact Funct Neurosurg*. 1996;66 Suppl 1:208–213.
181. Hill JC, Sealy R, Shackleton D, Stannard C, Korrubel J, Hering E, Loxton C. Improved iodine-125 plaque design in the treatment of choroidal malignant melanoma. *Br J Ophthalmol*. 1992;76:91–94.
182. Astrahan MA, Luxton G, Jozsef G, Liggett PE, Petrovich Z. Optimization of 125I ophthalmic plaque brachytherapy. *Med Phys*. 1990;17:1053–1057.
183. Shields CL, Shields JA, Karlsson U, Markoe AM, Brady LW. Reasons for enucleation after plaque radiotherapy for posterior uveal melanoma. Clinical findings. *Ophthalmology* 1989;96:919–923; discussion 924.
184. Muller RP, Busse H, Potter R, Kroll P, Haverkamp U. Results of high dose 106-ruthenium irradiation of choroidal melanomas. *Int J Radiat Oncol Biol Phys*. 1986;12:1749–1755.
185. Hermann RM, Pradier O, Lauritzen K, Ott M, Schmidberger H, Hess CF. Does escalation of the apical dose change treatment outcome in beta-radiation of posterior choroidal melanomas with 106Ru plaques? *Int J Radiat Oncol Biol Phys*. 2002;52: 1360–1366.
186. Caminal Mitjana JM, Quintana Casany M, Pera Fabregas J, Cinos Cope C, Guedea F. Resultado de la radioterapie con placas Iodo-125 en el tratamiento del melanoma del úvea. [Results of Iodine-125 radiotherapy in the treatment of uveal melanoma]. *Arch Soc Esp Oftalmol*. 2002;77:29–38.
187. Shields CL, Shields JA, De Potter P, Quaranta M, Freire J, Brady LW, Barrett J. Plaque radiotherapy for the management of uveal metastasis. *Arch Ophthalmol*. 1997;115: 203–209.
188. Summanen P, Immonen I, Kivela T, Tommila P, Heikkonen J, Tarkkanen A. Radiation related complications after ruthenium plaque radiotherapy of uveal melanoma. *Br J Ophthalmol*. 1996;80:732–739.
189. Lean EK, Cohen DM, Liggett PE, Luxton G, Langholz B, Lau R, Astrahan MA, Hyden EC, Petrovich Z. Episcleral radioactive plaque therapy: initial clinical experience with 56 patients. *Am J Clin Oncol*. 1990;13:185–190.
190. Gunduz K, Shields CL, Shields JA, Cater J, Freire JE, Brady LW. Radiation complications and tumor control after plaque radiotherapy of choroidal melanoma with macular involvement. *Am J Ophthalmol*. 1999;127:579–589.
191. Shields CL, Shields JA, Gunduz K, Freire JE, Mercado G. Radiation therapy for uveal malignant melanoma. *Ophthalmic Surg Lasers*. 1998;29:397–409.
192. Packer S, Stoller S, Lesser ML, Mandel FS, Finger PT. Long-term results of iodine 125 irradiation of uveal melanoma. *Ophthalmology* 1992;99:767–773; discussion 774.
193. Finger PT. Plaque radiation therapy for malignant melanoma of the iris and ciliary body. *Am J Ophthalmol*. 2001;132:328–335.
194. De Potter P, Shields CL, Shields JA, Cater JR, Brady LW. Plaque radiotherapy for juxtapapillary choroidal melanoma.Visual acuity and survival outcome. *Arch Ophthalmol*. 1996;114:1357–1365.
195. Reader S, Grigg J, Billson FA. Choroidal melanoma: a review of the experience of the Sydney Eye Hospital Professorial Unit 1979–1995. *Aust NZJ Ophthalmol*. 1997;25: 15–24.
196. Petrovich Z, Pike M, Astrahan MA, Luxton G, Murphree AL, Liggett PE. Episcleral plaque thermoradiotherapy of posterior uveal melanomas. *Am J Clin Oncol*. 1996;19: 207–211.

197. Shields CL, Cater J, Shields JA, Chao A, Krema H, Materin M, Brady LW. Combined plaque radiotherapy and transpupillary thermotherapy for choroidal melanoma: tumor control and treatment complications in 270 consecutive patients. *Arch Ophthalmol.* 2002;120:933–940.
198. Currie ZI, Rennie IG, Talbot JF. Retinal vascular changes associated with transpupillary thermotherapy for choroidal melanomas. *Retina.* 2000;20:620–626.
199. Ma D, Gerard RD, Li XY, Alizadeh H, Niederkorn JY. Inhibition of metastasis of intraocular melanomas by adenovirus-mediated gene transfer of plasminogen activator inhibitor type 1 (PAI-1) in an athymic mouse model. *Blood.* 1997;90:2738–2746.
200. Alizadeh H, Ma D, Berman M, Bellingham D, Comerford SA, Gething MJ, Sambrook JF, Niederkorn JY. Tissue-type plasminogen activator-induced invasion and metastasis of murine melanomas. *Curr Eye Res.* 1995;14:449–458.
201. Park SS, Li L, Korn TS, Mitra MM, Niederkorn JY. Effect of transforming growth factor-beta on plasminogen activator production of cultured human uveal melanoma cells. *Curr Eye Res.* 1996;15:755–763.
202. Cox G, O'Byrne KJ. Matrix metalloproteinases and cancer. *Anticancer Res.* 2001;21:4207–4219.
203. Seftor EA, Meltzer PS, Kirschmann DA, Pe'er J, Maniotis AJ, Trent JM, Folberg R, Hendrix MJ. Molecular determinants of human uveal melanoma invasion and metastasis. *Clin Exp Metastasis.* 2002;19:233–246.
204. Repesh LA. A new in vitro assay for quantitating tumor cell invasion. *Invasion Metastasis.* 1989;9:192–208.
205. Woodward JK, Nichols CE, Rennie IG, Parsons MA, Murray AK, Sisley K. An *in vitro* assay to assess uveal melanoma invasion across endothelial and basement membrane barriers. *Invest Ophthalmol Vis Sci.* 2002;43:1708–1714.
206. Mooy CM, De Jong PT. Prognostic parameters in uveal melanoma: a review. *Surv Ophthalmol.* 1996;41:215–228.
207. Lugassy C, Christensen L, Le Charpentier M, Faure E, Escande JP. Angio-tumoral laminin in murine tumors derived from human melanoma cell lines. Immunohistochemical and ultrastructural observations. *J Submicrosc Cytol Pathol.* 1998;30: 231–237.
208. Lugassy C, Christensen L, Le Charpentier M, Faure E, Escande JP. Ultrastructural and immunohistochemical observations concerning laminin in B16 melanoma. Is an amorphous form of laminin promoting a non hematogenous migration of tumor cells? *J Submicrosc Cytol Pathol* 1998;30:137–144.
209. Grossniklaus HE, Wilson MW, Barron BC, Lynn MJ. Anterior vs posterior intraocular melanoma. Metastatic differences in a murine model. *Arch Ophthalmol.* 1996;114: 1116–1120.
210. Dithmar S, Diaz CE, Grossniklaus HE. Intraocular melanoma spread to regional lymph nodes: report of two cases. *Retina.* 2000;20:76–79.
211. Tobal K, Sherman LS, Foss AJ, Lightman SL. Detection of melanocytes from uveal melanoma in peripheral blood using the polymerase chain reaction. *Invest Ophthalmol Vis Sci.* 1993;34:2622–2625.
212. Foss AJ, Guille MJ, Occleston NL, Hykin PG, Hungerford JL, Lightman S. The detection of melanoma cells in peripheral blood by reverse transcription-polymerase chain reaction. *Br J Cancer.* 1995;72:155–159.
213. Keilholz U, Willhauck M, Rimoldi D, Brasseur F, Dummer W, Rass K, De Vries T, Blaheta J, Voit C, Lethe B, Burchill S. Reliability of reverse transcription-polymerase chain reaction (RT-PCR)-based assays for the detection of circulating tumor cells: a quality-assurance initiative of the EORTC Melanoma Cooperative Group. *Eur J Cancer.* 1998;34:750–753.

214. Keilholz U, Willhauck M, Scheibenbogen C, De Vries TJ, Burchill S. Polymerase chain reaction detection of circulating tumor cells. EORTC Melanoma Cooperative Group, Immunotherapy Subgroup. *Melanoma Res.* 1997;7 Suppl 2:S133–141.
215. Kulik J, Nowecki ZI, Rutkowski P, Ruka W, Rochowska M, Skurzak H, Siedlecki JA. Detection of circulating melanoma cells in peripheral blood by a two-marker RT-PCR assay. *Melanoma Res.* 2001;11:65–73.
216. Hanekom GS, Stubbings HM, Johnson CA, Kidson SH. The detection of circulating melanoma cells correlates with tumor thickness and ulceration but is not predictive of metastasis for patients with primary melanoma. *Melanoma Res.* 1999;9:465–473.
217. Pepper MS. Lymphangiogenesis and tumor metastasis: myth or reality? *Clin Cancer Res.* 2001;7:462–468.
218. Pepper MS. Lymphangiogenesis and tumor metastasis: more questions than answers. *Lymphology.* 2000;33:144–147.
219. Karkkainen MJ, Makinen T, Alitalo K. Lymphatic endothelium: a new frontier of metastasis research. *Nat Cell Biol.* 2002;4:E2–5.
220. Partanen TA, Paavonen K. Lymphatic versus blood vascular endothelial growth factors and receptors in humans. *Microsc Res Tech.* 2001;55:108–121.
221. Eskelin S, Pyrhonen S, Summanen P, Prause JU, Kivelä T. Screening for metastatic malignant melanoma of the uvea revisited. *Cancer.* 1999;85:1151–1159.
222. Diener-West M, Hawkins BS, Markowitz JA, Schachat AP. A review of mortality from choroidal melanoma. II. A meta-analysis of 5-year mortality rates following enucleation, 1966 through 1988. *Arch Ophthalmol.* 1992;110:245–250.
223. Rajpal S, Moore R, Karakousis CP. Survival in metastatic ocular melanoma. *Cancer.* 1983;52:334–336.
224. Sieczkiewicz GJ, Hussain M, Kohn EC. Angiogenesis and metastasis. *Cancer Treat Res.* 2002;107:353–381.
225. Berman RS, Portera CA, Jr., Ellis LM. Biology of liver metastases. *Cancer Treat Res.* 2001;109:183–206.
226. Ma D, Niederkorn JY. Role of epidermal growth factor receptor in the metastasis of intraocular melanomas. *Invest Ophthalmol Vis Sci.* 1998;39:1067–1075.
227. Hurks HM, Metzelaar-Blok JA, Barthen ER, Zwinderman AH, De Wolff-Rouendaal D, Keunen JE, Jager MJ. Expression of epidermal growth factor receptor: risk factor in uveal melanoma. *Invest Ophthalmol Vis Sci.* 2000;41:2023–2027.
228. All-Ericsson C, Girnita L, Seregard S, Bartolazzi A, Jager MJ, Larsson O. Insulin-like growth factor-1 receptor in uveal melanoma: a predictor for metastatic disease and a potential therapeutic target. *Invest Ophthalmol Vis Sci.* 2002;43:1–8.
229. Niederkorn JY, Mellon J, Pidherney M, Mayhew E, Anand R. Effect of anti-ganglioside antibodies on the metastatic spread of intraocular melanomas in a nude mouse model of human uveal melanoma. *Curr Eye Res.* 1993;12:347–358.
230. Hendrix MJ, Seftor EA, Seftor RE, Trevor KT. Experimental co-expression of vimentin and keratin intermediate filaments in human breast cancer cells results in phenotypic interconversion and increased invasive behavior. *Am J Pathol.* 1997;150:483–495.
231. Repp AC, Mayhew ES, Howard K, Alizadeh H, Niederkorn JY. Role of fas ligand in uveal melanoma-induced liver damage. *Graefes Arch Clin Exp Ophthalmol.* 2001;239: 752–758.
232. Papetti M, Herman IM. Mechanisms of normal and tumor-derived angiogenesis. *Am J Physiol Cell Physiol.* 2002;282:C947–970.
233. Bashyam MD. Understanding cancer metastasis: an urgent need for using differential gene expression analysis. *Cancer.* 2002;94:1821–1829.

234. Kusters B, Leenders WP, Wesseling P, Smits D, Verrijp K, Ruiter DJ, Peters JP, Van Der Kogel AJ, De Waal RM. Vascular endothelial growth factor-A(165) induces progression of melanoma brain metastases without induction of sprouting angiogenesis. *Cancer Res.* 2002;62:341–345.
235. Folkman J, Hanahan D. Switch to the angiogenic phenotype during tumorigenesis. *Princess Takamatsu Symp.* 1991;22:339–347.
236. Bergers G, Brekken R, McMahon G, Vu TH, Itoh T, Tamaki K, Tanzawa K, Thorpe P, Itohara S, Werb Z, Hanahan D. Matrix metalloproteinase-9 triggers the angiogenic switch during carcinogenesis. *Nat Cell Biol.* 2000;2:737–744.
237. Giordano FJ, Johnson RS. Angiogenesis: the role of the microenvironment in flipping the switch. *Curr Opin Genet Dev.* 2001;11:35–40.
238. Strieth S, Hartschuh W, Pilz L, Fusenig NE. Angiogenic switch occurs late in squamous cell carcinomas of human skin. *Br J Cancer.* 2000;82:591–600.
239. Care A, Felicetti F, Meccia E, Bottero L, Parenza M, Stoppacciaro A, Peschle C, Colombo MP. HOXB7: a key factor for tumor-associated angiogenic switch. *Cancer Res.* 2001;61:6532–6539.
240. Fang J, Shing Y, Wiederschain D, Yan L, Butterfield C, Jackson G, Harper J, Tamvakopoulos G, Moses MA. Matrix metalloproteinase-2 is required for the switch to the angiogenic phenotype in a tumor model. *Proc Natl Acad Sci USA.* 2000;97: 3884–3889.
241. Wen S, Stolarov J, Myers MP, Su JD, Wigler MH, Tonks NK, Durden DL. PTEN controls tumor-induced angiogenesis. *Proc Natl Acad Sci USA.* 2001;98:4622–4627.
242. O'Reilly MS, Holmgren L, Chen C, Folkman J. Angiostatin induces and sustains dormancy of human primary tumors in mice. *Nat Med.* 1996;2:689–692.
243. Ribatti D, Vacca A, Nico B, De Falco G, Giuseppe Montaldo P, Ponzoni M. Angiogenesis and anti-angiogenesis in neuroblastoma. *Eur J Cancer.* 2002;38:750–757.
244. Shepherd FA. Angiogenesis inhibitors in the treatment of lung cancer. Lung *Cancer.* 2001;34 Suppl 3:S81–89.
245. Zogakis TG, Libutti SK. General aspects of anti-angiogenesis and cancer therapy. *Expert Opin Biol Ther.* 2001;1:253–275.
246. Kirsch M, Santarius T, Black PM, Schackert G. Therapeutic anti-angiogenesis for malignant brain tumors. *Onkologie.* 2001;24:423–430.
247. Ellis LM, Liu W, Fan F, Reinmuth N, Shaheen RM, Jung YD, Ahmad S. Role of angiogenesis inhibitors in cancer treatment. *Oncology (Huntingt).* 2001;15(7 Suppl 8):39–46.
248. Rajkumar SV. Current status of thalidomide in the treatment of cancer. *Oncology (Huntingt).* 2001;15:867–874; discussion 877–869.
249. Chen QR, Zhang L, Gasper W, Mixson AJ. Targeting tumor angiogenesis with gene therapy. *Mol Genet Metab.* 2001;74:120–127.
250. Robert EG, Hunt JD. Lipid messengers as targets for antiangiogenic therapy. *Curr Pharm Des.* 2001;7:1615–1626.
251. Baselga J. The EGFR as a target for anticancer therapy—focus on cetuximab. *Eur J Cancer.* 2001;37 Suppl 4:S16–22.
252. Buchsbaum DJ, Curiel DT. Gene therapy for the treatment of cancer. *Cancer Biother Radiopharm.* 2001;16:275–288.
253. Ellis LM, Liu W, Ahmad SA, Fan F, Jung YD, Shaheen RM, Reinmuth N. Overview of angiogenesis: Biologic implications for antiangiogenic therapy. *Semin Oncol.* 2001;28(5 Suppl 16):94–104.
254. Margolin K. Inhibition of vascular endothelial growth factor in the treatment of solid tumors. *Curr Oncol Rep.* 2002;4:20–28.

255. Kieran MW, Billett A. Antiangiogenesis therapy. Current and future agents. *Hematol Oncol Clin North Am.* 2001;15:835–851, viii.
256. Bence AK, Sheehan JB, Adams VR. Antiangiogenesis agents in clinical trials. *J Am Pharm Assoc (Wash).* 2001;41:893–895.
257. Pinedo HM. Advances in the use of angiogenesis inhibitors in cancer. *Cancer J.* 2001;7 Suppl 3:S107–108.
258. Xu XC. COX-2 inhibitors in cancer treatment and prevention, a recent development. *Anticancer Drugs.* 2002;13:127–137.
259. Rosen LS. Clinical experience with angiogenesis signaling inhibitors: focus on vascular endothelial growth factor (VEGF) blockers. *Cancer Control.* 2002;9(2 Suppl):36–44.
260. Li WW, Li VW, Brainerd N, Fagen SJ. Global development of angiogenesis inhibitors for cancer: principles, progress and new paradigms. *Gan To Kagaku Ryoho.* 2002;29 Suppl 1:50–58.
261. Ghilardi C, Bani MR, Giavazzi R. Anticancer therapy with angiogenesis inhibitors. *Tumori.* 2001;87:S14–16.
262. Prewett M, Huber J, Li Y, Santiago A, O'Connor W, King K, Overholser J, Hooper A, Pytowski B, Witte L, Bohlen P, Hicklin DJ. Antivascular endothelial growth factor receptor (fetal liver kinase 1) monoclonal antibody inhibits tumor angiogenesis and growth of several mouse and human tumors. *Cancer Res.* 1999;59:5209–5218.
263. Harmey JH, Bouchier-Hayes D.Vascular endothelial growth factor (VEGF), a survival factor for tumor cells: implications for anti-angiogenic therapy. *Bioessays.* 2002;24: 280–283.
264. Brekken RA, Thorpe PE.Vascular endothelial growth factor and vascular targeting of solid tumors. *Anticancer Res.* 2001;21:4221–4229.
265. Tosetti F, Ferrari N, De Flora S, Albini A. Angioprevention': angiogenesis is a common and key target for cancer chemopreventive agents. *FASEB J.* 2002;16:2–14.
266. Thun MJ, Henley SJ, Patrono C. Nonsteroidal anti-inflammatory drugs as anticancer agents: mechanistic, pharmacologic, and clinical issues. *J Natl Cancer Inst.* 2002;94: 252–266.
267. Gasparini G. Metronomic scheduling: the future of chemotherapy? *Lancet Oncol.* 2001;2:733–740.
268. Zhou S, Kestell P, Tingle MD, Paxton JW. Thalidomide in cancer treatment: a potential role in the elderly? *Drugs Aging.* 2002;19:85–100.
269. Sorokin P. New agents and future directions in biotherapy. *Clin J Oncol Nurs.* 2002;6: 19–24.
270. Rosen LS. Angiogenesis inhibition in solid tumors. *Cancer J.* 2001;7 Suppl 3:S120–128.
271. Burke PA, DeNardo SJ. Antiangiogenic agents and their promising potential in combined therapy. *Crit Rev Oncol Hematol.* 2001;39:155–171.
272. Yu JL, Rak JW, Coomber BL, Hicklin DJ, Kerbel RS. Effect of p53 status on tumor response to antiangiogenic therapy. *Science.* 2002;295:1526–1528.
273. Yu JL, Rak JW, Carmeliet P, Nagy A, Kerbel RS, Coomber BL. Heterogeneous vascular dependence of tumor cell populations. *Am J Pathol.* 2001;158:1325–1334.

ROBERT FOLBERG, JACOB PE'ER AND ANDREW J. MANIOTIS

# 11. Extravascular Matrix Patterns in Uveal Melanoma: Histogenesis, Structure, and Molecular Regulation*

## BACKGROUND

Uveal melanomas are among the few forms of cancer treated before a pathologist reviews tissue samples to assess the likely biological behavior of the lesion. When patients are managed by vision-sparing methods of tumor ablation such as radiation therapy, it is unlikely that tissue from the primary tumor will ever come to analysis—whether the analyses are morphological or molecular. The technique referred to by ophthalmic oncologists as a 'fine-needle aspiration biopsy'[1–4] is typically restricted to one pass or limited numbers of sampling points through the tumor, and is therefore considerably less representative of the lesion that similar biopsy techniques employed elsewhere in the body.[5] Tumors, including uveal melanomas, are characteristically heterogeneous in composition.[6,7] A pathologist cannot assure an oncologist that an ophthalmic limited sample needle biopsy will contain material that is representative of the most aggressive component of the tumor.

In 1984, our group sought to identify physical characteristics of ciliary body and choroidal melanomas that were related to outcome and that would be detectable by non-invasive imaging techniques. It eventually became clear that the clinical detection of cell types according to a modification of the Callender classification relating cellular morphology to outcome was unrealistic because an assessment of cell size and shape was clearly below any expected resolution of medical imaging devices,[8,9] and because the Callender classification, even among experienced ophthalmic pathologists, suffers from limitations in reproducibility.

Therefore, we began to identify histologic patterning within choroidal and ciliary body melanoma that was delimited by PAS-positive extracellular matrix. These matrix patterns were consistently traced back to blood vessels, and some regions the matrix patterning appeared to contain either red blood cells or plasma,[10,11] The hypothesis relating patterning to the tumor microcirculation was supported

* The work summarized herein was supported by a grant R01 EY10457 from the National Eye Institute, Bethesda, Maryland, USA.

by the observation that these patterns labeled, focally and segmentally, with the lectin, *Ulex europaeus* agglutinin I (UEAI).[12] We originally presumed that these patterns represented the remodeled tumor blood vessels, as implied in the titles of our earlier papers.[10,12] Indeed, in our early studies, it appeared that some of these patterns consisted ultrastructurally of thick extracellular matrix lined by cells that we presumed initially to be endothelium merely because we assumed that all cells in contact with blood in a small channel were, by virtue of location, endothelial cells.[10,13] This supposition has undergone radical reinterpretation by us as the histogenesis,[14,15] ultrastructure,[15] three-dimensional configuration,[16] and molecular regulation of pattern formation[14,15,17,18] was delineated.

## EXTRAVASCULAR MATRIX PATTERNS AS A MARKER OF MALIGNANT BEHAVIOR IN UVEAL MELANOMA

Postulating that the interconnecting patterned matrix may represent a new structural characteristic of uveal melanomas that is related to aggressive tumor behavior, we first described the prognostic relationship between what we initially perceived to be 'vascular' loops in two-dimensional sections of choroidal and ciliary body melanomas and outcome.[12] In a subsequent publication,[10] we described the presence of seven patterns of PAS-positive extracellular matrix (arcs without and with branching, loops, networks, parallel without and with cross-linking), the presence of normal pre-existing vessels within the tumors (vascular incorporation), and zone of avascularity, originally called the 'silent' pattern. The detection of these patterns is highly reproducible by pathologists from histological sections[10,19] and prognostic significance of these matrix patterns has been confirmed repeatedly by multiple independent laboratories.[19–23]

## ANGIOGENESIS AND UVEAL MELANOMA

Weidner et al.[24] called to the attention of pathologists the possibility that a focal high density of microvessels (presumably reflective of angiogenesis) in biopsy samples from patients with breast cancer might be predictive of mortality. Other investigators soon followed Weidner's hypothesis, applying the technique to other forms of cancer and utilizing a variety of putative markers for endothelial cells. A number of studies document the success of relating microvascular density (MVD) to outcome[25] but there are also numerous studies in which no relationship between outcome and microvascular density were identified (see review by Folberg et al.)[17].

Foss et al.[26,27] assessed vascularity in choroidal and ciliary body melanomas by staining these tumors for Factor VIII related antigen (F8rAg) and calculated the MVD by counting discrete foci of F8rAg staining in hot spots within the tumor following the methods of Weidner et al.[24] (who had studied the relationship of microvascular density to outcome breast cancer). Foss et al.[27] also recorded the presence of absence or looping patterns and concluded that (a) the patterns did not label with F8rAg and were therefore not vessels and could not contribute to perfusion; (b) the patterns were 'fibrovascular septa'; and (c) the patterns were not even independent prognostic indicators of metastasis.

Mäkitie et al.[19,28] who concluded that *both* MVD and PAS-positive patterns were independent predictors of metastasis discovered that Foss et al.[26,27] had underreported the incidence of PAS-positive patterns in uveal melanomas and thus concluded that Foss et al.[26,27] did not identify these patterns correctly—mistaking thick bundles of fibrovascular connective tissue for the PAS-positive looping patterns. In an ultrastructural study of looping patterns performed in an animal xenograft, Clarijs et al.[29] reported that the patterns were rich in collagen and contained blood vessels, leading to the conclusion that these patterns were fibrovascular septa and therefore a host response rather than being generated directly by aggressive tumor cells.[30] Fibrovascular septa no doubt exist in human uveal melanomas, but they are encountered uncommonly,[19,28] and as Foss et al. showed, they are not of prognostic significance, in contrast to the prognostic significance of PAS-positive patterns demonstrated by numerous independent groups.[19,20,22,23,31,32] Furthermore, recent data correlating the *in vitro* behavior of human uveal melanoma cells with human tissue samples refutes the assumption that we initially held—that these patterns represented blood vessels—and the assumption that these patterns represent a host response of fibrovascular septa.

## UNDERSTANDING THE HISTOGENESIS OF PATTERN GENERATION

Maniotis et al.[14,15,33] designed a series of experiments to reconstitute these patterns *in vitro*. Highly aggressive primary and metastatic uveal melanoma cells formed looping patterns rich in extracellular matrix in 3D cultures containing Matrigel or dilute Type I collagen (Type I collagen is the dominant choroidal collagen type). These patterns were identical morphologically to PAS-positive patterns in tumors of patients at high risk for metastasis. These patterns were formed by the aggressive melanoma cells in the absence of endothelial cells or fibroblasts. These *in vitro* observations were consistent with observations by us[14,15,17] and Foss et al.[26,27] that the looping patterns tend not to label with endothelial markers in tissue sections. Poorly aggressive uveal melanoma cells did not make these patterns under identical culture conditions, even after the addition of conditioned media from aggressive melanoma cell lines, soluble growth factors (including bFGF, TGF-β, VEGF-A, and PDGF) and relative regimes of hypoxia.[14,15] The formation of looping matrix-rich patterns by aggressive uveal melanoma cells is regulated by matrix thickness.[15] The generation of looping patterns by aggressive cell lines but not by non-aggressive cell lines was consistent with repeated observations from human tissue samples linking the presence of patterns to other aggressive tumor characteristics (e.g., cell type) and to metastasis.[19–23,31,32]

When aggressive uveal melanoma cells were co-cultured with a wide variety of endothelial cells, the endothelial cells survived only very briefly when in direct contact with the laminin-positive patterns but were lysed rapidly elsewhere.[15] This observation is not unexpected: if aggressive cancer cells are locally destructive of the host microenvironment, then one would not expect new endothelial cell sprouts to grow directly into the aggressive tumor cell compartment that generates laminin-positive, PAS-positive looping patterns. Thus, angiogenesis in uveal melanoma

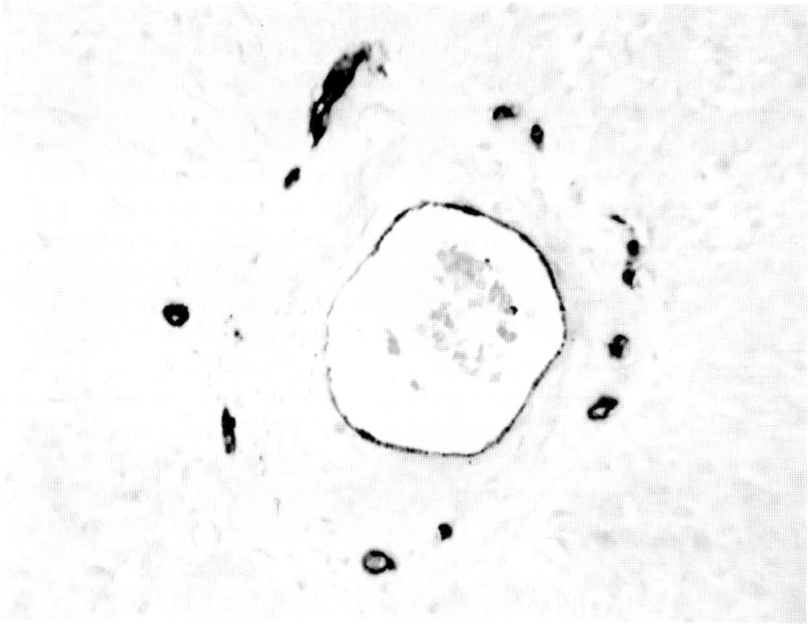

Fig. 11.1. Angiogenesis in retinoblastoma. Numerous small vessels are identified surrounding a larger vessel. As is typical of angiogenesis, the vessels appear as either circles (cross-sections of tubes) or ellipses (tangential sections of tubes). CD34, Vector Purple, ×20 original magnification.

may develop adjacent to highly aggressive tumor cell populations but most likely develops within less aggressive components of the tumor. This is consistent with the observation by Foss et al.[27] that looping fibrovascular septa in uveal melanoma are not associated with an aggressive clinical course. It is therefore important to distinguish between the host response—fibrovascular septa—and the laminin-rich, PAS-positive patterns generated by aggressive melanoma cells.

The ultrastructure of PAS-positive patterns was examined in detail using human primary uveal melanoma tissue that was fixed in glutaraldehyde. The patterns were found to be composed of a sandwich of electron dense material (consistent with laminin) on either side of tumor cells, remarkably consistent with the appearance of patterns formed by aggressive melanoma cells *in vitro.* Although the patterns may contain red blood cells, the patterns are, therefore, clearly not blood vessels.[15] Furthermore, the patterns in human tissue samples are not rich in Type I collagen ultrastructurally, nor do they contain fibroblasts,[15] data that contradicts observations made from the animal xenograft model[29] and challenges the assumption[30] that these patterns are host-derived 'fibrovascular septa.' Because the looping patterns are clearly not blood vessels (Fig. 11.1 illustrates angiogenesis in retinoblastoma) and are *extra* vascular, we now designate looping and interconnected PAS-positive patterns (Fig. 11.2) as *extravascular matrix patterns* or EMPs.

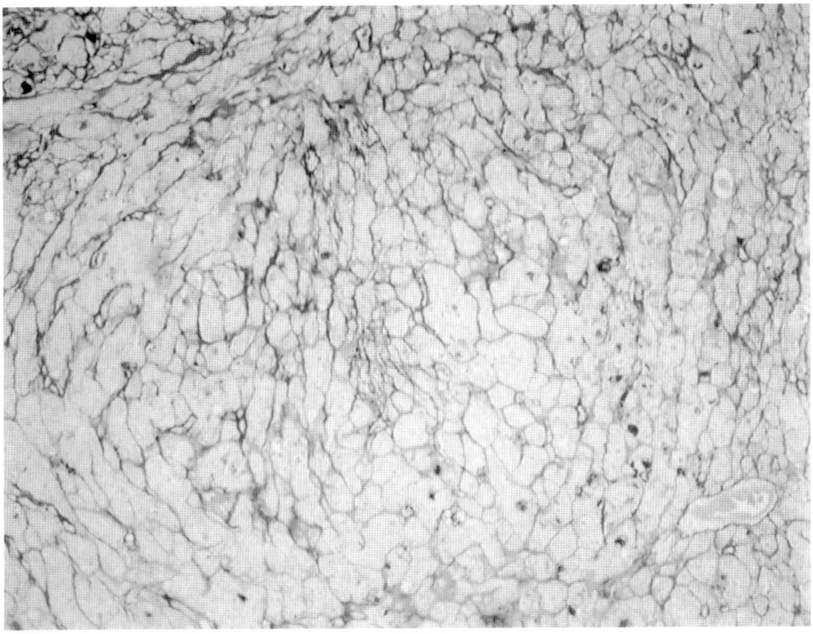

Fig. 11.2. Patterned matrix in melanoma forming networks of back-to-back loops. The matrix is thin and partitions the tumor into clusters which may represent spheroids three-dimensionally. PAS without hematoxylin, ×10 original magnification.

## EXTRAVASCULAR MATRIX PATTERNS AS A PERFUSION SYSTEM IN UVEAL MELANOMAS

In mature three-dimensional cultures, Maniotis et al.[14,15,17] also observed that the PAS-positive patterns formed *in vitro* were able to conduct dye over distances following *in vitro* microinjection. These observations suggested a radical idea—that the PAS-positive patterns detected in human tumors, in which red blood cells and plasma had been identified, might contribute to a functional tumor perfusion. Potgens et al. [34] observed tracer material within looping patterns of heparin sulfate proteoglycan (HSPG) in an animal model utilizing a xenograft of cutaneous melanoma. Most importantly, makers for endothelial cells did not co-localize to the looping HSPG patterns that conducted fluorescent tracer, suggesting that the HSPG patterns provided a mechanism for the distribution of fluid from the circulation throughout the tumor independent of endothelial cell lined blood vessels. This experiment was later repeated by Clarijs et al. [29] using a xenotransplant of uveal melanoma. Tumors contained looping EMPs perfused by plasma. Clarijs et al.[29] proposed that these PAS, laminin-positive[15] patterns formed a 'fluid-conducting meshwork.' Parenthetically, Mueller et al.[35] have since developed an orthotopic model of aggressive human uveal melanoma containing laminin-rich extravascular matrix patterns by injecting suspensions of uveal melanoma cells into the suprachoroidal space of SCID mice eyes.

To investigate the possibility that plasma circulates in EMPs in human tumors, we double labeled human uveal melanoma tissue for laminin and fibrinogen, using fibrinogen as a surrogate for plasma. Fibrinogen co-localized to the looping laminin-positive patterns that anastomosed to blood vessels.[15] It is not likely that the antibody directed to fibrinogen detected fibrin because transmission electron microscopy failed to demonstrate fibrin in the patterns (fibrin has a characteristic ultrastructural morphology).[36] Over-expression of TFPI 1,2 by aggressive uveal melanoma cells that generate the extravascular matrix patterns[37] may help to explain failure of fibrinogen to polymerize to fibrin.

Further evidence that these patterns play a role in providing a functional circulation came from studies in human patients performed by Mueller et al.[38,39] These investigators injected indocyanine green into the antecubital vein of patients with posterior choroidal melanomas and demonstrated the presence of looping channels in these tumors by means of laser scanning confocal angiography within 15 seconds after injection. In one clinicopathologic correlation, the presence of looping patterns angiographically was documented by the presence of looping PAS-positive matrix patterns after this tumor had been removed and microdissected in the same vicinity as the component of the tumor imaged angiographically; in another patient with posterior choroidal melanoma that lacked looping patterns angiographically, the histological sections through the imaged portion of the tumor revealed only normal choroidal vessels, matching the angiographic image.

The angiographic-histologic correlation studies suggested that confocal angiography might be useful in detecting looping patterns in uveal melanoma. Indeed, in a prospective evaluation of patients studied by indocyanine green confocal angiography, the detection of looping microcirculation patterns was the strongest predictor of tumor growth[40] and was shown in a subsequent study to be predictive of a rapid response of tumor to radiation therapy.[41]

The clinical detection of extravascular matrix patterns may present ophthalmologists with a non-invasive substitute for biopsy to permit patients to be classified into risk categories for metastasis, a development that may be increasingly important in an era of management that emphasizes vision-sparing treatments of uveal melanoma rather than enucleation. The analysis of raw radiofrequency data by ultrasound power spectrum analysis may provide a non-invasive means of detecting extravascular matrix patterns in patients that is independent of any perfusion properties held by the patterns.[42–44]

## VASCULOGENIC MIMICRY

In angiogenesis, new blood vessels are generated from existing vessels; in vasculogenesis, vessels are generated *de novo*. The generation of perfusable extravascular matrix patterns or perfusable tubes by aggressive tumor cells *de novo* is neither angiogenesis nor vasculogenesis: the structures formed are clearly not blood vessels and the process merely *mimics* the development of a vascular perfusion system *de novo*. We[14,17] developed the term 'vasculogenic mimicry' to describe the process by which aggressive tumor cells generate such a non-vascular perfusion system *de novo*. There are two forms of vasculogenic mimicry: extravascular matrix patterns (EMP) and tubes. Both may co-exist with incorporated vessels, mosaic vessels, and angiogenic vessels in tumors.[45]

A commentary by McDonald et al.,[46] published in the *American Journal of Pathology*, criticized the concept of vasculogenic mimicry. The journal's editor, however, published an essay,[47] conceding that critique by McDonald et al.[46] contained factual errors. McDonald et al.[46] claimed that our failure to label the extravascular matrix patterns with endothelial cell markers was an artifact (despite illustrating internal positive controls).[17] In four studies, others[29,34,48,49] also failed to label the patterned extravascular matrix with endothelial cell markers. McDonald and Foss[50] studied uveal melanomas by transmission electron microscopy and immunohistochemistry and concluded that 100% of tumor vessels are lined by endothelial cells. This claim was particularly intriguing because in the same year that McDonald and Foss[50] claimed that all tumor vessels were lined by endothelial cells, McDonald was the corresponding author of a paper[51] that used the term 'vessel lining cells' instead of endothelial cells: 'In the present study, we have cautiously referred to the lining cells of tumor vessels, rather than assuming that these cells are endothelial cells. Definitive identification of the lining cells, particularly the branched phenotype, awaits unambiguous ultrastructural localization with the appropriate cell markers. There is no consensus on the single best marker of endothelial cells.' How, then, can anyone state with certainty that *all* tumor blood vessels are lined by endothelial cells?

## THE AMBIGUITY ENDOTHELIAL CELL MARKERS: MICROVASCULAR DENSITY (MVD) REVISITED

There are precedents for being circumspect about the identity of cells lining tumor blood vessels. Ultrastructurally, thin branches of tumor cells may appear identical to endothelial cells.[52] Immunohistochemistry may also be inconclusive. We illustrated this by showing CD31 labeling uveal melanoma cells;[17] Hendrix et al.[53] showed expression of VE-cadherin by uveal melanoma cells. These findings are not unique. The ECV 304 line was used by investigators as an 'immortalized HUVEC' line because it expressed F8rAg, contained Weibel-Palade bodies, and formed tubes on Matrigel.[54,55] It was recently discovered that the ECV 304 line was derived from the bladder carcinoma line T14.[56]

In human uveal melanoma tissue sections, we[45] detected tumor cells positive for melanoma markers (eg., S100 protein, Melan-A) that also labeled with CD34, considered to be most reliable maker for the uveal melanoma microcirculation.[28] MVD is calculated by counting discrete staining for putative endothelial cell markers. We[45] stained 200 uveal melanomas for both CD34 and S100 protein and, like Foss et al.[26] and Mäkitie et al.[28] showed that MVD was an independent marker of metastatic behavior. However, as MVD increased, so did the co-localization of CD34 in S100-positive melanoma cells. Therefore, tumor MVD quantifies not only blood vessels, including angiogenic vessels, but also tumor cells that inappropriately label for endothelial cell markers.[45]

## THE HETEROGENEOUS COMPOSITION OF THE UVEAL MELANOMA MICROCIRCULATION

In the course of double-labeling human primary uveal melanoma tissue samples with endothelial cell markers and markers for melanoma cells, we[45] demonstrated the existence of mosaic vessels in these tumors: vessels which are lined in part by endothelial cells and in part by tumor cells. Hammersen et al.[57] illustrated tumor cells within the lining of blood vessels in melanoma xenografts previously. Recently, Chang et al.[58] documented that 15% of the vessels in animal models of colon carcinoma and in human colon biopsy specimens were lined by endothelial cells *and* tumor cells, a condition they termed 'mosaicism'. These findings were consistent with the shedding of $10^6$ tumor cells per day into the microcirculation and Folkman[59] commented that mosaicism might contribute significantly to metastasis.

Thus, the uveal melanoma microcirculation may be complex and heterogeneous in composition, including angiogenic vessels, mosaic vessels, and incorporated vessels. Skinner et al.[60] described the incorporation of pre-existing vessels into experimental rat colon carcinoma. Holash et al.[61] described incorporation of pre-existing vessels in an animal model of aggressive glioma and termed this process *co-option*. Recently, Passalidou et al.[62] described a form of human non-small cell carcinoma of the lung that derived its blood supply completely from incorporation of pre-existing alveolar capillaries. Leenders et al.[63] reported co-option in an animal model of cutaneous melanoma. There is abundant evidence for vessel incorporation in uveal melanocytic neoplasia. In a model of primary uveal melanocytic lesions induced by topical application of 7,12-dimethylbenz[a]anthracene (DMBA) to the rabbit eye, nevi and small melanomas were generated: the melanocytes expanded the choroid and grew around normal pre-existing vessels.[64,65] It has been known for many years that human choroidal nevi contain incorporated choroidal vessels.[66] Incorporated vessels are documented in 55–97% of primary human choroidal and ciliary body melanomas.[10,19]

To the list of these perfusion pathways—incorporated vessels, angiogenic vessels, and mosaic vessels—we add non-vascular extravascular matrix patterns, generated by the aggressive uveal melanoma cells through the pathway of vasculogenic mimicry. Although angiogenesis may be a very important mechanism by which uveal melanomas acquire a vasculature, strategies that either target the vasculature as a means of therapy or that exploit the vasculature to deliver therapeutic agents must take into account *all* pathways by which human uveal melanomas establish and maintain perfusion[63]—including perfusable extravascular matrix patterns.

## EVIDENCE OF VASCULOGENIC MIMICRY IN CANCERS OTHER THAN UVEAL MELANOMA

Rummelt et al.[67] had suggested that the histologic presence of PAS-positive networks in conjunctival melanoma was associated with an adverse outcome. Stenback et al.[68] had described looping patterns of extracellular matrix in cutaneous melanoma, and there was a report of PAS-positive loops in a focus of metastatic cutaneous melanoma.[69] Warso et al.[70] discovered that networks, loops and parallel with cross-linking patterns was significantly associated with decreased disease-free survival in cutaneous melanoma, a finding subsequently confirmed by Thies et al.[71]

Vasculogenic mimicry has been reported in inflammatory breast cancer.[48,49,72] There is also now evidence of vasculogenic mimicry in ovarian carcinoma,[73] prostate cancer,[74] synovial sarcoma, and alveolar rhabdomyosarcoma.[75]

## THE TOPOLOGY OF PERFUSED EXTRAVASCULAR MATRIX PATTERN: IMPLICATIONS FOR DIAGNOSTICS AND THERAPEUTICS

The topology of the patterned extravascular matrix is far different from blood vessels. In two dimensional tissue sections, these PAS and laminin-positive patterns may be divided into two hierarchical morphological groupings: a curved group that includes arcs, arcs with branching, loops and networks of back to back loops, and a straight group that includes straight, parallel and cross-linking parallel patterns.[76] There was considerable speculation about the three-dimensional configuration of these patterns[77]: we[16] and others[46] proposed that the curved patterns in two dimensions represented sections through spheroidal nests of tumor cells that were surrounded by PAS-positive/laminin-positive material. The hypothesis of a spheroidal configuration did not account for the existence of the straight hierarchy of patterns including the parallel with cross-linking pattern.

Recently, the extravascular matrix patterns in human uveal melanoma were reconstructed from serial sections labeled for laminin and studied by laser scanning confocal microscopy in a three-dimensional immersive environment. These preliminary reconstructions clearly distinguished blood vessels (which anastomose to these patterns) from the patterns themselves, and showed the patterns to represent wrappings around cylindrical rather than spheroidal nests of tumor cells. Moreover, the cylinders of tumor cells divide and branch.[16] The cylindrical arrangement of the laminin-positive material is consistent with the *in vitro* generation of these patterns in thick matrix and with the appearance of both looping patterns and parallel and cross-linking parallel patterns in two-dimensional tissue sections. The co-localization of fibrinogen to these cylindrical wrappings[16] suggests that the perfused surface area in extravascular matrix patterns may be significantly greater than the area provided by tumor blood vessels.

## EXTRAVASCULAR MATRIX PATTERNS: ADDITIONAL IMPLICATIONS AND FUTURE DIRECTIONS

Few patients die of uveal melanoma without the primary tumor containing looping EMPs.[10] Moreover, EMPs are present in all sites of metastatic uveal melanoma.[78] Nevertheless, one may argue that the presence of these patterns is merely a marker of aggressive tumor cells and that the patterns play no role in metastasis. The following observations, however, support a mechanistic role for the patterns in metastasis. Tumor cells are embedded within the looping matrix patterns which connect to tumor vessels.[15] Aggressive melanoma cells migrate along laminin-positive looping scaffolds.[79] Thus, the extravascular matrix patterns, in which aggressive tumor cells are embedded, are scaffolds along which tumor cells migrate toward blood vessels. Folkman[59] stated that the exposure of tumor cells to the circulation in mosaic vessels (tumor vessels lined by both endothelial cells and tumor cells)[58] facilitates metastasis. Therefore, by analogy, metastasis would be facilitated by melanoma cells contained within the plasma-perfused extravascular matrix patterns. Primary uveal melanomas contain vessels that are incorporated into the tumor, angiogenic and mosaic vessels, and extravascular patterned matrix.[45] Treatment targeting only perfusion pathway (e.g., angiogenic vessels) may still permit hematogenous dissemination through other paths including the extravascular matrix patterns (present in 88% of primary tumors of patients who die of metastatic uveal melanoma).[10] Moreover, the discovery that these patterns conduct plasma and blood raises the possibility of exploiting this system to deliver drugs and other therapeutic agents to aggressive primary tumors and their metastases.

## REFERENCES


1. Augsburger JJ, Shields JA, Folberg R, Lang WR, O'Hara BJ, Claricci JD. Fine needle aspiration biopsy in the diagnosis of intraocular cancer cytologic–histologic correlations. *Ophthalmology* 1985;92:39–49.
2. Char DH, Kroll SM, Stoloff A, Kaleta-Michaels S, Crawford JB, Miller TR, Howes EL, Jr., Ljung BM. Cytomorphometry of uveal melanoma. Comparison of fine needle aspiration biopsy samples with histologic sections. *Anal Quant Cytol Histol.* 1991;13:293–299.
3. Shields JA, Shields CL, Ehya H, Eagle RC, Jr., De Potter P. Fine-needle aspiration biopsy of suspected intraocular tumors. The 1992 Urwick Lecture. *Ophthalmology.* 1993;100:1677–1684.
4. Eide N, Syrdalen P, Walaas L, Hagmar B. Fine needle aspiration biopsy in selecting treatment for inconclusive intraocular disease. *Acta Ophthalmol Scand.* 1999;77:448–452.
5. DeMay RM. *The Art and Science of Cytopathology.* 1996; Chicago: ASCP Press.
6. Hart IR, Fidler IJ. The implications of tumor heterogeneity for studies on the biology and therapy of cancer metastasis. *Biochim Biophys Acta.* 1981;651:37–50.
7. Yoon SS, Fidler IJ, Beltran PJ, Bucana CD, Wang YF, Fan D. Intratumoral heterogeneity for epigenetic modulation of MDR-1 expression in murine melanoma. *Melanoma Res.* 1997;7:275–287.
8. Coleman DJ, Silverman RH, Rondeau MJ, Lizzi FL, McLean IW, Jakobiec FA. Correlations of acoustic tissue typing of malignant melanoma and histopathologic features as a predictor of death. *Am J Ophthalmol.* 1990;110:380–388.
9. Coleman DJ, Silverman RH, Rondeau MJ, Coleman JA, Rosberger D, Ellsworth RM, Lizzi FL. Ultrasonic tissue characterization of uveal melanoma and prediction of patient survival after enucleation and brachytherapy. *Am J Ophthalmol.* 1991;112:682–688.
10. Folberg R, Rummelt V, Parys-Van Ginderdeuren R, Hwang T, Woolson RF, Pe'er J, Gruman LM. The prognostic value of tumor blood vessel morphology in primary uveal melanoma. *Ophthalmology.* 1993;100:1389–1398.
11. Folberg R, Mehaffey M, Gardner LM, Meyer M, Rummelt V, Pe'er J. The microcirculation of choroidal and ciliary body melanomas. *Eye.* 1997;11:227–238.
12. Folberg R, Pe'er J, Gruman LM, Woolson RF, Jeng G, Montague PR, Moninger TO, Yi H, Moore KC. The morphologic characteristics of tumor blood vessels as a marker of tumor progression in primary human uveal melanoma: a matched case-control study. *Hum Pathol.* 1992;23:1298–1305.

13. Rummelt V, Folberg R, Rummelt C, Gruman LM, Hwang T, Woolson RF, Yi H, Naumann GOH. Microcirculation architecture of melanocytic nevi and malignant melanomas of the ciliary body and choroid. A comparative histopathologic and ultrastructural study. *Ophthalmology* 1994;101:718–727.
14. Maniotis AJ, Folberg R, Hess A, Seftor EA, Gardner LMG, Pe'er J, Trent JM, Meltzer PS, Hendrix MJC. Vascular channel formation by human melanoma cells *in vivo* and *in vitro*: vasculogenic mimicry. *Am J Pathol.* 1999;155:739–752.
15. Maniotis AJ, Chen X, Garcia C, DeChristopher PJ, Wu D, Pe'er J, Folberg R. Control of melanoma morphogenesis, endothelial survival, and perfusion by extracellular matrix. *Lab Invest.* 2002;82:1031–1043.
16. Chen X, Ai Z, Rasmussen M, Bajesy P, Auvil L, Welge M, Leach L, Vangveeravongs S, Maniotis AJ, Fohlberg R. Three-dimensional reconstruction of extravascular matrix patterns and blood vessels in human uveal melanoma tissue: techniques and preliminary findings. *Invest Ophthalmol Vis Sci.* 2003;44:2834–2840.
17. Folberg R, Hendrix MJ, Maniotis AJ. Vasculogenic mimicry and tumor angiogenesis. *Am J Pathol.* 2000;156:361–381.
18. Seftor EA, Meltzer PS, Kirschmann DA, Pe'er J, Maniotis AJ, Trent JM, Folberg R, Hendrix MJC, Molecular determinants of human uveal melanoma invasion and metastasis. *Clin Exp Metastasis.* 2002;19: 233–246.
19. Mäkitie T, Summanen P, Tarkannen A, Kivelä T. Microvascular loops and networks as prognostic indicators in choroidal and ciliary body melanomas. *J Natl Cancer Inst.* 1999;91:359–367.
20. Sakamoto T, Sakamoto M, Yoshikawa H, Hata Y, Ishibashi T, Ohnishi Y, Inomata H. Histologic findings and prognosis of uveal malignant melanoma in Japanese patients. *Am J Ophthalmol.* 1996;121:276–283.
21. Schaling DF, Van der Pol JP, Schlingemann RO, Parys-Van Ginderdeuren R, Ruiter DJ, Jager MJ. Vascular density and vascular patterns in the prognosis of choroidal melanoma. In: Schaling DF, ed. *Radionucleotides and Radiolabelled Antibodies in Choroidal Melanoma (Diagnosis and Therapy).* Thesis, Leiden: Rijksuniversiteit te Leiden, 1996, pp. 1–64.
22. McLean IW, Keefe KS, Burnier MN. Uveal melanoma: comparison of the prognostic value of fibrovascular loops, mean of the ten largest nucleoli, cell type and tumor size. *Ophthalmology.* 1997;104:777–780.
23. Seregard S, Spangberg B, Juul C, Oskarsson M. Prognostic accuacy of the mean of the largest nucleoli, vascular patterns, and PC-10 in posterior uveal melanoma. *Ophthalmology.* 1998; 105:485–491.
24. Weidner N, Semple JP, Welch WR, Folkman J. Tumor angiogenesis and metastasis—correlation in invasive breast carcinoma. *N Engl J Med.* 1991;324:1–8.
25. Weidner N. Tumoral vascularity as a prognostic factor in cancer patients—the evidence continues to grow. *J Pathol.* 1998;184:119–122.
26. Foss AJE, Alexander RA, Jefferies LW, Hungerford JL, Harris AL, Lightman S. Microvessel count predicts survival in uveal melanoma. *Cancer Res.* 1996;56:2900–2903.
27. Foss AJE, Alexander RA, Hungerford JL, Harris AL, Cree IA, Lightman S. Re-assessment of the PAS patterns in uveal melanoma. *Br J Ophthalmol.* 1997;81:240–246.
28. Mäkitie T, Summanen P, Tarkkanen A, Kivelä T. Microvascular density in predicting survival of patients with choroidal and ciliary body melanoma. *Invest Ophthalmol Vis Sci.* 1999;40:2471–2480.
29. Clarijs R, Otte-Höller I, Ruiter DJ, De Waal RM. Presence of a fluid-conducting meshwork in xenografted cutaneous and primary human uveal melanoma. *Invest Ophthalmol Vis Sci.* 2002;43:912–918.

30. Ruiter D, Bogenrieder T, Elder D, Herlyn M. Melanoma-stroma interactions: structural and functional aspects. *Lancet Oncol.* 2002;3:35–43.
31. Schaling DF, Oosterhuis JA, Jager MJ, Kakebeeke-Kemme H, Pauwels EKJ. Possibilities and limitations of radioimmunoscintigraphy and conventional diagnostic modalities in choroidal melanoma. *Br J Ophthalmol.* 1994;78:244–248.
32. Loeffler KU, McLean IW. Membrane patterns, Factor VIII staining and prognosis in 100 cases of human uveal melanoma. *Invest Ophthalmol Vis Sci.* 2001;42 (suppl)[4]:S216.
33. Folberg R, Chen X, Boldt HC, Pe'er J, Brown CK, Woolson RF, Maniotis, AJ. Microcirculation patterns other than loops and networks in choroidal and ciliary body melanomas. *Ophthalmology.* 2001;108:996–1001.
34. Potgens AJG, Van Altena MC, Lubsen NH, Ruiter DJ, De Waal RMW. Analysis of the tumor vasculature and metastatic behavior of xenografts of human melanoma cell lines transfected with vascular permeability factor. *Am J Pathol.* 1996;148:1203–1217.
35. Mueller AJ, Maniotis AJ, Freeman WR, Bartsch DU, Schaller UC, Bergeron-Lynn G, Cheng L, Taskintura I, Chen X, Kan-Mitchell J, Folberg R. An orthotopic model for human uveal melanoma in SCID mice. *Microvasc Res.* 2002;64:207–213.
36. Nagy JA, Brown LF, Senger DR, Lanir N, Van de Water L, Dvorak AM, Dvorak HF. Pathogenesis of tumor stroma generation: a critical role for leaky blood vessels and fibrin deposition. *Biochim Biophys Acta.* 1989;948: 305–326.
37. Seftor EA, Meltzer PS, Kirschmann DA, Pe'er J, Maniotis AJ, Trent JM, Folberg R, Hendrix MJC. Molecular determinants of uveal melanoma metastasis. *Clin Exp Metastasis.* 2002;19:233–246.
38. Mueller AJ, Freeman WR, Folberg R, Bartsch DU, Scheider A, Schaller U, Kampik A. Evaluation of microvascularization pattern visibility in human choroidal melanomas: comparison of confocal fluorescein with indocyanine green angiography. *Graefes Arch Clin Exp Ophthalmol.* 1999;237:448–456.
39. Mueller AJ, Bartsch DU, Folberg R, Mehaffey MG, Boldt HC, Meyer M, Gardner LM, Goldbaum MH, Peer J, Freeman WR. Imaging the microvasculature of choroidal melanomas with confocal indocyanine green scanning laser ophthalmoscopy. *Arch Ophthalmol.* 1998;116:31–39.
40. Mueller AJ, Schaller U, Freeman W, Folberg R, Kampik A. Complex microcirculation patterns detected by confocal Indocyanine green angiography predict time to growth of small choroidal melanocytic tumors. MuSIC-Report II. *Ophthalmology.* 2002;109: 2207–2214.
41. Schaller UC, Mueller AJ, Bartsch DU, Schaumberger M, Freeman WR, Kampik A. Correlation of networks in the ICG angiography with regression rate of uveal melanomas after brachytherapy. *Ophthalmologe.* 2002;99:545–548.
42. Coleman DJ, Rondeau MJ, Silverman RH, Folberg R, Rummelt V, Woods SM, Lizzi FL. Correlation of microcirculation architecture with ultrasound parameters of uveal melanoma. *Eur J Ophthalmol.* 1995;5:96–106.
43. Silverman RH, Folberg R, Boldt HC, Rondeau MJ, Lloyd HO, Mehaffey MG, Lizzi FL, Coleman DJ. Correlation of ultrasound parameter imaging with microcirculatory patterns in uveal melanomas. *Ultrasound Med Biol.* 1997;23:573–581.
44. Silverman RH, Folberg R, Rondeau MJ, Boldt HC, Lloyd HO, Chen X, Lizzi FL, Weingeist TA, Coleman DJ. Detection of prognostically significant histologic features in uveal melanoma with backscatter spectrum analysis. *Ultrasound Med Biol.* In press.
45. Chen X, Maniotis AJ, Majumdar D, Pe'er J, Folberg R. Uveal melanoma cell staining for CD34 and assessment of tumor vascularity. *Invest Ophthalmol Vis Sci.* 2002;43: 2533–2539.

46. McDonald DM, Munn L, Jain RK.Vasculogenic mimicry: how convincing, how novel, and how significant? *Am J Pathol.* 2000;156:383–388.
47. Fausto N.Vasculogenic mimicry in tumors. Fact or artifact? *Am J Pathol.* 2000;156:359.
48. Shirakawa K, Tsuda H, Heike Y, Kato K, Asada R, Inomata M, Sasaki H, Kasumi F, Yoshimoto M, Iwanaga T, Konishi F, Terada M, Wakasugi H. Absence of endothelial cells, central necrosis, and fibrosis are associated with aggressive inflammatory breast cancer. *Cancer Res.* 2001;61:445–451.
49. Shirakawa K, Kobayashi H, Heike Y, Kawamoto S, Brechbiel MW, Kasumi F, Iwanaga T, Konishi F, Terada M, Wakasugi H. Hemodynamics in vasculogenic mimicry and angiogenesis of inflammatory breast cancer xenograft. *Cancer Res.* 2002;62:560–566.
50. McDonald DM, Foss AJE. Endothelial cells of tumor vessels: Abnormal but not absent. *Cancer Metastasis Rev.* 2000;19:109–120.
51. Hashizume H, Baluk P, Morikawa S, McLean JW, Thurston G, Roberge S, Jain RK, McDonald DM. Openings between defective endothelial cells explain tumor vessel leakiness. *Am J Pathol.* 2000;156:1363–1380.
52. Konerding MA, Steinberg F, Budach V. The vascular system of xenotransplanted tumors–scanning electron and light microscopic studies. *Scanning Microsc.* 1989;3: 327–335.
53. Hendrix MJ, Seftor EA, Meltzer PS, Gardner LM, Hess AR, Kirschmann DA, Schatteman GC, Seftor RE. Expression and functional significance of VE-cadherin in aggressive human melanoma cells: role in vasculogenic mimicry. *Proc Natl Acad Sci USA.* 2001;98:8018–8023.
54. Takahashi K, Sawasaki Y, Hata J, Mukai K, Goto T. Spontaneous transformation and immortalization of human endothelial cells. *In Vitro Cell Dev Biol.* 1990;26:265–274.
55. Hughes SE. Functional characterization of the spontaneously transformed human umbilical vein endothelial cell line ECV304: use in an *in vitro* model of angiogenesis. *Exp Cell Res.* 1996;225:171–185.
56. Lucas M, Rose PE, Morris AG. Contrasting effects of HSP72 expression on apoptosis in human umbilical vein endothelial cells and an angiogenic cell line, ECV304. *Br J Haematol.* 2000;110:957–964.
57. Hammersen F, Endrich B, Messmer K. The fine structure of tumor blood vessels. I. Participation of non-endothelial cells in tumor angiogenesis. *Int J Microcirc Clin Exp.* 1985;4:31–43.
58. Chang YS, di Tomaso E, McDonald DM, Jones R, Jain RK, Munn LL. Mosaic blood vessels in tumor: frequency of cancer cells in contact with flowing blood. *Proc Nat. Acad Sci USA.* 2000;97:14608–14613.
59. Folkman J. Can mosaic tumor vessels facilitate molecular diagnosis of cancer? *Proc Natl Acad Sci USA.* 2001;98:398–400.
60. Skinner SA, Tutton PJM, O'Brien PE. Microvascular architecture of experimental colon tumors in the rat. *Cancer Res.* 1990;50:2411–2417.
61. Holash J, Maisonpierre PC, Compton D, Boland P, Alexander CR, Zagzag D, Yancopoulos GD, Wiegand SJ. Vessel cooption, regression, and growth in tumors mediated by angiopoietins and VEGF. *Science.* 1999;284:1994–1998.
62. Passalidou E, Trivella M, Singh N, Ferguson M, Hu J, Cesario A, Granone P, Nicholson AG, Goldstraw P, Ratcliffe C, Tetlow M, Leigh I, Harris AL, Gatter KC, Pezzella F. Vascular phenotype in angiogenic and non-angiogenic lung non-small cell carcinomas. *Br J Cancer.* 2002;86:244–249.
63. Leenders WPJ, Kusters B, De Waal RMW. Vessel co-option: How tumors obtain blood supply in the absence of sprouting angiogenesis. *Endothelium.* 2002;9:83–87.

64. Folberg R, Baron J, Reeves RD, Stevens RH, Tse DT. Primary melanocytic lesions of the rabbit choroid following topical application of 7,12-dimethylbenz[a]anthracene: preliminary observations. *J Toxicol Cutan Ocul Toxicol.* 1990;9:313–334.
65. Pe'er J, Folberg R, Massicotte SJ, Baron J, Parys-Van Ginderdeuren R, Zimmerman B, Meyer ML, Worsey H. Clinicopathologic spectrum of primary uveal melanocytic lesions in an animal model. *Ophthalmology.* 1992; 99:977–986.
66. Naumann G, Yanoff M, Zimmerman LE. Histogenesis of malignant melanomas of the uvea I Histopathologic characteristics of nevi of the choroid and ciliary body. *Arch Ophthalmol.* 1966;76:784–796.
67. Rummelt V, Axmacher K, Folberg R et al. Microcirculation patterns as prognostc factor in conjunctival melanoma. *Invest Ophthalmol Vis Sci.* 1997;38: S807.
68. Stenback F, Wasenius VM. Occurrence of basement membranes in pigment cell tumors of the skin, relation to cell type and clinical behavior. *J Cutan Pathol.* 1986;13:175–186.
69. Nowak MA, Fatteh SM, Campbell TE. Glycogen-rich malignant melanomas and glycogen-rich balloon cell malignant melanomas—frequency and pattern of PAS posivity in primary and metastatic melanomas. *Arch Pathol Lab Med.* 1998;122:353–360.
70. Warso MA, Maniotis AJ, Chen X, Majumdar D, Patel MK, Shilkaitis A, Gupta TK, Folberg R. Prognostic significance of periodic acid-Schiff-positive patterns in primary cutaneous melanoma. *Clin Cancer Res.* 2001;7:473–477.
71. Thies A, Mangold U, Moll I, Schumacher U. PAS-positive loops and networks as a prognostic indicator in cutaneous malignant melanoma. *J Pathol.* 2001;195:537—542.
72. Shirakawa K, Wakasugi H, Heike Y, Watanabe I, Yamada S, Saito K, Konishi F. Vasculogenic mimicry and pseudo-comedo formation in breast cancer. *Int J Cancer.* 2002;99:821–828.
73. Sood AK, Seftor EA, Fletcher MS, Gardner LMG, Heidger PM, Buller RE, Seftor REB, Hendrix MJC. Molecular determinants of ovarian cancer plasticity. *Am J Pathol.* 2001;158:1279–1288.
74. Sharma N, Seftor RE, Seftor EA, Gruman LM, Heidger PM, Jr., Cohen MB, Lubaroff DM, Hendrix MJ. Prostatic tumor cell plasticity involves cooperative interactions of distinct phenotypic subpopulations: role in vasculogenic mimicry. *Prostate.* 2002;50: 189–201.
75. Hao X, Sun B, Zhang S, Zhao X. Microarray study of vasculogenic mimicry in bi-directional differentiation malignant tumor. *Zhonghua Yi Xue Za Zhi.* 2002;82: 1298–1302.
76. Folberg R, Chen X, Boldt HC, Pe'er J, Brown CK, Woolson RF, Maniotis, AJ. Microcirculation patterns other than loops and networks in choroidal and ciliary body melanomas. *Ophthalmology.* 2001;108:996–1001.
77. Barinaga M. A face-off over tumor blood supply. *Science.* 2000;287:783–785.
78. Rummelt V, Mehaffey MG, Campbell RJ, Peer J, Bentler SE, Woolson RF, Naumann GOH, Folberg R. Microcirculation architecture of metastases from primary ciliary body and choroidal melanomas. *Am J Ophthalmol.* 1998; 126:303–305.
79. Lugassy C, Christensen L. Melanoma and extravascular migratory metastasis. *J Cutan Pathol.* 2000;27:481.

RUUD CLARIJS, DIRK J. RUITER, ROBERT M.W. DE WAAL

# 12. Fluid-Conducting Meshworks in Uveal Melanoma

## INTRODUCTION

The formation of a neovasculature (i.e., angiogenesis) induced by tumor cells is essential for outgrowth and metastasis in many cancer types.[1] The role of the vasculature in mediating metastasis has been supported by studies demonstrating that microvascular density is a negative prognostic factor.[2,3] However, in primary uveal melanoma, the most common malignant intraocular tumor with a poor prognosis once metastasized,[4] conflicting reports exist on the validity of this prognostic factor.[5–7] Remarkably, dissemination of primary intraocular and posterior uveal melanoma cells occurs exclusively by a hematogenous route[4] which is generally explained by the absence of lymphatic channels in the normal eye and its derived melanoma.[8]

Various patterns of extracellular matrix deposition detected by conventional periodic acid-Schiff (PAS) histochemistry have been described both in uveal and cutaneous melanoma.[9–13] Specific subtypes which contained PAS-positive patterns arranged in arcs, loops and networks proved to be related to the rate of metastasis and, hence, prognosis.[9,10,12,14] Recently, the presence of blood-conducting channels lined by tumor cells which were in close contact to the blood vasculature and associated with arcs, loops and network patterns in uveal melanoma was reported.[13] This newly described phenomenon was assigned the term 'vasculogenic mimicry.'

So, the nature of blood conducting structures in uveal melanoma appears to be rather complicated and incompletely understood. Initially, it was assumed that the presence of blood vessels and the absence of lymphatic vessels determine the metastatic properties of the tumor, but the finding of blood-conducting (i.e., vascular) channels challenges this view. Furthermore, a tumor containing vascular channels is not fully dependent on angiogenesis for growth and it would be less sensitive to drugs aimed at endothelial cells. Therefore, anti-angiogenic therapeutic interventions would have limited effectivity in such cases. Indeed, the presence of vascular channels might explain the disagreement on the value of microvascular density as a negative prognostic factor in the literature.[5–7]

The nature of the PAS-positive patterns and the existence of vasculogenic mimicry have been issues of extensive discussion in the literature. In this review, we will summarize part of this discussion and provide some additional data[15] to further elucidate the nature of the extracellular matrix patterns. Finally, we propose that the PAS-positive arcs, loops and network patterns represent a 'fluid-conducting extracellular matrix meshwork'.[15,16]

## WHAT ARE THE PAS-POSITIVE PATTERNS?

Initially, nine different patterns of microvessel architecture in uveal melanoma were reported by Robert Folberg et al.[10] These patterns were identified by using fluorescein-conjugated *Ulex europaeus* I, an endothelial marker, and PAS-histochemistry[9,10] that highlighted the basement membrane and collagen deposits.

The patterns were re-assessed by Foss et al. using PAS histochemistry, connective tissue stainings and endothelial vWF immunostaining.[17] They concluded that the PAS-positive patterns consisted of connective tissue. In this connective tissue, blood vessels were embedded, forming the so-called fibrovascular tissue. Although Foss et al. could explain their different findings by tissue autofluorescence, it was questioned whether the patterns described by Foss et al. were identical to the patterns studied by Folberg et al.[6,7,18] So, perhaps, there exist two types of PAS-positive patterning in uveal melanoma?

PAS-histochemistry highlights the extracellular matrix patterns by staining basement membranes and collagen.[10,19] The PAS patterns can be enhanced by omitting haematoxylin counterstaining and the use of a green filter during microscopical analysis.[13] We evaluated the extracellular matrix patterns in human primary uveal melanomas using different matrix stainings including PAS, elastin-von-Masson, and Azan histochemistry and found that these stainings detected identical patterns. In addition, detailed morphological analysis in combination with immunostainings using a panel of endothelial markers showed that a part of these patterns could be classified as blood vessels. Additional immuno-electron microscopy of arcs, loops and network patterns in xenografted melanoma using an endothelial marker confirmed our initial observations: the PAS-positive patterns consisted of solid bundles of mainly collagen and laminin in which blood vessels were embedded. Therefore our results are in line with the observations by Foss et al.[17]

## DOES VASCULOGENIC MIMICRY EXIST?

Doubt was raised about the existence of vascular channels[11,13] present in the arcs, loops and network PAS-positive patterns.[20,21] Main criticism by McDonald and co-workers implied that the data delivered by Maniotis et al.[13] were unconvincing. So, we took advantage of the discrete visualization of erythrocytes and extracellular matrix patterns by Azan histochemistry. Combined with a parallel immunostaining for an endothelial marker, these analyses demonstrated that erythrocytes were exclusively associated with lumina positive for endothelial markers and not present in the extracellular matrix patterns. Similar results were obtained in xenografted melanoma lesions in nude mice, also containing arcs, loops and network patterns. In this animal model, an intravenously injected tracer was distributed in- and outside the endothelial marker-positive lumina along curved sheets of extracellular matrix patterns (demonstrated by confocal microscopy). In more detail, our tracer data implied that oxygen and other nutrients can relatively rapidly be transported via the arcs, loops and network patterns (manuscript submitted). Additional (immuno-) electron microscopy supported the nature of endothelial cells lining the endothelial marker-positive lumina. However, different types of cells were associated with the patterns, including macrophages.[22,23] So, we were not able to observe evident tumor cell-lined blood-conducting channels in the PAS-positive extracellular matrix patterns both in primary uveal and xenografted melanoma.

To explain the differences between the findings of Maniotis et al.[13] and ours, the following considerations can be made. In addition to issues raised in prior discussions,[20,21] it must be questioned whether PAS-histochemistry can be used as a reliable technique to detect all extracellular matrix components. Indeed, PAS-staining highlights mainly glycogen and polysaccharides and to a lesser extent the matrix components fibrin and collagen. So, it might well be possible that part of the lumina observed by Maniotis et al. in fact represented a very weak or absent PAS staining of part of the extracellular matrix. This idea is supported by the need of a green filter for a reliable detection of the PAS-positive patterns.[9,10,13,17] Furthermore, the presence of erythrocytes in small lumina is more difficult to establish by PAS immunohistochemistry as compared to Azan histochemistry (which stains erythrocytes intensely red). Maniotis et al. observed immunostaining of melanoma cells for endothelial markers which was supported by a recent report showing that melanoma cells express a variety of endothelial and other markers.[13] In their study, tumor cells lining blood-conducting channels were identified using double immuno-staining for endothelial and melanoma markers. Thus it appears that expression of endothelial markers by melanoma cells hampers a reliable detection of endothelial cells in uveal melanoma lesions. Indeed, extensive review pointed at the sometimes difficult detection of endothelial cells based on the presence of endothelial markers and morphology in tumors.[21,24] So, are the endothelial marker-positive cells lining vascular channels tumor, endothelial and/or mosaics of tumor and endothelial cells? The final possibility is supported by a recent study demonstrating that approximately 4% of the total vascular surface area in a colon carcinoma xenograft mouse model is occupied by tumor cells in direct contact with blood flow.[25] This observation could explain the observations of Maniotis et al.,[13] indicating that vascular channels were, in fact, blood vessels lined by a mixture of mainly endothelial and a few tumor cells. Using an animal model combined with xenografted melanoma of human origin, the difficult detection of blood vasculature due to the expression of endothelial markers by tumor cells may be overcome. Since it is not likely that human melanoma cells express murine endothelial markers, endothelial cells can be detected by immunohistochemistry and immuno-electron microscopy. Using this approach, we concluded that the endothelial marker-positive cells lining erythrocyte-containing lumina are, in fact, endothelial cells. One must however realize that, although evident similarities in distribution of laminin, collagen and macrophages in the extracellular matrix patterns the relevance of conclusions drawn from an animal model for primary uveal melanoma are relevant for the human situation can always be questioned.

In summary, data from our animal model indicated absence of vascular channels in uveal melanoma. However, our study pointed at the existence of a fluid-stream outside the blood vasculature along the arcs, loops and network–extracellular matrix patterns.

## THE PAS-POSITIVE PATTERNS MAY REPRESENT A FLUID-CONDUCTING MESHWORK

In melanoma lesions containing arcs, loops and network patterns, extracellular matrix is distributed as curved septa surrounding nests of tumor cells[20] (our study). An intravenously injected tracer was distributed in- and outside the vasculature, indicating that a fluid stream leaves the blood vessels and enters the extracellular matrix. This flow is explained by the presence of interstitial spaces between bundles of collagen and laminin in the extracellular matrix tissue allowing it to serve as a fluid-conducting meshwork.

In general, fluid movement across vessel walls is governed by differences between blood pressure and local interstitial fluid pressure (IFP). Fluid can leave the blood stream and form an exudate. This fluid movement is induced by the local higher arterial pressure compared to the IFP which is elevated in tumors.[26–29] The exudate may be conducted by the meshwork towards the venous microvasculature, where pressure is likely to be lower than the elevated IFP. This difference in pressure would allow re-entry of the interstitial fluid into veins. Alternatively, interstitial fluid may leak into surrounding pre-existent tissue (which has an IFP of approximately 0 mm Hg[27,29] or into the vitreous body (oozing out) in case of uveal melanoma. High IFP is maintained by the absence of lymphatics[8] and by a limited drainage capacity of the fibrous vascular network. This hypothetical mechanism is depicted schematically in Figure 12.1.

As discussed, besides the transport of exudate-like fluid along the extracellular matrix patterns, these patterns harbored different types of cells, mainly macrophages. Thus, it may serve as a gateway for cells to enter or leave the tumor (which is in line with the reported high malignancy containing the matrix patterns[9,10,12,14]). Fluid-transportation outside the blood vasculature is normally a function of the lymphatic system. As noted above, no lymphatics are present in uveal melanoma.[8] Therefore, the fluid-conducting meshwork may represent an alternative lymphatic system: indeed, both exudate-like fluid and inflammatory and tumor cells may be transported along this structure.

## CONCLUSIONS

In contrast to Maniotis et al.,[13] we did not observe conductance of blood outside the blood vasculature.[15,16] Although the existence of vascular mimicry in primary human uveal melanoma cannot be ruled out yet due to technical limitations, we propose the existence of a fluid-conducting meshwork as a functional alternative for the concept of vascular channels. The presence of a fluid-conducting meshwork indeed explains the functional data of Maniotis et al. regarding the intratumoral transportation of intravenous fluorescent dye.[13] There are strong indications that the arcs and loops forming the extracellular matrix are involved in inflammatory

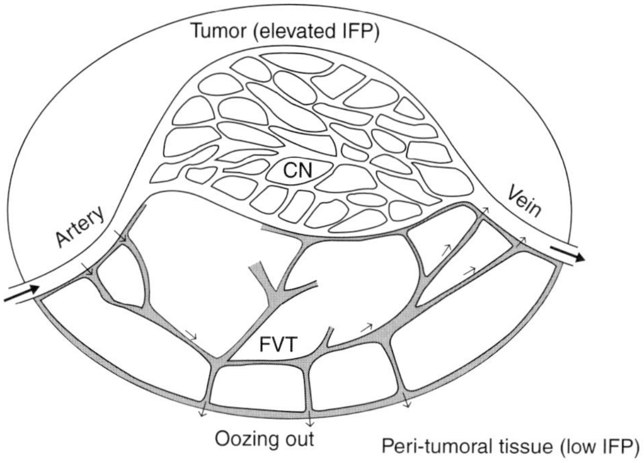


Fig. 12.1. Schematic drawing of the role of fibrovascular tissue tumor perfusion. Blood flow is conducted via the artery, the capillary network (CN) towards the venous vessel (large arrows). Exudate-like fluid (containing no non-migratory blood cells) moves across an arterial microvessel wall (small arrows) into the fibrovascular tissue (FVT) in tumor areas where arterial pressure exceeds the IFP. The fibrovascular tissue conducts the exudate-like fluid towards the venous microvasculature (small arrows) where the blood pressure is lower than the IFP, causing absorbance into the blood stream. Also, leakage into the peri-tumoral tissue (in which IFP is approximately 0 mm Hg) or the vitreous body in case of uveal melanoma (i.e., oozing out) may occur.

cell invasion, nutrition of tumor cells, regulation of local tissue fluid flow and, possibly, metastasis. These patterns may, in fact, represent a surrogate lymphatic vascular system.

## ACKNOWLEDGEMENT

This work was supported by grant 98-1816 from the Dutch Cancer Society.

## REFERENCES

1. Folkman, J. What is the evidence that tumors are angiogenesis dependent? *J Natl Cancer Inst.* 1990;82:4–6.
2. Weidner, N, Semple JP, Welch WR, Folkman J. Tumor angiogenesis and metastasis—correlation in invasive breast carcinoma. *N Engl J Med.* 1991;324:1–8.
3. Weidner, N. Intratumoral microvessel density as a prognostic factor in cancer. *Am J Pathol.* 1995;147:9–19.
4. Kath R, Hayungs J, Bornfeld N, Sauerwein W, Hoffken K, Secber S. Prognosis and treatment of disseminated uveal melanoma. *Cancer.* 1993;72:2219–2223.
5. Foss AJ, Alexander RA, Jefferies W, Hungerford JL, Harris AL, Lightman S. Microvessel count predicts survival in uveal melanoma. *Cancer. Res.* 1996;56:2900–2903.
6. Mäkitie T, Summanen P, Tarkkanen A, Kivelä T. Microvascular density in predicting survival of patients with choroidal and ciliary body melanoma. *Invest Ophthalmol Vis Sci.* 1999;40:2471–2480.

7. Lane AM, Egan KM, Yang J, Saornil MA, Abroy J, Albert D, Gragoudas ES. An evaluation of tumour vascularity as a prognostic indicator in uveal melanoma. *Melanoma Res.* 1997;7:237–242.
8. Clarijs R, Schalkwijk L, Ruiter DJ, De Waal RM. Lack of lymphangiogenesis despite coexpression of VEGF-C and its receptor Flt-4 in primary uveal melanoma. *Invest Ophthalmol Vis Sci.* 2001;42:1422–1428.
9. Folberg R, Pe'er J, Gruman LM, Woolson RF, Jeng G, Montague PR, Moninger TO, Yi H, Moore KC. The morphologic characteristics of tumor blood vessels as a marker of tumor progression in primary human uveal melanoma. *Hum Pathol.* 1992;23: 1298–1305.
10. Folberg R, Rummelt V, Parys-Van Ginderdeuren R, Hwang T, Woolson RF, Pe'er J, Gruman LM. The prognostic value of tumor blood vessel morphology in primary uveal melanoma. *Ophthalmology.* 1993;100:1389–1398.
11. Folberg R, Hendrix MJC, Maniotis AJ. Vasculogenic mimicry and tumor angiogenesis. *Am J Pathol.* 2000;156:361–381.
12. Warso MA, Maniotis AJ, Chen X, Maguindar D, Patewl MK, Shilkaitis A, Gupter TK, Folberg R. Prognostic significance of periodic acid-Schiff-positive patterns in primary cutaneous melanoma. *Clin Cancer Res.* 2001;7:473–477.
13. Maniotis AJ, Folberg R, Hess A, Seftor EA, Gardner LMG, Pe'er J, Trent JM, Melzer PS, Hendrix MJC. Vascular channel formation by human melanoma cells in vivo and in vitro: vasculogenic mimicry. *Am J Pathol.* 1999;155:739–752.
14. Mäkitie T, Summanen P, Tarkkanen A, Kivelä T. Microvascular loops and networks as prognostic indicators in choroidal and ciliary body melanomas. *J Natl Cancer Inst.* 2000;91:359–367.
15. Clarijs R, Otte-Höller I, Ruiter DJ, De Waal RM. Presence of a fluid-conducting meshwork in xenografted cutaneous and primary human uveal melanoma. *Invest Ophthalmol Vis Sci.* 2002;43: 912–918.
16. Clarijs R, Ruiter DJ, De Waal RM. Pathophysiological implications of stroma pattern formation in uveal melanoma. *J Cell Physiol.* 2003;194:267–271.
17. Foss AJ, Alexander RA, Hungerford JL, Harris AL, Cree IA, Lightman S. Reassessment of the PAS patterns in uveal melanoma. *Br J Ophthalmol.* 1997;81:240–246.
18. Folberg R. Discussion of paper by Foss et al. *Br J Ophthalmol.* 1997;81:240–246.
19. Rummelt V, Gardner LM, Folberg R, Beck S, Knosp B, Moninger TO, Moore KC. Three-dimensional relationships between tumor cells and microcirculation with double cyanine immunolabeling, laser scanning confocal microscopy, and computer-assisted reconstruction: an alternative to cast corrosion preparations. *J Histochem Cytochem.* 1994;42:681–686.
20. McDonald DM, Munn L, Jain RK. Vasculogenic mimicry: how convincing, how novel and how significant? *Am J Pathol.* 2000;156:383–388.
21. McDonald DM, Foss AJ. Endothelial cells of tumor vessels: abnormal but not absent. *Cancer Metastasis Rev.* 2000;19:109–120.
22. Mäkitie T, Summanen P, Tarkkanen A, Kivelä T. Tumor-infiltrating macrophages (cd68(+) cells) and prognosis in malignant uveal melanoma. *Invest Ophthalmol Vis Sci.* 2001;42:1414–1421.
23. Mäkitie T, Tarkkanen A, Kivelä T. Comparative immunohistochemical oestrogen receptor analysis in primary and metastatic uveal melanoma. *Graefes Arch Clin Exp Ophthalmol.* 1998;236:415–419.
24. Meltzer P, Chen Y, Jiang Y, Seftor E, Hendrix M, et al. Molecular classification of cutaneous malignant melanoma by gene expression profiling. *Nature.* 2000;406: 536–540.

25. Chang YS, di Tomaso E, McDonald DM, Jones R, Jain RK, Munn LL. Mosaic blood vessels in tumors: frequency of cancer cells in contact with flowing blood. *Proc Natl Acad Sci USA*. 2000;97:14608–14613.
26. Gutmann R, Leunig M, Feyh J, Goetz AE, Messmer K, Kastenbauer E, Jain RK. Interstitial hypertension in head and neck tumors in patients: correlation with tumor size. *Cancer Res*. 1992;52:1993–1995.
27. Roh HD, Boucher Y, Kalnicki S, Buchsbaum R, Bloomer WD, Jain RK. Interstitial hypertension in carcinoma of uterine cervix in patients: possible correlation with tumor oxygenation and radiation response. *Cancer Res*. 1991;51:6695–6698.
28. Boucher Y, Baxter LT, Jain RK. Interstitial pressure gradients in tissue-isolated and subcutaneous tumors: implications for therapy. *Cancer Res*. 1990;50:4478–4484.
29. Boucher Y, Kirkwood JM, Opacic D, De Santis M, Jain RK. Interstitial hypertension in superficial metastatic melanomas in humans. *Cancer Res*. 1991;51:6691–6694.

PÄIVI TOIVONEN, TEEMU MÄKITIE AND TERO KIVELÄ*

# 13. Microvessels and Macrophages in Choroidal and Ciliary Body Melanoma[1]

ABSTRACT: Microvascular factors and tumor-infiltrating macrophages, identified by labelling for the CD68 epitope, are reported to predict prognosis of patients with malignant uveal melanoma. We studied microvascular factors and macrophages at different stages of tumor progression in 134 enucleated choroidal and ciliary body melanomas, in 33 metastases originating from these primary tumors, and in 36 unrelated primary tumors treated with brachytherapy, which were secondarily enucleated because of local tumor recurrence and treatment complications. Microvascular loops and networks were identified from bleached, uncounterstained sections with the periodic acid-Schiff stain. Microvascular density (MVD) in areas of densest vascularisation and the number and morphologic type of tumor-infiltrating macrophages were determined with antibodies to the CD34 and CD68 epitopes, respectively. Metastases had a higher MVD than primary tumors overall (53 vs. 40 vessels/0.313 mm$^2$; $p = 0.033$). As compared to the primary tumors, the corresponding metastases showed a trend toward higher MVD ($p = 0.072$ pairwise comparison). Irradiated primary tumors had a significantly lower MVD (18 vs. 35 vessels/0.313 mm$^2$; $P < 0.001$) than the enucleated tumors, but equal numbers of macrophages ($p = 0.35$). The frequency of microvascular loops and networks tended to be smaller in irradiated tumors ($p = 0.093$) and higher in metastases overall ($p = 0.015$), but not if primary tumors and corresponding metastases were compared pairwise ($p = 0.80$). Microvascular loops and networks, MVD, presence of epithelioid cells and largest basal tumor diameter independently predicted prognosis, controlling for the number of macrophages. According to this study, MVD is both associated with death from uveal melanoma and it increases and decreases in a logical way with tumor progression and regression, respectively. Microvascular loops and networks independently predict metastasis and thus likely reflect different processes in tumor progression. Tumor-infiltrating macrophages are ubiquitous both before and after irradiation of uveal melanoma.

## INTRODUCTION

It is well known that the eye and orbit lack lymphatic vessels, a fact that recently was explicitly confirmed as regards uveal malignant melanoma,[1] the most common intraocular malignancy. Consequently, it should not be surprising that, unlike

[1] Supported by grants from the Helsinki University Central Hospital (TYH8217, TYH1217), the Finnish Medical Research Fund, and the Finnish Eye Foundation.

* To whom correspondence should be addressed.

most other cancers including skin melanoma, uveal melanoma metastasises predominantly hematogenously.[2,3] Only if it extends through the anterior sclera to infiltrate the conjunctiva, uveal melanoma can gain access to lymphatic vessels, and metastasis to the cervical lymph nodes can then take place.[4,5]

Given the almost exclusively hematogenous dissemination, it is astonishing that serious attention focused on vascularisation of uveal melanoma only recently and almost by chance. In 1992, Robert Folberg with his group searched for light microscopic features of uveal melanoma that would be both associated with life prognosis and large enough to be visualised by noninvasive methods.[6] They noticed that the arrangement of microvessels varied from tumor to tumor, and classified these vascular patterns in nine categories. Some patterns were found to be associated with high risk of metastasis, most notably the patterns of microvascular loops and networks, arcs with branching, and parallel vessels with cross-linking.[6–10] Even though challenged initially, their observations have now been confirmed beyond reasonable doubt.[11–15]

Another line of research focused on microvascular density (MVD), a measure of the number of microvessels in malignant tumors, which in 1991 was for the first time linked with risk of metastasis, initially in patients with breast cancer.[16,17] Especially areas of densest vascularisation, or 'hot spots', might be involved in hematogenous metastasis. In 1996, Alexander Foss and colleagues noted that high MVD as measured from hot spots was associated with survival also after enucleation for uveal melanoma.[18,19] Although the role of MVD was challenged in smaller reports,[11,20] these were not based on analysis of hot spots, and the observations of Foss have now also been independently confirmed.[21]

These two observations have changed the previous neglect of microvascular factors into a heated debate on the role of microvessels in uveal melanoma. In one extreme, microvascular patterns are postulated to be formed by tumor cells by a process known as microvascular mimicry,[22,23] whereas in the other they are merely a marker of aggressive melanoma without direct involvement in the metastatic process.[24] Be as it may, mortality from uveal melanoma must be a function of several parameters, which include the ability of tumor cells and microvessels to interact so that neoplastic cells can escape the eye, the ability of tumor cells to grow in the target organs, and the ability of immune surveillance and other host defences to keep tumor cells under control. Microvessels may be important also in the latter regard, because they provide conduits through which leukocytes, macrophages and other effector cells gain access to primary and metastatic uveal melanoma.

Tumor-infiltrating macrophages have long been known to reside in uveal melanoma,[25–29] but they have been regarded as a relatively inconspicuous cell population. More recently, immunohistochemistry has identified macrophage-like cells to be a ubiquitous component of uveal melanoma, even when treated with primary enucleation.[30] While high numbers of macrophages are linked with increased uveal melanoma-specific mortality,[30] it is unknown whether these cells are causally related to tumor progression, for example by secreting growth-promoting cytokines, or whether they are mere scavengers that reflect high cell turnover rate in more rapidly growing, aggressive melanomas.[30] We summarise here some current evidence relevant to this problem.

When initially looking for the presence of tumor-infiltrating macrophages in primary uveal melanoma, we analysed a series of 167 choroidal and ciliary body tumors enucleated from 1972 to 1981. During this period, prompt enucleation was the standard treatment for all but the smallest uveal melanomas in Finland. The analysis presented here is based on a subset of 134 eyes in which microvascular factors could be assessed (inclusion ratio, 80%).[15,21]

Of the nine microvascular patterns, we evaluated those two that have been most consistently associated with poor prognosis, namely microvascular loops and networks.[6,7,13–15,31] This was to minimise statistical problems related to multiple comparisons of variables that also may be partially interrelated. Because networks consist of three or more back-to-back loops,[6] loops and networks were analysed as an ordered three-category variable (no loops, loops without networks, loops forming networks), which considers networks to be an advanced stage of loops. Thus, only one log-rank test instead of two was needed to assess prognostic significance.

The patterns were independently assessed by two observers under a dark green filter from sections first bleached with potassium permanganate and oxalic acid and then stained with periodic acid-Schiff without counterstain, according to the original method of Folberg.[7]

The monoclonal antibody (mAb) QBEND/10 to the CD34 epitope of vascular endothelial cells was used to label microvessels.[21] To enable evaluation of immunoreaction in pigmented tumors, the peroxidase reaction was developed with 3,3′-diaminobenzidine tetrahydrochloride, and melanin was subsequently bleached with hydrogen peroxide and disodium hydrogen phosphate.[32] This sequence obviates any change in antigenicity that may occur if bleaching is done prior to immunostaining.

The hot spot was identified under low magnification. Microvessels were counted from the most highly vascularised area in each tumor using an eyepiece with an etched graticule corresponding to 0.313 $mm^2$ at ×200.[18,21] Any immunolabeled vessel, separate from an adjacent one and either totally inside the graticule or touching its top or left border, was counted as a microvessel. MVD was divided in quartiles for univariate analysis, and square root transformed for multivariate analysis to achieve normal distribution.[18]

At least one closed microvascular loop was detected in 80 (60%) of 134 primarily enucleated uveal melanomas, and networks were found in 47 of them (35%; Table 13.1). MVD of the 134 enucleated uveal melanomas, based on the globally highest vessel count ('hot spot'), varied from 5 to 121 vessels/0.313 $mm^2$. MVD was higher if loops and networks were present ($p < 0.001$, Kruskal–Wallis test), but overlap between categories was notable (Fig. 13.1).

It is useful to remember that MVD as measured from hot spots is only a rough measure of the overall degree of vascularisation, and that what exactly corresponds to MVD at the cellular level is debated. Whereas tumor microvessels traditionally are thought to be of endothelial origin and generated by angiogenesis, evidence has also been provided as mentioned that in uveal melanoma they might be formed by

Table 13.1. Comparison of 134 enucleated primary choroidal and ciliary body melanomas to 33 metastatic and 36 irradiated primary melanomas that were later enucleated.

| Variable | Primary enucleated | Compared against: Metastasis | P | Irradiated | P |
|---|---|---|---|---|---|
| Microvascular loops and networks, *n* (%) | | | | | |
| No loops | 54 (40) | 6 (18) | 0.015[a] | 15 (43) | 0.093[a] |
| Loops without networks | 33 (25) | 9 (27) | | 16 (46) | |
| Networks | 47 (35) | 18 (55) | | 4 (11) | |
| Median microvascular density, vessels/0.313 $mm^2$ (range) | 40 (5–121) | 53 (18–91) | 0.033[b] | 18 (0–63) | < 0.001[b] |
| Number of infiltrating macrophages, *n* (%) | | | | | |
| Few | 23 (18) | – | | 6 (17) | 0.35[a] |
| Moderate numbers | 62 (50) | – | | 23 (64) | |
| Many | 40 (32) | – | | 7 (19) | |
| Type of infiltrating macrophages, *n* (%) | | | | | |
| Predominantly dendritic | 30 (24) | – | | 1 (3) | 0.011[c] |
| Intermediate | 70 (56) | – | | 23 (64) | |
| Predominantly round | 25 (20) | – | | 12 (33) | |

[a]Kruskal–Wallis test, two-sided.
[b]Mann–Whitney *U*-test, two-sided.
[c]Pearson's chi-square test, two-sided.

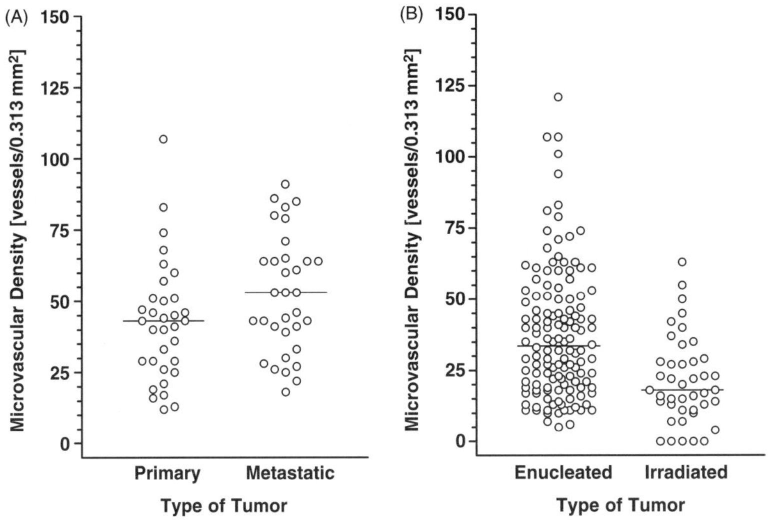


Fig. 13.1. Microvascular density in primary enucleated uveal melanomas as compared to corresponding metastases (A), and in primarily enucleated uveal melanomas as compared to those secondarily enucleated after brachytherapy (B). Bar = median.

aggressive melanoma cells in the absence of endothelium.[22,23] Such unconventional vasculogenesis is not necessarily unique to this cancer.[23]

Monoclonal antibody PG-M1 was used to recognise the CD68 epitope of macrophages.[33] MAb PG-M1 performed best as compared to two other anti-macrophage mAbs, including KP1 which also detects the CD68 epitope.[33] The number of tumor-infiltrating macrophages in non-necrotic areas was graded semi-quantitatively as few, moderate and many according to published standard photographs.[30] The tumors were also divided according to standard photographs into those with predominantly dendritic, intermediate-shaped and round macrophages.[30] The intermediate class included tumors in which macrophages either appeared intermediate in shape between dendritic and round, or about equal numbers of dendritic and round ones were found. Confluent areas of macrophages in necrotic areas did not influence the grading.

Few macrophages were found in 18%, moderate numbers in 50%, and high numbers in 32% of enucleated primary melanomas (Table 13.1). They infiltrated the tumor diffusely, but some were arranged along loops, networks, and other microvascular patterns. The number of macrophages was associated with MVD ($p = 0.0011$, Mann–Whitney $U$-test) but not with presence of loops and networks ($p = 0.53$, Jonckheere–Terpstra test). Most infiltrating macrophages were intermediate in shape (Table 13.1). The predominant morphologic type of macrophages was not associated with MVD ($p = 0.84$, Mann–Whitney $U$-test).

The presence of tumor-infiltrating macrophages in uveal melanomas is not surprising, because macrophages have been long known to occur in many cancers.[34] Their presence in uveal melanoma has been appreciated previously, but it appears that their frequency has been underestimated.[25–29] Theoretically, macrophages might mediate both anti-tumor functions, such as tumor cytotoxicity,[35–37] and pro-tumor functions, including promotion of angiogenesis[38–40] and degradation of the tumor stroma to promote invasion.[41,42] Interestingly, macrophages in uveal melanoma were mostly distributed diffusely and along microvascular patterns, whereas they are usually thought to accumulate in poorly vascularised and hypoxic areas of tumors.[43,44]

## ASSOCIATION WITH MELANOMA-SPECIFIC SURVIVAL

The median follow-up time after enucleation was 22 years (range, 18–26). Melanoma-specific mortality (Fig. 13.2) was associated with presence of microvascular loops and networks ($p = 0.0012$, log-rank test for linear trend), MVD ($p = 0.0001$), and number of infiltrating macrophages ($p = 0.0012$). No loops and few macrophages were associated with better prognosis than loops ($p = 0.043$ log-rank test, Bonferroni correction), networks ($p = 0.043$), moderate ($p = 0.043$) and high numbers of macrophages ($p = 0.003$). No difference was noted between melanomas with loops as compared to those with networks, and those with moderate and high numbers of macrophages ($p > 0.10$).

By Cox multivariate regression, adjusted for the effect of macrophages, presence of microvascular loops and networks, presence of epithelioid cells, largest basal tumor diameter, and MVD retained independent statistical significance

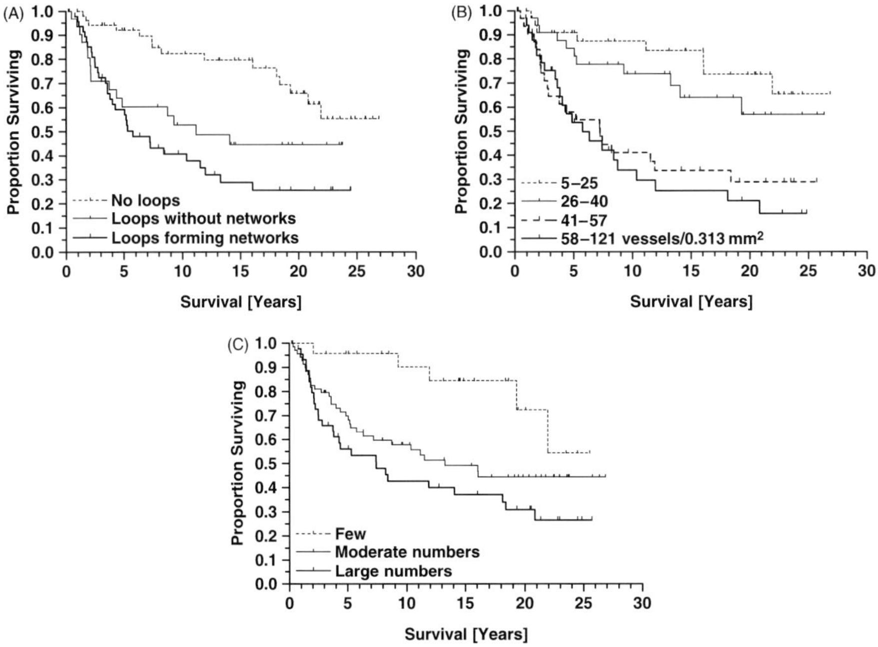


Fig. 13.2. Melanoma-specific survival according to presence of microvascular loops and networks (A), microvascular density (B) and number of tumour-infiltrating macrophages (C).

Table 13.2 Cox proportional hazards regression of melanoma-specific survival among 134 patients who had an eye enucleated because of a primary choroidal and ciliary body melanoma[a].

| Independent variable | Coefficient (Standard error) | Hazard ratio (95% Confidence interval) | *P* |
|---|---|---|---|
| Epithelioid cells[b] | 0.678 (0.277) | 1.97 (1.14–3.39) | 0.014 |
| Largest basal diameter[c] | 0.127 (0.039) | 1.14 (1.05–1.23) | 0.0013 |
| Loops and networks[d] | 0.338 (0.159) | 1.40 (1.03–1.91) | 0.030 |
| Microvascular density[e] | 0.213 (0.075) | 1.24 (1.07–1.43) | 0.0049 |

[a] Model stratified by number of infiltrating macrophages (few vs. moderate to many).
[b] Categories: No = 0, Yes = 1.
[c] Continuous variable, in mm.
[d] Categories: No loops = 0, Loops without networks = 1, Loops forming networks = 2.
[e] Continuous variable: log(microvessels/0.313 $mm^2$), in log units.

(Table 13.2). The number of macrophages did not fulfil the assumption of proportional hazards and was thus modelled by stratification. The stratified model was preferred to a competing, nonstratified model that disregarded the effect of macrophages (likelihood ratio, 243.6 vs. 187.9, $P < 0.001$ chi-squared test, 1 df).

In order to try to gain a better idea into the possible role of microvascular factors and macrophages in uveal melanoma, we thought it informative to compare them between primary and metastatic uveal melanomas (tumor progression) and between primary melanomas managed by enucleation and brachytherapy (tumor regression).

## TUMOR PROGRESSION: SYSTEMIC METASTASIS

Of the 80 tumor deaths, 64 (80%) were histopathologically confirmed and 33 specimens were large enough to allow determination of microvascular factors (inclusion ratio, 52%).

Loops were found in 27 (82%) and networks in 18 (55%) of the 33 metastases (Table 13.1). In five patients (15%), these patterns were observed only in the primary tumor and in four patients (12%) only in the metastasis. Loops and networks were significantly more common in metastatic than in primary uveal melanoma overall (Table 13.1; $p = 0.015$, Kruskal–Wallis test). When primaries and corresponding metastases were compared pairwise, however, the distributions of the two patterns were similar ($p = 0.80$, Stuart–Maxwell test). Quantitatively, microvascular networks could be more or less pronounced in metastases than in the corresponding primary (Fig. 13.3).

The MVD of the metastases varied from 18 to 91 vessels/0.313 $mm^2$ (Table 13.1). The MVD of metastases was significantly higher than that of the 134 primary melanomas overall (Table 13.1; $p = 0.033$, Mann–Whitney $U$-test), and it tended to be higher also when the metastasis and corresponding primary tumor were compared pairwise (median, 53 vs. 43 vessels/0.313 $mm^2$; $p = 0.072$, Wilcoxon signed rank test; Figs. 13.1 and 13.2). In metastases MVD was not significantly associated with microvascular loops and networks ($p = 0.58$, Kruskal–Wallis test).

In addition to tumor progression, a higher MVD of metastases might reflect differences between the intraocular and extraocular environment.

## TUMOR REGRESSION: BRACHYTHERAPY

We ascertained 43 consecutive irradiated patients who had an eye removed because of suspected local recurrence or treatment complications between 1982 and 2001. During this period, our center was responsible for more than 90% of brachytherapies in Finland. The series is thus essentially unselected and representative of all uveal melanomas so treated.

In seven eyes microvascular factors could not be evaluated because of tumor destruction, leaving 36 irradiated tumors in analysis (inclusion ratio, 84%). Of the 36 evaluable primary melanomas removed after brachytherapy, loops were observed in 20 (57%) and networks in 4 (11%). These patterns tended to be less frequent among irradiated than among primarily enucleated intraocular melanomas (Table 13.1; $p = 0.093$, Kruskal–Wallis test).

Among irradiated primary melanomas, the MVD varied from 0 to 63 vessels/ 0.313 $mm^2$ (Table 13.1). The MVD of irradiated, secondarily enucleated melanomas was significantly lower than that of primarily enucleated tumors (median,

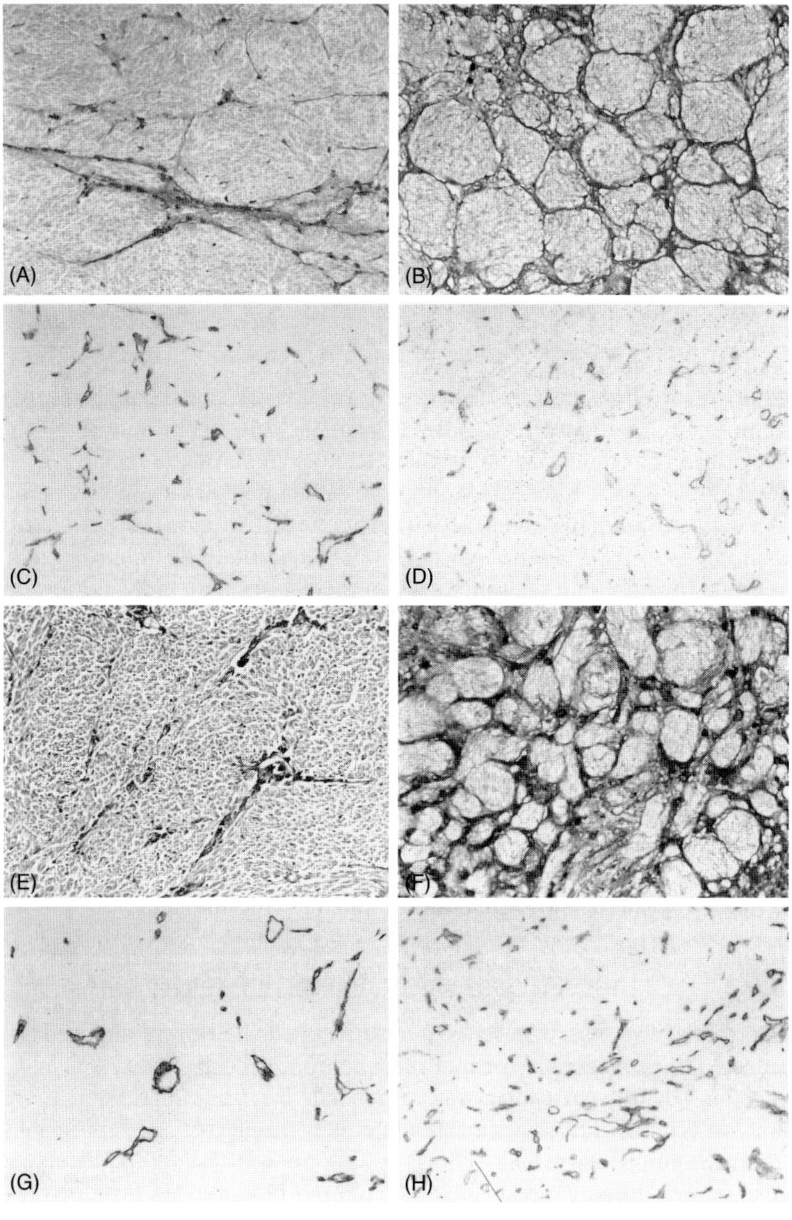


Fig. 13.3. Microvascular factors in primary (A, C, E, G) and metastatic uveal melanoma (B, D, F, H). Microvascular loops and indistinct networks in a primary tumor (A) with more pronounced, well formed networks in a corresponding metastasis (B). The microvascular density in a hot spot of the primary tumor (C) and metastasis (D) are comparable. In a second primary tumor, the microvascular pattern of arcs with branching is present, but loops and networks were not detected (E). In a corresponding metastasis, well formed networks have developed; note relatively thick patterns with extracellular material (F). In this primary tumor, the microvascular density is low (G), but in the corresponding metastasis it is high (H).

18 vs. 40 vessels/0.313 mm$^2$; $p < 0.001$, Mann–Whitney $U$-test; Fig. 13.1). The MVD of irradiated tumors ($p = 0.95$) was not significantly associated with presence of microvascular loops and networks.

Whether formed by endothelial or tumor cells, irradiation would be expected to reduce tumor microvessels and cause a reduction in MVD. However, the alternative possibility remains that brachytherapy may have selected for enucleation and for melanomas that originally had a lower than average MVD. If tumors with low MVD were more resistant to radiation, they would leave behind larger residual masses, which potentially could spawn more frequent recurrences and more pronounced radiation-related complications, both of which would more likely lead to enucleation. In contrast, if tumors with high MVD were more radiosensitive they might regress without recurrence and complications.

The number of macrophages was small in 17%, moderate in 64% and high in 19% of irradiated primary melanomas (Table 13.1), and these proportions were comparable to those of primary enucleated uveal melanomas overall ($p = 0.35$, Kruskal–Wallis test). Most macrophages were intermediate in shape. The rest in enucleated tumors were equally often dendritic and round in shape, whereas in irradiated tumors round macrophages predominated over dendritic ones ($p = 0.011$, Pearson's chi-square test).

The finding that the number of macrophages was comparable to primarily enucleated tumors casts doubt on claims that they would be indicative of treatment effect in conservatively managed uveal melanoma.[45,46] One explanation might be that resident macrophages died along with tumor cells after brachytherapy and 'mummified' within the tumor. Macrophages might also continuously enter and exit the tumor, falsely suggesting a stationary population. Indeed, macrophages repopulate irradiated experimental neoplasms.[47]

The more frequent presence of round as compared to dendritic macrophages in irradiated uveal melanomas would be consistent with phagocytosis of degenerating tumor cells. A limitation of the present study is that only tumors that necessitated secondary enucleation could be studied. The results are not necessarily representative of those irradiated melanomas which do not recur or cause complications.

## SUMMARY AND CONCLUSIONS

Of the two microvascular factors analysed, MVD was higher among metastatic than among primary uveal melanomas, and significantly lower in irradiated as compared to primarily enucleated uveal melanomas. These differences suggest an association between MVD and progression of uveal melanoma, which is also in line with the observation that high MVD in uveal melanoma is independently associated with high risk of metastasis.[18,19,21]

The presence of microvascular loops and networks has been linked with aggressiveness of uveal melanoma as well.[22] We found that loops and networks were, in general, significantly more common in metastatic than in primary uveal melanomas, which would be in support of this theory. However, when metastases were compared pairwise with the primaries that had spawned them, the difference diminished. We also noted that metastases from primary tumors that had loops and networks could sometimes lack them, and unlike the case in a previous analysis of 19 metastases from uveal melanoma,[48] we found that several metastases contained neither loops nor networks.

As regards tumors enucleated after brachytherapy, the data suggested some reduction in the frequency of networks and more frequent absence of loops as compared to primary enucleation. It is not surprising that the difference, if real, would be less marked than that in MVD, because microvascular patterns are composed in part of extracellular matrix,[23] which likely takes some time to be remodelled. The argument might also be raised that the study design might have selected disproportionate numbers of tumors with no loops and networks for study.

In summary, progression to metastasis and regression after brachytherapy are associated with corresponding changes in MVD, but microvascular loops and networks either are less rapidly remodelled or they are less affected by tumor progression and regression. The role of macrophages in uveal melanoma remains an intriguing open question that merits more attention. In particular, the factors that control their presence[49,50] and the mediators they contribute remain to be determined. It is important to be aware of their presence, because infiltrating macrophages may react with antibodies to growth factors and other antigens that also may be secreted by tumor cells.[28,51,52] This may lead to errors of interpretation on the part of ophthalmic pathologists.

## REFERENCES


1. Clarijs R, Schalkwijk L, Ruiter DJ, De Waal RM. Lack of lymphangiogenesis despite coexpression of VEGF-C and its receptor Flt-4 in uveal melanoma. *Invest Ophthalmol Vis Sci.* 2001;42:1422–1428.
2. Didolkar MS, Elias EG, Barber NA, Moore RH. Biologic behavior of ocular malignant melanoma and comparison with melanoma of the head and neck. *Am J Surg.* 1980; 140:522–526.
3. Folberg R. Tumor progression in ocular melanomas. *J Invest Dermatol.* 1993;100:326S–331S.
4. Tojo D, Wenig BL, Resnick KI. Incidence of cervical metastasis from uveal melanoma: implications for treatment. *Head Neck.* 1995;17:137–139.
5. Dithmar S, Diaz CE, Grossniklaus HE. Intraocular melanoma spread to regional lymph nodes: report of two cases. *Retina.* 2000;20:76–79.
6. Folberg R, Pe'er J, Gruman LM, Woolson RF, Jeng G, Montague PR, Moninger TO, Yi H, Moore KC. The morphologic characteristics of tumor blood vessels as a marker of tumor progression in primary human uveal melanoma: a matched case-control study. *Hum Pathol.* 1992;23:1298–1305.
7. Folberg R, Rummelt V, Parys-Van Ginderdeuren R, Hwang T, Woolson RF, Pe'er J, Gruman LM. The prognostic value of tumor blood vessel morphology in primary uveal melanoma. *Ophthalmology.* 1993;100:1389–1398.
8. Rummelt V, Folberg R, Woolson RF, Hwang T, Pe'er J. Relation between the microcirculation architecture and the aggressive behavior of ciliary body melanomas. *Ophthalmology.* 1995;102:844–851.
9. Mehaffey MG, Gardner LM, Folberg R. Distribution of prognostically important vascular patterns across multiple levels in ciliary body and choroidal melanomas. *Am J Ophthalmol.* 1998;126:373–378.

10. Folberg R, Chen X, Boldt HC, Pe'er J, Brown CK, Woolson RF, Maniotis AJ. Microcirculation patterns other than loops and networks in choroidal and ciliary body melanomas. *Ophthalmology.* 2001;108:996–1001.
11. Schaling DF, Van der Pol JP, Schlingemann RO, Parys-Van Ginderdeuren R, Ruiter DJ, Jager MJ. Vascular density and vascular patterns in the prognosis of choroidal melanoma. In: Schaling DF, ed. *Radionuclides and Radiolabelled Antibodies in Choroidal Melanoma (Diagnosis and Therapy).* Thesis, Leiden; Rijksuniversiteit te Leiden, 1996; 43–54.
12. Sakamoto T, Sakamoto M, Yoshikawa H, Hata Y, Ishibashi T, Ohnishi Y, Inomata H. Histologic findings and prognosis of uveal malignant melanoma in Japanese patients. *Am J Ophthalmol.* 1996;121:276–283.
13. McLean IW, Keefe KS, Burnier MN. Uveal melanoma: comparison of the prognostic value of fibrovascular loops, mean of the ten largest nucleoli, cell type, and tumor size. *Ophthalmology.* 1997;104:777–780.
14. Seregard S, Spångberg B, Juul C, Oskarsson M. Prognostic accuracy of the mean of the largest nucleoli, vascular patterns, and PC-10 in posterior uveal melanoma. *Ophthalmology.* 1998;105:485–491.
15. Mäkitie T, Summanen P, Tarkkanen A, Kivelä T. Microvascular loops and networks as prognostic indicators in choroidal and ciliary body melanomas. *J Natl Cancer Inst.* 1999;91:359–367.
16. Weidner N, Semple JP, Welch WR, Folkman J. Tumor angiogenesis and metastasis–correlation in invasive breast carcinoma. *N Engl J Med.* 1991;324:1–8.
17. Weidner N, Folkman J, Pozza F, Bevilacqua P, Allred EN, Moore DH. Tumor angiogenesis: a new, significant, and independent prognostic indicator in early staged breast carcinoma. *J Natl Cancer Inst.* 1992;84:1875–1887.
18. Foss AJE, Alexander RA, Jefferies LW, Hungerford JL, Harris AL, Lightman S. Microvessel count predicts survival in uveal melanoma. *Cancer Res.* 1996;56: 2900–2903.
19. Foss AJE, Alexander RA, Hungerford JL, Harris AL, Cree IA, Lightman S. Reassessment of the PAS patterns in uveal melanoma. *Br J Ophthalmol.* 1997;81:240–246.
20. Lane AM, Egan KM, Yang J, Saornil MA, Alroy J, Albert D, Gragoudas ES. An evaluation of tumour vascularity as a prognostic indicator in uveal melanoma. *Melanoma Res.* 1997;7:237–242.
21. Mäkitie T, Summanen P, Tarkkanen A, Kivelä T. Microvascular density in predicting survival of patients with choroidal and ciliary body melanoma. *Invest Ophthalmol Vis Sci.* 1999;40:2471–2480.
22. Maniotis AJ, Folberg R, Hess A, Seftor EA, Gardner LMG, Pe'er J, Trent JM, Meltzer PS, Hendrix MJC. Vascular channel formation by human melanoma cells in vivo and in vitro: Vasculogenic mimicry. *Am J Pathol.* 1999;155:739–752.
23. Folberg R, Hendrix MJC, Maniotis AJ. Vasculogenic mimicry and tumor angiogenesis. *Am J Pathol.* 2000;156:361–381.
24. McDonald DM, Munn L, Jain RK. Vasculogenic mimicry: How convincing, how novel, and how significant? *Am J Pathol.* 2000;156:383–388.
25. Davidorf FH, Lang JR. Lymphocytic infiltration in choroidal melanoma and its prognostic significance. *Trans Ophthalmol Soc UK.* 1977;97:394–401.
26. Fuchs U, Kivelä T, Tarkkanen A, Laatikainen L. Histopathology of enucleated intraocular melanomas irradiated with cobalt and ruthenium plaques. *Acta Ophthalmol (Copenh).* 1988;66:255–266.
27. Tobal K, Deuble K, McCartney A, Lightman S. Characterization of cellular infiltration in choroidal melanoma. *Melanoma Res.* 1993;3:63–65.

28. Mäkitie T, Tarkkanen A, Kivelä T. Comparative immunohistochemical oestrogen receptor analysis in primary and metastatic uveal melanoma. *Graefes Arch Clin Exp Ophthalmol.* 1998;236:415–419.
29. The Collaborative Ocular Melanoma Study Group. Histopathologic characteristics of uveal melanomas in eyes enucleated from the Collaborative Ocular Melanoma Study. COMS report no. 6. *Am J Ophthalmol.* 1998;125:745–766.
30. Mäkitie T, Summanen P, Tarkkanen A, Kivelä T. Tumor-infiltrating macrophages ($CD68^+$ cells) and prognosis in malignant uveal melanoma. *Invest Ophthalmol Vis Sci.* 2001;42:1414–1421.
31. Folberg R, Mehaffey M, Gardner LM, Meyer M, Rummelt V, Pe'er J. The microcirculation of choroidal and ciliary body melanomas. *Eye.* 1997;11:227–238.
32. Kivelä T. Immunohistochemical staining followed by bleaching of melanin: a practical method for ophthalmic pathology. *Br J Biomed Sci.* 1995;52:325–326.
33. Pulford KA, Rigney EM, Micklem KJ, Jones M, Stross WP, Gatter KC, Mason DY. KP1: a new monoclonal antibody that detects a monocyte/macrophage associated antigen in routinely processed tissue sections. *J Clin Pathol.* 1989;42:414–421.
34. Van Ravenswaay Claasen HH, Kluin PM, Fleuren GJ. Tumor infiltrating cells in human cancer. On the possible role of CD16+ macrophages in antitumor cytotoxicity. *Lab Invest.* 1992;67:166–174.
35. Urban JL, Shepard HM, Rothstein JL, Sugarman BJ, Schreiber H. Tumor necrosis factor: a potent effector molecule for tumor cell killing by activated macrophages. *Proc Natl Acad Sci USA.* 1986;83:5233–5237.
36. Hibbs JB, Jr., Taintor RR, Vavrin Z, Rachlin EM. Nitric oxide: a cytotoxic activated macrophage effector molecule. *Biochem Biophys Res Commun.* 1988;157:87–94.
37. Pozzi LA, Weiser WY. Human recombinant migration inhibitory factor activates human macrophages to kill tumor cells. *Cell Immunol.* 1992;145:372–379.
38. Shimizu T, Abe R, Nakamura H, Ohkawara A, Suzuki M, Nishihira J. High expression of macrophage migration inhibitory factor in human melanoma cells and its role in tumor cell growth and angiogenesis. *Biochem Biophys Res Commun.* 1999;264: 751–758.
39. Etoh T, Shibuta K, Barnard GF, Kitano S, Mori M. Angiogenin expression in human colorectal cancer: the role of focal macrophage infiltration. *Clin Cancer Res.* 2000;6: 3545–3551.
40. Sunderkotter C, Steinbrink K, Goebeler M, Bhardwaj R, Sorg C. Macrophages and angiogenesis. *J Leukoc Biol.* 1994;55:410–422.
41. Davies B, Waxman J, Wasan H, Abel P, Williams G, Krausz T, Neal D, Thomas D, Hanby A, Balkwill F. Levels of matrix metalloproteases in bladder cancer correlate with tumor grade and invasion. *Cancer Res.* 1993;53:5365–5369.
42. Lah TT, Kalman E, Najjar D, Gorodetsky E, Brennan P, Somers R, Daskal I. Cells producing cathepsins D, B, and L in human breast carcinoma and their association with prognosis. *Hum Pathol.* 2000;31:149–160.
43. Lewis JS, Landers RJ, Underwood JC, Harris AL, Lewis CE. Expression of vascular endothelial growth factor by macrophages is up-regulated in poorly vascularized areas of breast carcinomas. *J Pathol.* 2000;192:150–158.
44. Turner L, Scotton C, Negus R, Balkwill F. Hypoxia inhibits macrophage migration. *Eur J Immunol.* 1999;29:2280–2287.
45. Messmer E, Bornfeld N, Foerster M, Schilling H, Wessing A. Histopathologic findings in eyes treated with a ruthenium plaque for uveal melanoma. *Graefes Arch Clin Exp Ophthalmol.* 1992;230:391–396.

46. Schurmans LRHM, Blom DJR, De Waard-Siebinga I, Keunen JEE, Prause JU, Jager MJ. Effects of transpupillary thermotherapy on immunological parameters and apoptosis in a case of primary uveal melanoma. *Melanoma Res.* 1999;9:297–302.
47. Stephens TC, Currie GA, Peacock JH. Repopulation of gamma-irradiated Lewis lung carcinoma by malignant cells and host macrophage progenitors. *Br J Cancer.* 1978;38: 573–582.
48. Rummelt V, Mehaffey MG, Campbell RJ, Pe'er J, Bentler SE, Woolson RF, Naumann GO, Folberg R. Microcirculation architecture of metastases from primary ciliary body and choroidal melanomas. *Am J Ophthalmol.* 1998;126:303–305.
49. Manor RS, Livni E, Joshua H, Ben-Sira I. Inhibition of macrophage migration by choroidal malignant melanoma-associated antigens in patients with uveal melanoma. *Invest Ophthalmol Vis Sci.* 1978;17:684–687.
50. Repp AC, Mayhew ES, Apte S, Niederkorn JY. Human uveal melanoma cells produce macrophage migration-inhibitory factor to prevent lysis by NK cells. *J Immunol.* 2000;165:710–715.
51. Scholes AG, Hagan S, Hiscott P, Damato BE, Grierson I. Overexpression of epidermal growth factor receptor is restricted to macrophages in uveal melanoma. *Arch Ophthalmol.* 2001;119:373–377.
52. All-Ericsson C, Girnita L, Seregard S, Bartolazzi A, Jager MJ, Larsson O. Insulin-like growth factor-1 receptor in uveal melanoma: a predictor for metastatic disease and a potential therapeutic target. *Invest Ophthalmol Vis Sci.* 2002;43:1–8.

RITA PARYS-VAN GINDERDEUREN

# 14. Clinical Relevance of PAS Patterns in Uveal Melanomas

## INTRODUCTION

It has already been known for a long-time that the presence of vessels plays a role in the prognosis and the development of metastatic disease in tumors. This is also known for melanomas of the uvea which have no lymphatics, and metastatic uveal melanoma is thus an example of a tumor that spreads purely hematogeneously.

Since the first publication of the group of Folberg in 1992,[1] it has been accepted that the morphology of vascular patterns, highlighted by the PAS stain, is important for the prognosis[2–8] in patients with a uveal melanoma.

In the first study[1] about the morphology of vessels in uveal melanomas, nine morphologic patterns were identified by two methods. Using the first method, tissue sections were stained by *Ulex europaeus* I and vascular patterns were described by using laser scanning confocal microscopy. The second technique was a modified PAS stain, which can be prepared by routine laboratory techniques: the sections were first bleached if needed because of the sometimes heavy pigmentation, and stained with a routine PAS stain without counterstain. The slides were reviewed with a green filter to highlight the contrast (Fig. 14.1). The magenta colour of the PAS stain has a maximum absorption peek in green light at 544 nm.

## FURTHER STUDIES

In the study of Folberg in Human Pathology in 1992,[1] 40 choroidal and ciliary body melanoma cases were investigated for the presence of the PAS patterns. A group of 20 melanoma cases was compared to another group of 20 cases by tumor size and location; one group consisted of tumors from patients who died from metastatic disease and the other group of patients who survived at least 15 years, free of metastatic melanoma. There was a clear association between the presence of loops and survival. Of the 20 patients who were still alive after 15 years, only three of the tumors had loops and 17 did not contain loops. In the tumors of the 20 patients who died of metastatic disease 18 contained loops and two did not, but these two had intravascular invasion. In this study, closed loops were associated with other

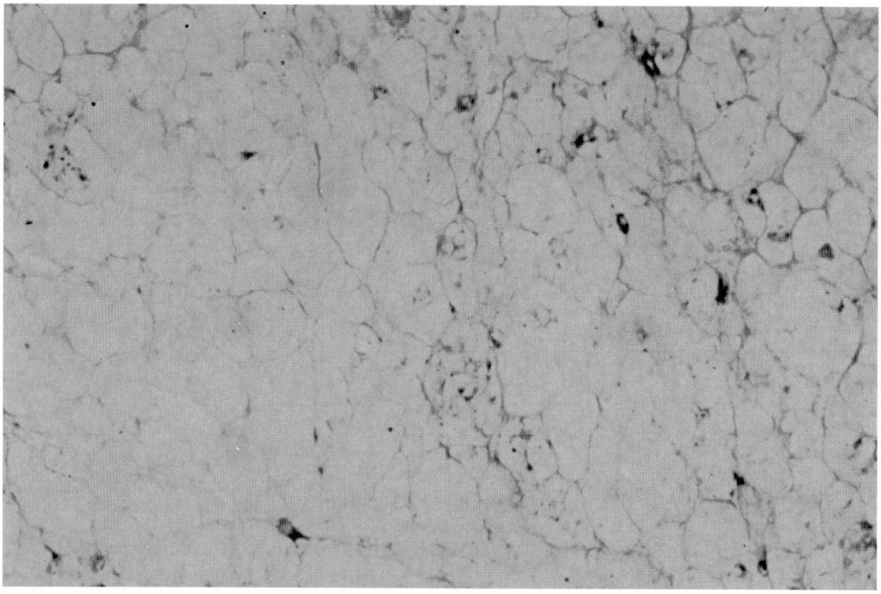

Fig. 14.1. PAS patterns in uveal melanoma, viewed with green filter: multiple loops forming a network are visible in a choroidal melanoma.

histologic features that are predictive of an unfavorable outcome: epithelioid cells and mitotic figures.

In 1993, a larger study of 234 eyes removed for ciliary body or choroidal melanomas was published in Ophthalmology.[2] Of the 234 tumors, 56% contained loops and 44% did not; 46% of the tumors contained networks. The tumors which did not contain loops or networks had a very high survival rate: 91% and 88%, respectively. But if loops or networks were present the chance for survival was only 51 and 55%. In this study the presence of vascular networks was the feature most strongly associated with death from metastatic disease. Other significant prognostic factors in a Cox model included, in descending order of importance, largest tumor dimension, number of mitoses, parallel with cross-linking pattern and age.

In the study of McLean in Ophthalmology in 1997,[3] a comparison was made of the prognostic value of fibrovascular loops, the mean of the ten largest nucleoli, cell type and tumor size in uveal melanomas with a follow up time of 15 years. However, they performed a standard PAS stain without looking through a green filter and the prevalence of loops was much lower than in the former studies. Loops were found in only 24% of tumors, but if they were present, 66% of patients died of metastatic disease. If loops were not present, the death rate was 33% after 15 years. With these results they concluded that the presence of loops was an indicator of poor prognosis but less than shown in the former studies. Even so, they advised to put the results in the final pathologic report.

In the study of Seregard in 1998 in Ophthalmology,[4] a comparison was made between the prognostic value and predictive accuracy of the PC-10 cell-cycling marker, the largest tumor diameter, the mean of the largest nucleoli, and vascular patterns in posterior uveal melanoma. In this study on 132 patients with a melanoma, 55% died of metastatic disease and 45% was alive after 10 or more years. Only 38% of these tumors contained loops and only in 19% of cases networks were detected. All of these parameters, i.e., vessel patterns, expression of PC-10, and largest tumor diameter were independently associated with outcome. However, each had only a poor-to-moderate predictive accuracy. They proposed a prognostic index combining two or more indicators to improve the predictive precision. The sensitivity of networks was low but the specificity was very high.

In the study of Mäkitie in 1999,[5] 167 melanomas of choroid or ciliary body were analysed. They could investigate the vascular patterns in 134 cases. In this study, loops were present in 60% of tumors and networks in 35%. If the tumor did not contain loops the patient survival rate was 83%. In the presence of networks the survival rate diminished to 41%. They decided that these patterns were the strongest univariate prognostic factor. Next was the presence of epithelioid cells, then came largest basal diameter and involvement of the ciliary body.

It is known that ciliary body melanomas have a worse prognosis and give rise to metastases more frequently; the vascular patterns and the aggressive behaviour of ciliary body melanomas were compared in order to investigate their relation.[9] Regardless of location, ciliary body or choroid, the presence of vascular networks is related to a shorter survival. The tumor location looses its significance when the vascular patterns are added. The aggressive behaviour of ciliary body melanomas appeared to be related to the tendency for vascular networks to develop in this location.

Recently, these vascular patterns were investigated in relation to other locations of the tumor; melanomas confined to the iris are characterised by a low rate of proliferation and histologic absence of loops and networks; while the prevalence was higher in choroidal and even more in ciliary body tumors.[10] The prevalence of the vascular patterns was correlated to prognosis by location.

The distribution of these patterns across multiple levels in melanomas was studied and it was concluded that these vessels may be consistent throughout the depth of the tumor, which eliminates the need for sectioning the tumor at multiple levels.[11]

There is a relative importance of the amount of area occupied by these patterns, but the most dramatic increase in prognostic information is provided by determination of the presence or absence of specific microvascular patterns.[12]

## CONCLUSION

In conclusion, all these studies show that the presence of the PAS patterns loops and networks are an independent prognostic factor in uveal melanoma. If networks or loops are present, the death rate is between 45 and 66%; in the absence of loops, the survival rate is very high (from 92 to 67%); this prediction can be even higher by combining other prognostic factors.

## REFERENCES


1. Folberg R, Pe'er J, Gruman LM, Woolson RF, Jeng G, Montague PR, Moninger TO, Yi H, Moore KC. The morphologic characteristics of tumor blood vessels as a marker of tumor progression in primary human uveal melanoma: a matched case-control study. *Hum Pathol.* 1992;23:1298–1305.
2. Folberg R, Rummelt V, Parys-Van Ginderdeuren R, Hwang T, Woolson RF, Pe'er J, Gruman LM. The prognostic value of tumor blood vessel morphology in primary uveal melanoma. *Ophthalmology.* 1993;100:1389–1398.
3. McLean IW, Keefe KS, Burnier MN. Uveal melanoma. Comparison of the prognostic value of fibrovascular loops, mean of the ten largest nucleoli, cell type, and tumor size. *Ophthalmology.* 1997;104:777–780.
4. Seregard S, Spangberg B, Juul C, Oskarsson M. Prognostic accuracy of the mean of the largest nucleoli, vascular patterns, and PC-10 in posterior uveal melanoma. *Ophthalmology.* 1998;105:485–491.
5. Makitie T, Summanen P, Tarkkanen A, Kivela T. Microvascular loops and networks as prognostic indicators in choroidal and ciliary body melanomas. *J Natl Cancer Inst.* 1999;17:359–367.
6. Pe'er J, Rummelt V, Mawn L, Hwang T, Woolson RF, Folberg R. Mean of the ten largest nucleoli, microcirculation architecture, and prognosis of ciliochoroidal melanomas. *Ophthalmology.* 1994;101:1227–1235.
7. Foss AJ, Alexander RA, Hungerford JL, Haris AL, Cree IA, Lightman S. Reassessment of the PAS patterns in uveal melanoma. *Brit J Ophthalmol.* 1997;81:240–246.
8. Sakamato T, Sakamato M, Yoshikawa H, Hata Y, Ishibashi T, Ohnishi Y, Inomata H. Histologic findings and prognoses of uveal malignant melanoma in Japanese patients. *Am J Ophthalmol.* 1996;121:276–283.
9. Rummelt V, Folberg R, Woolson RF, Hwang T, Pe'er J. Relation between the microcirculation architecture and the aggressive behavior of ciliary body melanomas. *Ophthalmology.* 1995;102(5):844–851.
10. Chowers I, Folberg R, Livni N, Pe'er J. Comparison of microcirculation patterns and MIB-1 immunoreactivity in iris and posterior uveal melanoma. *Ophthalmology.* 2001; 108:367–371.
11. Mehaffey MG, Gardner LM, Folberg R. Distribution of prognostically important vascular patterns across multiple levels in ciliary body and choroidal melanomas. *Am J Ophthalmol.* 1998;126:373–378.
12. Mehaffey MG, Folberg R, Meyer M, Bentler SE, Hwang T, Woolson R, Moore KC. Relative importance of quantifying area and vascular patterns in uveal melanomas. *Am J Ophthalmol.* 1997;123:798–809.

A.J. MUELLER, D.-U. BARTSCH, U. SCHALLER, W.R. FREEMAN AND A. KAMPIK

# 15. Frequency of Microcirculation Patterns in Human Choroidal Melanomas Using Simultaneous Confocal Sodium-Fluorescein/Indocyanine Green Angiography

## INTRODUCTION

The uveal melanoma is the most common primary intraocular tumor of the adult with an age-adjusted incidence of six tumors in one million patients.[1] A variety of therapeutical options are currently available.[2–16] However, many authors recommend to wait for definite tumor growth in smaller melanomas mainly to distinguish them from so-called 'pseudomelanomas'.[17–36]

Several years ago a large histopathologic study demonstrated various microcirculation patterns (MCP) in uveal melanomas, some of which were highly significantly correlated with metastatic disease from uveal melanoma.[37–42] These results have been confirmed in several independent studies.[43–48] So-called silent zones, the normal and the parallel without cross-linking MCP was correlated with a favorable prognosis, while networks and the parallel with cross-linking MCP was correlated with a high risc of metastatic disease.

We[49–52] and others (*Ophthalmologe* 95 (Suppl 1): 53; 1998) demonstrated previously that all microcirculation patterns that were described histologically can be imaged by indocyanine green angiography (Fig. 15.1). We confirmed the presence of various ICG angiographically imaged microcirculation patterns in direct angiographic/histopathologic comparisons in humans and in newly developed human melanoma animal models that were specifically designed for this purpose.[50,51] Microcirculation patterns do demonstrate specific changes after brachtherapy that are also imageable.[53] We also demonstrated that the identification of microcirculation patterns using confocal ICG is superior to fluorescein angiograms using a conventional acquisition technique with a fundus camera[52] (Fig. 15.2). It is well known that conventional fluorescein angiography using a fundus camera does not show a pathognomonic fluorescence pattern (FA) in choroidal melanomas[54–58] nor are microcirculation patterns consistently seen. Size and pigmentation of the tumor has a considerable influence on the appearance of the fluorescein angiogram. The effect of the tumor on adjacent ocular structures, particularly the retinal pigment epithelium, also contributes significantly to its fluorescein angiographic appearance. If the overlying retinal pigment epithelium is completely intact, a fairly normal fluorescein

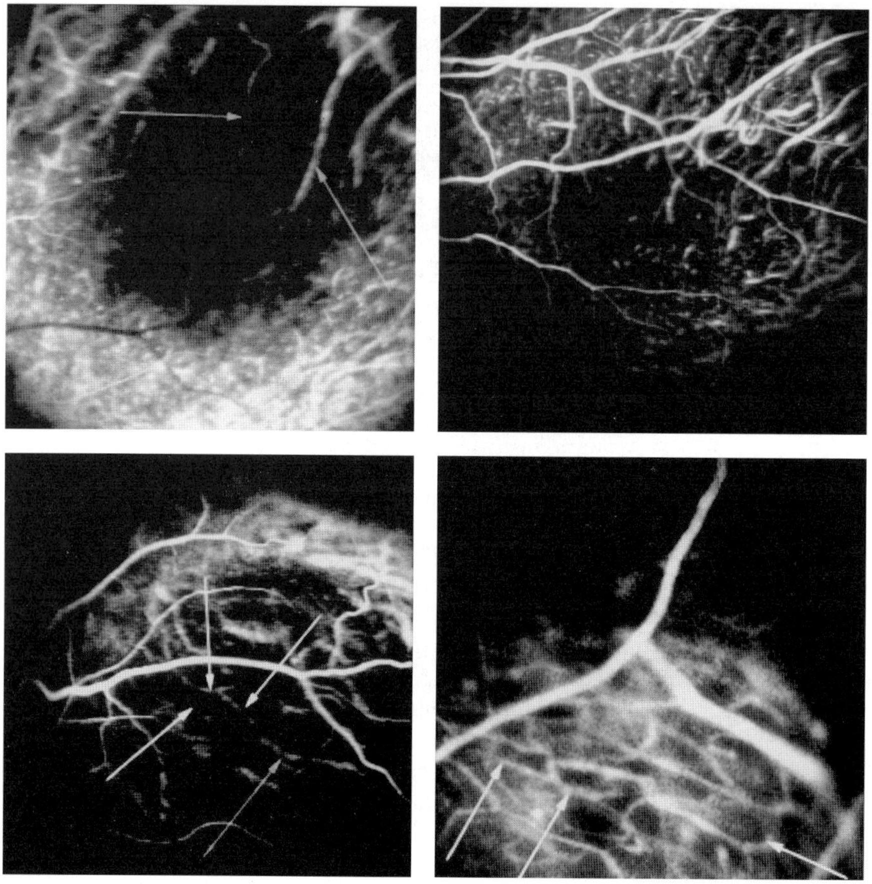

Fig. 15.1. ICG-angiographical appearance of the following microcirculation patterns: normal (top left), arcs with branching (top right), parallel with cross-linking (bottom left), and network (bottom right) containing three or more back-to-back loops.

angiogram may result. Overlying retinal vessels are usually easily visible during all phases. However, the so-called double or tumor circulation (simultaneous visualization of retinal and choroidal circulation) is often difficult to image. Usually it is only visible when the tumor is amelanotic or has broken through Bruch's membrane. Additionally, this sign is usually constricted to the very early phase of the FA. In later phases leakage of dye may mask these phenomenon (Fig. 15.3). Clearly, the absence of this finding does not indicate lack of extensive tumor microcirculation.

Indocyanine green angiography is a method which was primarily developed for imaging choroidal vessels *in vivo*.[11,59–62] Because the near-infrared light used for indocyanine green angiography penetrates the pigmented layers of the fundus more easily than the short wavelength light used in fluorescein angiography (Fig. 15.1), indocyaninegreen angiography has been primarily used to study leakage of dye in choroidal neovascularization during the late phase and thereby to detect changes

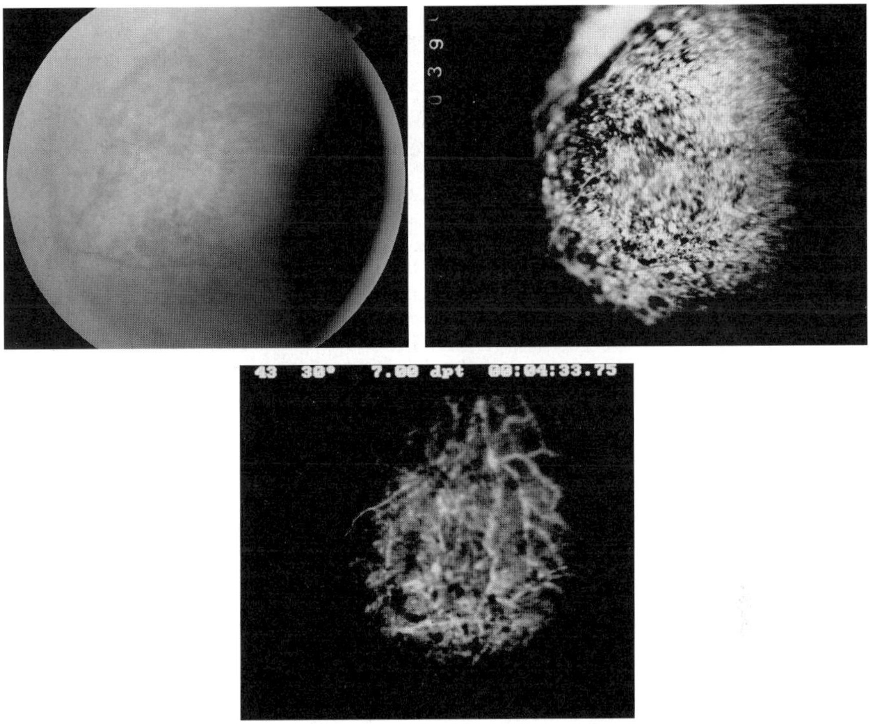


Fig. 15.2. Left: Female patient with a densely pigmented choroidal melanoma located in the upper temporal quadrant of the left eye. The maximum apical tumor height is 4.9 mm according to standardized ultrasound. Right: Fluorescein angiogram reveals the typical mottled hyperfluorescence, but due to the heavy pigmentation no internal microcirculation is imageable. Bottom: Indocyanine green angiography of the same area. Note the localization of the retinal vessel corresponding to the one in the fluorescein angiogram. Multiple dilated tumor vessels with anastomoses are seen.

in the vascular permeability of these vessels. Recently, our group described the confocal scanning laser technology to perform indocyanine green angiography[63] and later simultaneous FA/ICG angiography.[49] This technique uses sensitive digital image acquisition and processing. The horizontal image resolution has considerably improved to below 20 μm. The size of the reported histologic microcirculation patterns falls in this range and thus, we hypothesized, that the patterns should therefore be imageable with the above described technique. In this report we sought to determine the frequency of microcirculation patterns in 100 consecutive human choroidal melanomas using a simultaneous fluorescein/indocyanine green angiography.

## PATIENTS

We studied 100 patients with a newly diagnosed prominent choroidal mass diagnosed as choroidal melanoma. Diagnosis of choroidal melanoma was established by indirect ophthalmoscopy based on the characteristic appearance of this tumor

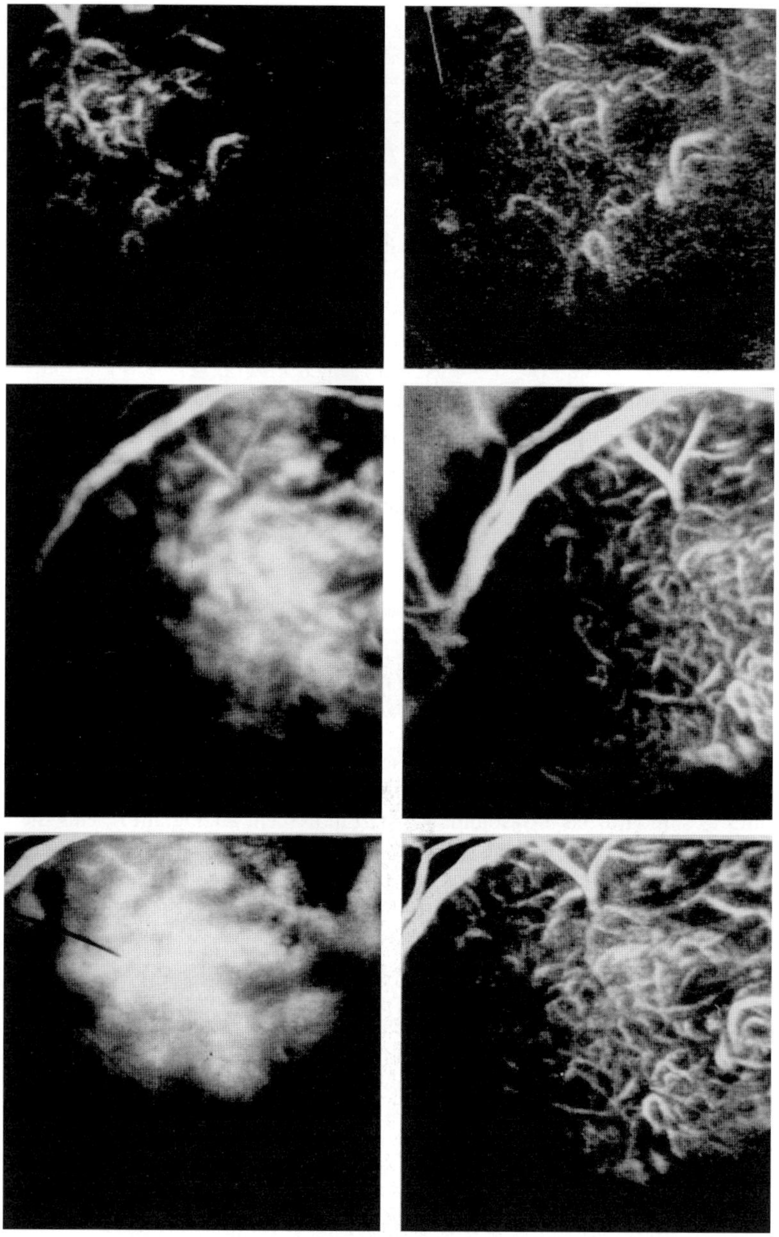

Fig. 15.3. Simultaneous confocal fluorescein (left column) and indocyanine green (right column) angiography of an amelanotic choroidal melanoma (top row: early phase, middle row: middle phase, bottom row: late phase). While the early phase clearly reveals signs of a double circulation in both angiograms, the tumor microcirculation is masked in the middle and late phase in the fluorescein channel due to diffuse leakage of the dye. In contrast, in the indocyanine green channel the microcirculation pattern can be consistently identified throughout all phases.

and confirmed using standardized ultrasound A- and B-scan. Only tumors with a maximum apical height of more than 1.5 mm and low or low to medium internal reflectivity (2 to 60% retinal spike height) according to standardized ultrasound A-scan were enrolled. Thereafter, simultaneous fluorescein/indocyanine green angiography was obtained using a confocal scanning laser ophthalmoscope (Heidelberg Retina Angiograph (HRA), Heidelberg Engineering, Heidelberg (Germany)). The instrument has been described in detail previously.[49]

The optics of this instrument allowed for spherical aberration compensation between −12 and +12 diopters (D). By automatically adjusting the focal plane, confocal serial optical sections were obtained (Fig. 15.4). This was performed to facilitate visualization of deep tumor vessels. The simultaneous fluorescein/indocyanine green angiograms were compared for the visibility of the so-called double or tumor circulation. Tumor circulation was defined by the presence of tubular structures that were filling with dye during the early (arterial) phase and that appeared empty in the late phase of the angiogram (Fig. 15.5). In addition, it was required that the filling pattern of these vessels was separate from that of the overlying retinal circulation.

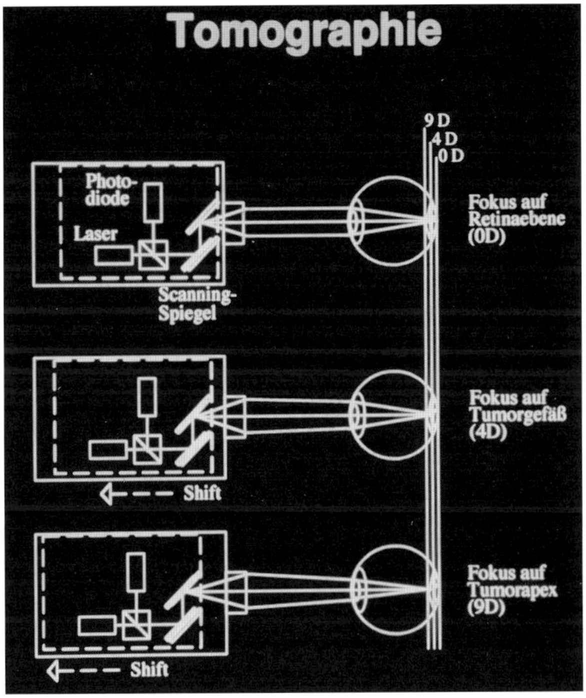


Fig. 15.4. Schematic drawing illustrating an optical sectioning series in a tumor of 3 mm height in an emmetropic eye. In this series, the scanning laser beam would be rapidly and consecutively focused in 1 D steps from 0 D (tumor basis) to 9 D (tumor apex). The following steps are shown: focusing on the plane of adjacent retina (top, 0 D), on a tumor vessel (middle, 4 D) and on the tumor apex (bottom, 9 D).

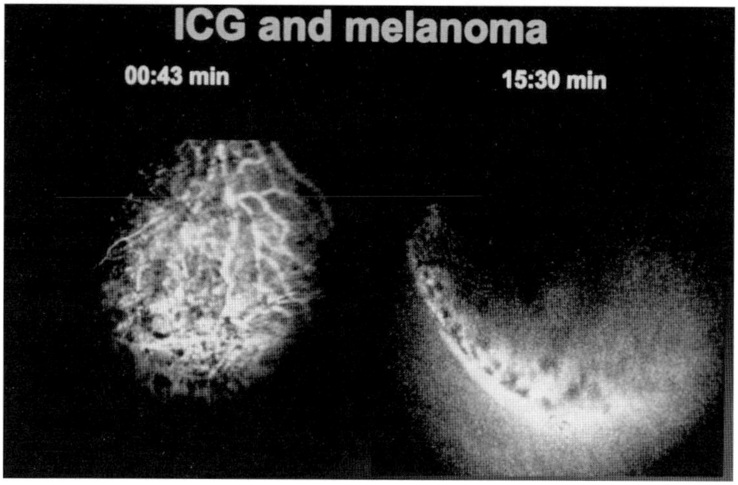


Fig. 15.5. Same patient as in Figure 15.2. Tumor circulation was defined by the presence of tubular structures that were filling with dye during the early (arterial) phase (left) and that appeared empty in the late phase of the angiogram (right).

When tumor vessels were visible in the fluorescein or indocyanine green angiogram, the microcirculation pattern of the tumor circulation was classified in a second step. The angiographic appearance of the microcirculation patterns was classified according to the histologic description: normal, silent, straight, parallel with and without cross-linking, arcs with and without branching, loops, networks.[38,39] If a tumor did not show any sign of localized or diffuse hyperfluorescence within the tumor borders the microcirculation pattern was classified as silent. However, some tumor angiograms disclosed multiple microcirculation pattern in different as well as in the same confocal optical sections which were described histologically. Thus, it was possible to classify multiple microcirculation pattern within one tumor (Fig. 15.1).

## INDOCYANINE GREEN ANGIOGRAMS

Confocal series of fluorescein and indocyanine green angiograms of 100 consecutive patients with untreated choroidal melanomas were analysed. Six patients (6%) had an amelanotic melanoma. The other tumors were pigmented. The median maximal apical tumor height according to standardized A-scan was 3.5 mm with a 95% CI of 2.0 to 7.7 mm. The median maximal diameter of the tumor basis was 10 mm with a 95% CI of 4.5 to 14 mm. The internal reflectivity according to standardized A-scan was low in 34 tumors (68%) and low to medium in the other 16 (32%) tumors.

In the confocal fluorescein angiograms tumor vessels could be detected in 24 (24%) of the 100 patients. In contrast, confocal indocyanine green angiography revealed tubular structures within the melanoma which were identified as tumor vessels based on their angiographic appearance in 94 (94%) of the studied 100 patients. The difference between the presence of visible tumor vessels in the confocal fluorescein (24%) and indocyanine green angiograms (94%) was statistically highly significant ($p = 0.001$, Fisher's exact test).

Traces of microcirculation patterns could be detected in six (6%) of the 100 examined patients in the confocal fluorescein angiogram. In all six cases it was only possible because the images were taken in the very early arterial phase and in three cases the microcirculation pattern was masked in later frames due to leakage of the dye (Fig. 15.3). In contrast, microcirculation patterns were identified in the confocal indocyanine green angiograms of all 94 patients in which tumor vessels were identified. Moreover, identification of microcirculation patterns was easily possible throughout the whole arterial venous phase and not limited to the early arterial phases (Fig. 15.3).

## SUMMARY OF FINDINGS

In summary, in 52 areas the microcirculation was classified as 'normal,' in 40 as 'silent,' in 82 as 'straight,' in 12 as 'parallel without cross-linking,' in 48 as 'parallel with cross-linking,' in 28 as 'arcs without branching,' in 28 as 'arcs with branching,' in 24 as 'loops' and in 24 more areas as 'networks' (Fig. 15.6). None of the cases with multiple microcirculation pattern contained the 'silent' or 'parallel without cross-linking' pattern together with the 'parallel with cross-linking' pattern or 'networks.'

## DISCUSSION

The accuracy of diagnosing a choroidal melanoma has considerably increased over the last 25 years.[64] Several well established treatment options are currently available, most of them capable of sufficiently controlling the primary tumor. However, it appears that none of these approaches is able to prevent late metastasis. Because none of the currently available treatment options seems to influence the rate of metastasis, it is desirable to identify clinically patients with high and low risk of developing metastases. For patients with low risk of developing metastases frequent clinical observation might be the best management of the tumor, especially if the tumor is small and does not show any growth. In contrast, several recent publications have suggested a possible role of active immunotherapy for the prevention or adjuvant chemotherapy for the treatment of overt metastases.[65,66] Some of the used substances are toxic and certainly not suitable for all patients with choroidal melanomas. Thus, it is also desirable to identify clinically patients with high risk of developing metastatic disease who might qualify for these new therapies. Although highly desirable, the role of tumor markers for identifying patients with a high risk of developing metastatic disease is currently under investigation but still remains to be established.[67]

Recently it has been shown that certain histologically identified microcirculation patterns are an independent risk factor for the metastatic behavior of choroidal melanomas. Especially complex microcirculation patterns such as 'parallel with cross-linking' and 'networks' indicate a high probability for metastatic disease whereas the presence of 'silent' and 'parallel without cross-linking' microcirculation patterns indicated a better prognosis for the patients.[37–42] Because this study was

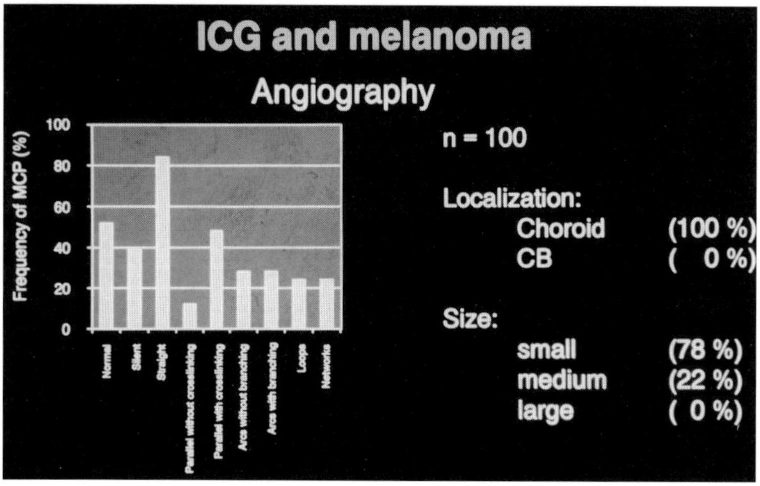


Fig. 15.6. Relative frequency of microcirculation patterns detected using confocal indocyanine green angiography in 100 consecutive small and medium-sized choroidal melanomas.

clearly confirmed by other independent histopathology labs[44,47,48] these important findings motivated us to determine whether it is possible to image and identify prognostically significant microcirculation patterns of choroidal melanomas *in vivo* using conventional fluorescein and indocyanine green angiography with a new confocal scanning ophthalmoscope.[63] We have found that confocal indocyanine green angiography is capable of detecting microcirculation pattern and superior to fluorescein angiography using a conventional fundus camera. Because of the commercial availability of a simultaneous fluorescein/indocyanine green angiograph[41] we now routinely use this instrument to study microcirculation patterns in human choroidal melanomas.

When comparing the visibility of tumor microcirculation in fluorescein with confocal indocyanine green angiograms, both taken simultaneously with the same confocal scanning laser ophthalmoscope, we found that tumor microcirculation was imaged in 94 (94%) of the examined 100 patients using confocal indocyanine green angiography. In the remaining six patients the tumor appeared indocyanine angiographically as empty. In these patients the microcirculation pattern was classified as silent. Hence, indocyanine green angiographically determined counterparts of histologically described microcirculation pattern could be determined in all patients in various confocal optical sections. Specifically we were able to image 'parallel with cross-linking' in 48 areas and 'networks' in 24 areas. The microcirculation pattern 'silent' was imaged in 40 areas and 'parallel without cross-linking' in 12 areas. All four microcirculation patterns have been demonstrated to be highly correlated with a specific risk for the patient of developing metastatic disease. In none of our cases high risk microcirculation patterns ('networks', 'parallel with cross-linking') were seen together with low risk microcirculation patterns ('silent', 'parallel without cross-linking').

In contrast, simultaneously taken confocal fluorescein angiography was able to reveal signs of tumor vessels in only 24 (24%) of the studied 100 patients. Moreover, in only six of the latter cases, traces of microcirculation patterns could be identified in the confocal fluorescein angiograms. However, this was only possible in the very early arterial phase of the angiogram. In the later phases the microcirculation pattern was masked due to leakage of the dye.

## CONCLUSION

Our study demonstrates that indocyanine green angiography using a confocal scanning laser ophthalmoscope is superior to fluorescein angiography even when using the same instrument in imaging microcirculation patterns. The angiographically seen microcirculation patterns appear to be identical to patterns that have been identified histologically and that have prognostic significance in choroidal melanomas. Thus, this minimally-invasive technique has the potential to be used as a 'non-invasive biopsy.' This method may also play a future role in monitoring patients with choroidal melanomas who will undergo anti-angiogenesis therapy. Although this is not a standard treatment yet, there are currently at least 20 anti-angiogenesis drugs under clinical investigation[68] and some of these have already entered phase III trials. In this scenario, confocal ICG could be helpful in monitoring the anti-angiogenetic effect *in vivo*.

## ACKNOWLEDGEMENTS

Supported by Deutsche Forschungsgemeinschaft (DFG) Mu1204/1-1,1-2, Whitaker Foundation (D.-U.B.), and Stern Foundation (W.R.F.).

## REFERENCES

1. Egan K, Seddon J, Glynn R, Gragoudas E, Albert D. Epidemiologic aspects of uveal melanoma. *Surv Ophthalmol.* 1988;32:239–251.
2. Bonnett D, Kacperek A, Sheen M, Goodall R, Saxton T. The 62 MeV proton beam for the treatment of ocular melanoma at Clatterbridge. *Br J Radiol.* 1993;66:907–914.
3. Char DH, Kroll S, Quivey JM, Castro J. Long term visual outcome of radiated uveal melanomas in eyes eligible for randomisation to enucleation versus brachytherapy. *Br J Ophthalmol.* 1996;80:117–124.
4. Char DH, Kroll SM, Castro J. Long-term follow-up after uveal melanoma charged particle therapy. *T Am Ophthal Soc.* 1997;95:171–187.
5. Char DH, Kroll SM, Castro J. Ten-year follow-up of helium ion therapy for uveal melanoma. *Am J Ophthalmol.* 1998;125:81–89.
6. Collaborative ocular melanoma study group T. Factors predictive of growth and treatment of small choroidal melanoma: COMS Report No. 5. The Collaborative Ocular Melanoma Study Group [see comments]. *Arch Ophthalmol.* 1997;115:1537–1544.
7. Damato B. An approach to the management of patients with uveal melanoma. *Eye.* 1993; 7:388–397.
8. De Potter P, Shields CL, Shields JA, Cater JR, Brady LW. Plaque radiotherapy for juxtapapillary choroidal melanoma. Visual acuity and survival outcome. *Arch Ophthalmol.* 1996;114:1357–1365.

9. Gragoudas E, Goitein M, Koehler A. Proton irradiation of small choroidal malignant melanomas. *Am J Ophthalmol.* 1977;83:665–673.
10. Gragoudas E, Goitein M, Verhey L, Munzenreider J, Suit H, Koehler A. Proton beam irradiation. An alternative to enucleation for intraocular melanomas. *Ophthalmology.* 1980;87:571–581.
11. Hochheimer B. Angiography of the retina with Indocyanine green. *Arch Ophthalmol.* 1971;86:564–565.
12. Lommatzsch P, Vollmar R. Ein neuer Weg zur konservativen Therapie intraokularer Tumoren mit Betastrahlen (106Ru/106Rh) unter Erhaltung der Sehfähigkeit. *Klin Monatsbl Augenh.* 1966;148:682–699.
13. Mueller AJ, Talies S, Schaller UC, Hoops JP, Schriever S, Kampik A, Wowra B, Horstmann G, Mack A. Die stereotaktische Präzisionsbestrahlung grosser uvealer Melanome mit dem Gamma-knife. *Ophthalmologe.* 2000;97:537–545.
14. Mueller AJ, Talies S, Schaller UC, Horstmann G, Wowra B, Kampik A. Stereotactic radiosurgery of large uveal melanomas with the gamma-knife. *Ophthalmology.* 2000; 107:1381–1387; discussion 1387–1388.
15. Shields J. Current approaches to the diagnosis and management of choroidal melanomas. *Surv Ophthalmol.* 1977;21:443–463.
16. Shields J, Shields C. *Intraocular Tumors.* Philadelphia, Saunders 1988.
17. Zehetmayer M, Menapace R, Kitz K, Ertl A, Strenn K, Ruhswurm I. Stereotactic irradiation of uveal melanoma with the Leksell gamma unit. *Front Radiat Ther On.* 1997;30:47–55.
18. Augsburger J, Gonder J, Amsel J, Shields J, Donoso L. Growth rates and doubling times of posterior uveal melanoma. *Ophthalmology.* 1984;91:1709–1715.
19. Augsburger J, Schroeder R, Territo C, Gamel J, Shields J. Clinical parameters predictive of enlargement of melanocytic choroidal lesions. *Br J Ophthalmol.* 1989;73:911–917.
20. Barr C, Sipperley J, Nicholson D. Small melanomas of the choroid. *Arch Ophthalmol.* 1978;96:1580–1582.
21. Butler P, Char DH, Zarbin M, Kroll S. Natural history of indeterminate pigmented choroidal tumors. *Ophthalmology.* 1994;101:710–716; discussion 717.
22. Chang AE, Karnell LH, Menck HR. The National Cancer Data Base report on cutaneous and noncutaneous melanoma: a summary of 84,836 cases from the past decade. The American College of Surgeons Commission on Cancer and the American Cancer Society. *Cancer.* 1998;83:1664–1678.
23. Char D, Hogan M. Management of small elevated pigmented choroidal lesions. *Br J Ophthalmol.* 1977;61:54–58.
24. Davidorf F, Lang J. Small malignant melanomas of the choroid. *Am J Ophthalmol.* 1974;78:788–793.
25. Davidorf F, Lang J. The natural history of malignant melanoma of the choroid: small vs large tumors. *T Am Acad Ophthalmol.* 1975;79:310–320.
26. Ganley J, Comstock G. Benign nevi and malignant melanomas of the choroid. *Am J Ophthalmol.* 1973;76:19–25.
27. Gass J. Problems in the differential diagnosis of choroidal nevi and malignant melanomas. *Am J Ophthalmol.* 1977;83:299–323.
28. Gass J. Observation of suspected choroidal and ciliary body melanomas for evidence of growth prior to enucleation. *Ophthalmology.* 1980;87:523–528.
29. Melia M, Diener WM, Schachat A. Mortality in patients with small choroidal melanoma. COMS report No. 4. *Arch Ophthalmol.* 1997;115:886–893.
30. Murray T. Small choroidal melanoma. *Arch Ophthalmol.* 1997;115:1577–1578.
31. Packard R. In malignant choroidal melanoma will a delay in radical treatment influence prognosis. *Trans Ophthal Soc UK.* 1983;103:49–53.

32. Shields C, Shields J, Kiratli H, De PP, Cater J. Risk factors for growth and metastasis of small melanocytic lesions. *Ophthalmology.* 1995;102:1351–1361.
33. Shields J. Lesions simulating malignant melanoma of the posterior uvea. *Arch Ophthalmol.* 1973;89:466–471.
34. Shields J, Augsburger J, Brown G, Stephens R. The differential diagnosis of posterior uveal melanoma. *Ophthalmology.* 1980;87:518–522.
35. Thomas J, Green W, Maumenee A. Small choroidal melanomas. A long-term follow-up study. *Arch Ophthalmol.* 1979;97:861–864.
36. Zimmerman L, McLean I. Do growth and onset of symptoms of uveal melanomas indicate subclinical metastasis. *Ophthalmology.* 1984;91:685–691.
37. Folberg R, Mehaffey M, Gardner L, Meyer M, Rummelt V, Pe'er J. The microcirculation of choroidal and ciliary body melanomas. *Eye.* 1997;11:227–238.
38. Folberg R, Pe'er J, Gruman L, Woolson R, Jeng G, Montague P, Moninger T, Yi H, Moore K. The morphologic characteristics of tumor blood vessels as a marker of tumor progression in primary human uveal melanoma: a matched case-control study. *Hum Pathol.* 1992;23:1298–1305.
39. Folberg R, Rummelt V, Parys, Van GR, Hwang T, Woolson R, Pe'er J, Gruman L. The prognostic value of tumor blood vessel morphology in primary uveal melanoma. *Ophthalmology.* 1993;100:1389–1398.
40. Rummelt V, Folberg R, Rummelt C, Gruman L, Hwang T, Woolson R, Hong YM, Naumann G. Microcirculation architecture of melanocytic nevi and malignant melanomas of the ciliary body and choroid. *Ophthalmology.* 1994;101:718–727.
41. Rummelt V, Folberg R, Woolson R, Hwang T, Pe'er J. Relation between the microcirculation architecture and the aggressive behavior of ciliary body melanomas. *Ophthalmology.* 1995;102:844–851.
42. Rummelt V, Gardner L, Folberg R, Beck S, Knosp B, Moninger T, Moore K. Three-dimensional relationships between tumor cells and microcirculation with double cyanine immunolabeling, laser scanning confocal microscopy, and computer-assisted reconstruction: an alternative to cast corrosion preparations. *J Histochem Cytochem* 1994;42:681–686.
43. Anastassiou G, Schilling H, Djakovic S, Bornfeld N. Expression of VLA-2, VLA-3 and αv integrin receptors in uveal melanoma: association with microvascular architecture of the tumour and prognostic value. *Br J Ophthalmol.* 2000;84:899–902.
44. Char D, Kroll S, Crawford J, O'Brien J, Lattman J. Uveal melanoma cycling, vascular patterns and prognosis. *Invest Ophthalmol Vis Sci.* 1994;35:17–21.
45. Mäkitie T, Summanen P, Kivelä T. Fibrovascular loops and networks in choroidal and ciliary body melanomas. *Ophthalmmic Res.* 1997;29:136–136.
46. McLean I, Keefe K, Burnier M. Uveal Melanoma. Comparison of the prognostic value of fibrovascular loops, mean of the ten largest nucleoli, cell type, and tumor size. *Ophthalmology.* 1997;104:777–780.
47. Sakamoto T, Sakamoto M, Yoshikawa H, Hata Y, Ishibashi T, Ohnishi Y, Inomata H. Histologic findings and prognosis of uveal malignant melanoma in japanese patients. *Am J Ophthalmol.* 1996;121:276–283.
48. Seregard S, Spanberg B, Juul C, Osskarsson M. Prognostic accuracy of the mean of the largest nucleoli, vascular patterns, and PC-10 in posterior uveal melanoma. *Ophthalmology.* 1998;105:485–491.
49. Freeman WR, Bartsch DU, Mueller AJ, Banker AS, Weinreb RN. Simultaneous indocyanine green and fluorescein angiography using a confocal scanning laser ophthalmoscope. *Arch Ophthalmol.* 1998;116:455–463.

50. Mueller AJ, Bartsch DU, Folberg R, Mehaffey MG, Boldt HC, Meyer M, Gardner LM, Goldbaum MH, Pe'er J, Freeman WR. Imaging the microvasculature of choroidal melanomas with confocal indocyanine green scanning laser ophthalmoscopy. *Arch Ophthalmol.* 1998;116:31–39.
51. Mueller AJ, Folberg R, Freeman W, Bartsch D-U, Bergeron-Lynn G, Mehaffey M, Kan-Mitchell J, X. H, Jian G, Avila C, Taskintuna I, Wang J. Evaluation of the human choroidal melanoma rabbit model for microvascularization patterns. *Exp Eye Res.* 1999;68:671–678.
52. Mueller AJ, Freeman W, Folberg R, Bartsch D-U, Scheider A, Schaller U, Kampik A. Evaluation of microvascularization pattern visibility in human choroidal melanomas comparing simultaneously taken confocal Fluorescein with Indocyanine green angiograms. *Graefes Arch Clin Exp Ophthalmol.* 1999;237:448–456.
53. Schaller U, Mueller AJ, Bartsch D-U, Freeman W, Kampik A. Choroidal melanoma microcirculation with confocal indocyanine green angiography before and 1 year after radiation brachytherapy. *Retina.* 2000;20:627–632.
54. Edwards MG, Schachat AP. Tumors in the posterior pole. *Int Ophthalmol Clin.* 1995;35:123–135.
55. Flindall R, Gass J. A histopathologic fluorescein angiographic correlative study of malignant melanomas of the choroid. *Can J Ophthalmol.* 1971;6:258–267.
56. Lommatzsch P, Ballin R, Helm W. Fluorescein angiography in the follow-up study of choroidal melanoma after 106Ru/106Rh plaque therapy. *Retina.* 1987;7:148–155.
57. Pettit T, Barton A, Foos R, Christensen R. Fluorescein angiography of choroidal melanomas. *Arch Ophthalmol.* 1970;83:27–38.
58. Tarkkanen A, Laatikainen L. Fluorescein angiography in the long-term follow-up of choroidal melanoma after conservative treatment. *Acta Ophthalmol.* 1985;63:73–79.
59. Flower R. Infrared absorption angiography of the choroid and some observations on the effects of high intraocular pressures. *Am J Ophthalmol.* 1972;74:600–614.
60. Flower R. Injection technique for indocyanine green and sodium fluorescein dye angiography of the eye. *Invest Ophthalmol Vis Sci.* 1973;12:881–895.
61. Flower R, Hochheimer B. Clinical infrared absorption angiography of the choroid. *Am J Ophthalmol.* 1972;73:458–459.
62. Flower R, Hochheimer B. Indocyanine green dye fluorescence and infrared absorption choroidal angiography performed simultaneously with fluorescein angiography. *Johns Hopkins Med J.* 1976;138:3–42.
63. Bartsch DU, Weinreb R, Zinser G, Freeman W. Confocal scanning infrared laser ophthalmoscopy for indocyanine green angiography. *Am J Ophthalmol.* 1195;20:642–651.
64. Albert D, Marcus D. Accuracy of diagnosis of choroidal melanomas in the collaborative ocular melanoma study. *Arch Ophthalmol.* 1990;108:1268–1273.
65. Mitchell M, Harel W, J. K-M, LeMay L, Goedegebuure P, Huang X, Hofman F, Groshen S. Active specific immunotherapy of melanoma with allogeneic cell lysates. Rationale, results, and possible mechanisms of action. *Ann NY Acad Sci.* 1993;690:153.
66. Quan W, Mitchell M. Phase II trial of carbetimer in metastatic melanoma. *Invest New Drug.* 1993;11:231–233.
67. Schaller UC, Bosserhoff AK, Neubauer AS, Buettner R, Kampik A, Mueller AJ. Melanoma inhibitory activity (MIA): a novel serum marker for uveal melanoma. *Mel Res.* 2002;12:593–599.
68. Casey R, Li W. Factors controlling ocular angiogenesis. *Am J Ophthalmol.* 1997;124: 521–529.

JERRY Y. NIEDERKORN

# 16. Immune Privilege and Intraocular Tumors

## IMMUNE PRIVILEGE OF THE EYE

It has been recognized for over 100 years that the anterior chamber of the eye is endowed with remarkable qualities that permit the long-term survival of foreign tissue and tumor grafts.[1] The capacity of histoincompatible tumor and tissue grafts to survive in the anterior chamber (AC), but not at other sites, spawned the notion that a unique privilege was extended to foreign tissues placed into this compartment of the eye. In the 1940s Greene and Lund took advantage of this property and used the AC as a site for propagating various human and animal tumors and for evaluating the metastatic potential of tumor biopsy specimens.[2] The conspicuous absence of patent lymphatic vessels draining the AC of the eye led to the conclusion that tissue and tumor grafts were sequestered from the peripheral lymphoid apparatus and thereby escaped immunologic recognition.

It was not until the late 1970s that this notion was changed when Kaplan and Streilein discovered that antigenic cells placed into the AC were not only perceived by the systemic immune apparatus, but in fact, elicited a dynamic down-regulation of alloimmune responses.[3,4] AC injection of alloantigenic lymphoid cells aroused the humoral arm of the immune response resulting in the generation of hemagglutinating antibodies against donor histocompatibility antigens. However, the cell-mediated component was impaired as demonstrated by the significant delay in the rejection of orthotopic donor-specific skin allografts in the AC-primed hosts.[3,4] Subsequent studies demonstrated that the lesion in the cell-mediated arm of the immune response was primarily in the generation and expression of systemic delayed-type hypersensitivity (DTH) responses to the antigens introduced into the AC. The other major form of cell-mediated immunity, cytotoxic T lymphocyte (CTL) activity, remained intact. The simultaneous activation of humoral immunity and down-regulation of DTH was termed 'lymphocyte-induced immune deviation'.[3,4] Subsequent studies from our lab indicated that the immune deviation induced by AC priming was not a function of lymphoid cells per se, but was a characteristic of the AC.[5,6] Accordingly, we coined the term 'anterior chamber-associated immune deviation' (ACAID) to emphasize the dynamic nature of this phenomenon and the fact that it required the participation of the AC.[5]

Since the original observations by Kaplan and Streilein, [3,4] hundreds of publications have confirmed the presence of ACAID using a wide range of antigens including: viral proteins,[7] soluble proteins,[8,9] histocompatibility antigens,[6,10–12] hapten-derivatized cells,[13] and important for this discussion, tumor antigens.[14]

In addition to ACAID, multiple factors contribute to the immune privilege of the intraocular environment. The aqueous humor (AH) contains a potpourri of immunomodulatory factors. Among these is transforming growth factor-beta (TGF-β), a cytokine that has pleiotropic effects that dampen both the adaptive and innate immune responses. TGF-β down regulates co-stimulatory molecule expression on antigen presenting cells (APC);[15] inhibits IL-12 production by APC;[16] promotes IL-10 production by APC;[16] down regulates MHC Class I and Class II expression on APC,[17,18] and inhibits the production of perforin and granzyme mRNA, two molecules crucial for the cytolytic function of CTL.[19] TGF-β also alters the function of ocular APC causing them to present antigen in a manner that leads to the generation of ACAID.[20] TGF-β is also a potent inhibitor of natural killer (NK) cells.[21]

The AH is also richly endowed with a variety of neuropeptides that exert anti-inflammatory and immunosuppressive effects. These include α-melanocyte stimulating hormone, calcitonin gene-related protein, somostatin, and vasoactive intestinal peptide.[22,24] Not only do these molecules possess anti-inflammatory properties, but they also promote the generation of T regulatory cells that suppress the development and expression of antigen-specific Thl immune responses.

The immune privilege of the eye is augmented by the extensive expression of Fas ligand (FasL) on the corneal endothelium, iris, ciliary body, and retinal cells. Inflammatory cells that enter the eye and come into contact with FasL subsequently undergo apoptosis.[25] Thus, the immune privilege of the eye is a superb example of biological redundancy in which multiple, overlapping mechanisms and molecules collaborate to prevent the induction and expression of antigen-specific and antigen-non-specific inflammation.

## WHAT IS THE EVIDENCE THAT IMMUNE PRIVILEGE INFLUENCES INTRAOCULAR TUMORS?

On first blush, it would seem axiomatic that the immune privilege of the eye would promote intraocular tumorigenesis. However, the incidence of uveal melanoma, the most common intraocular tumor in adults, is 16 times less than the incidence of skin melanomas. However, the low incidence of uveal melanoma compared to skin melanoma could be due to multiple parameters unrelated to the immunobiology of the tumor. Prospective studies in animals lend support to the proposition that ocular immune privilege protects intraocular tumors from the host's immune surveillance apparatus. As far back as the 1940s, Greene and Lund demonstrated that human tumor xenografts survived in the eyes of rabbits. More refined, contemporary studies in mouse models have revealed that highly immunogenic, syngeneic tumors that are routinely rejected at extraocular sites enjoy a prolonged, sometimes permanent, residence in the eye.[6,26] Using a syngeneic mouse adenovirus-transformed embryonic tumor model, Schurmans and co-workers[26] found that highly immunogenic tumors grew in the eyes of C57BL/6 mice for at least six weeks, while tumor inocula 30 times greater than the intraocular tumor inocula, failed to produce demonstrable tumors following subcutaneous transplantation. However, this privilege was limited as the highly immunogenic tumors were vulnerable to immunologic elimination if the hosts were infused with tumor-specific CTL. Immune rejection resulted in complete tumor resolution without producing collateral damage to juxtaposed normal ocular tissues.[26] Thus, the intraocular tumors were weakly immunogenic within the eye, but were highly antigenic and as a result, they were recognized by the adoptively transferred immune cells.

Perhaps an even more remarkable example of how immune privilege protects intraocular tumors from robust, systemic anti-tumor effector mechanisms is found in the P815 intraocular tumor model. P815 mastocytoma cells grow progressively in the eyes of allogeneic BALB/c mice, but fail to produce detectable tumors following subcutaneous transplantation, even at doses 100 times higher than the intraocular inocula.[27] The survival of the intraocular P815 tumors is directly attributable to the induction of ACAID.[27,28] The importance of immune privilege in general, and ACAID in specific, in sustaining the survival of intraocular tumors was demonstrated in experiments in which the induction of ACAID was prevented by splenectomy. The spleen is critical for the induction of ACAID; splenectomy up to seven days after intraocular tumor transplantation prevents the induction of ACAID and results in DTH-mediated rejection of intraocular P815 tumors.

## CONCOMITANT IMMUNITY: THE PARADOX OF OCULAR IMMUNE PRIVILEGE

Intraocular P815 mastocytomas disseminate rapidly from the eye to multiple organs including the spleen, lymph nodes, lungs, thymus, liver, and brain. Within four days of intraocular transplantation, viable P815 mastocytoma metastases can be cultured from the spleen, and by seven days, tumor cells can be cultured from the spleen, thymus, lymph nodes, lungs, and brain.[27] Although tumor cells can be cultured from the various organs for at least 21 days, the micrometastases are held in check as euthymic mice never develop fulminant metastases. Moreover, the micrometastases disappear within seven days of enucleation of the tumor-containing eye. The disappearance of the metastatic tumor cells is a T cell-mediated process as progressively growing metastases develop in athymic nude mice or in animals whose immune system is suppressed by whole-body gamma irradiation.[27] These results indicate that intraocular P815 tumor cells continuously disseminate to peripheral organs, but are swiftly eliminated by a T cell-dependent immune process that is effective in killing small numbers of micrometastases, yet is incapable of eliminating the primary intraocular tumor. This concomitant immunity is yet one more example of how the immune privilege of the eye shields the intraocular tumor from a robust systemic tumor-specific immune response.

## CIRCUMVENTION OF OCULAR IMMUNE PRIVILEGE AND SPONTANEOUS TUMOR RESOLUTION

The presence of immune privilege in the eye is irrefutable. However, ocular immune privilege is neither immutable nor universal. The induction of ACAID requires collaboration between the eye and the spleen. Ocular APC emigrate from the eye and transmit an antigen-specific signal to lymphoid cells in the spleen resulting in the generation of regulatory cells that inhibit the induction and expression of DTH. Using the P815 intraocular tumor model, we have shown that premature removal of the spleen before or shortly after tumor cells are introduced into the AC results in the abrogation of ACAID, the appearance of tumor-specific DTH, and the immune rejection of intraocular P815 tumors.[5] Interestingly, intraocular tumor rejection takes on the appearance of a DTH lesion and is characterized by ischemic necrosis of the tumor en masse and extensive damage to innocent bystander cells in the eye. Not all tumors induce ACAID. A highly immunogenic mutant of P815 mastocytoma, designated P91, induces strong DTH responses following intraocular transplantation in syngeneic DBA/2 mice.[29] The P91 tumors grow transiently in the DBA/2 mouse eye and induce DTH responses to the tumor-specific antigens. The acquisition of DTH coincides with the onset of tumor resolution. The histopathological features of intraocular P91 tumor resolution strongly resemble those found in P815 tumors undergoing immune rejection when ACAID is abrogated in splenectomized BALB/c mice. In both cases, tumor regression culminates in ischemic necrosis and phthisis of the affected eye.

Intraocular tumor rejection can also occur via a CTL-mediated process that does not culminate in phthisis. We have previously demonstrated that a highly immunogenic, syngeneic, UV-induced tumor (UV5C25) undergoes immune rejection following intraocular transplantation in syngeneic BALB/c mice.[30] Tumor rejection is T cell-dependent as it does not occur in athymic nude mice or mice rendered leukopenic by whole-body gamma irradiation. The resolving tumor lesions display a moth-eaten appearance characterized by the presence of tumor-infiltrating lymphocytes (TIL) and piecemeal necrosis of the intraocular tumors.[30] Using a 'Koch's postulates-like' approach, we tested the hypothesis that this form of intraocular tumor regression was mediated by tumor-specific CTL.[31] *In situ* immunohistochemical staining confirmed that the TIL expressed the CD8 molecule, the most common surface marker for CTL. The TIL were isolated and found to kill the UV5C25 tumor cells in an antigen-specific manner *in vitro*. Adoptive transfer of the TIL demonstrated that they were able to recapitulate the regression of intraocular UV5C25 tumors in third party hosts. That is, TIL were expanded *in vitro* and co-injected with tumor cells into the eyes of immunoincompetent hosts where they produced intraocular tumor resolution that mimicked the original phenotype, both clinically and histopathologically.

Results from two other studies lend support to the hypothesis that $CD8^+$ CTL can mediate intraocular tumor rejection.[26,32] Using an adenovirus-induced tumor model in syngeneic C57BL/6 mice, Schurmans and co-workers demonstrated that intravenously injected tumor-specific CTL entered the intraocular tumors and produced tumor resolution in a manner reminiscent of the aforementioned UV5C25 tumor rejection.[26] That is, tumor resolution occurred in a non-necrotizing manner that culminated in tumor rejection and minimal damage to normal ocular tissues. An almost identical pattern of intraocular tumor resolution was observed in an SV40 large T antigen transgenic retinal pigmented epithelial (RPE) tumor model in FVB/N mice.[32] Tumor resolution was accompanied by infiltration with $CD8^+$

TIL that displayed tumor-specific cytolytic activity *in vitro* and that produced intraocular tumor rejection following adoptive transfer to third party hosts. Thus, immunogenic intraocular tumors can undergo immune rejection in the eye by two distinct patterns. In one pattern, the mechanism involves ischemic necrosis by a DTH-like process that carries a heavy burden of innocent bystander damage. A second pattern is characterized by piecemeal necrosis of the tumor cells by CTL and does not inflict significant damage to normal ocular tissues.

## INTRAOCULAR SILENCING OF NATURAL KILLER CELLS

The notion that the immune system might be capable of recognizing and eliminating neoplasms was first articulated by the eminent microbiologist Paul Ehrlich and later modified by Burnet.[33] In the thirty years since Burnet's proposal of the immune surveillance theory, most research has centered on the role of T cells and cytokines in tumor immunity. However, in addition to T cell-mediated tumor immunity, natural resistance mechanisms may also be important.[34] Natural resistance mechanisms involve macrophages, natural killer (NK) cells, and granulocytes. NK cells seem particularly suited for the surveillance of neoplasms as these cells do not require priming or clonal expansion in order to exert anti-tumor effects. Like T cells, NK cells produce cell-mediated cytotoxicity and secrete a diverse array of cytokines and chemokines. However, unlike B and T cells, NK cell development and function does not require gene rearrangement.[34] Results from animal studies over the past two decades have provided compelling evidence that NK cells play an important role in limiting the growth and metastasis of various rodent tumors, especially skin melanomas. However, the role of NK cells in controlling the growth of intraocular melanomas is less clear and may turn out to be significantly different than what occurs in skin melanomas. *In vitro* studies have shown that uveal melanomas are susceptible to NK cell mediated lysis *in vitro*.[35,36] However, NK-sensitive uveal melanomas grow progressively when transplanted into the eyes of athymic nude mice that possess normal or even slightly elevated systemic NK cell activity. By contrast, the same NK-sensitive tumors, which grow progressively in the eye, are rejected when transplanted to subcutaneous sites, even at doses 50-fold higher than the intraocular inocula.[37] The intraocular silencing of NK cell activity appears to reside at least in part in the constituents of the AH. TGF-β is a pleiotropic cytokine that is present within both the anterior and posterior compartments of the eye. Among its many functions, TGF-β inhibits NK cell-mediated cytotoxicity.[21] *In vitro* studies have demonstrated that the optimal concentration of TGF-β for inhibiting NK cell-mediated cytolytic activity is the same as the normal physiological concentration within the aqueous humor of the eye (i.e., 2 ng/ml).[21,38] Other results have shown that AH inhibits NK cell-mediated cytolysis; however, unlike TGF-β, which requires 18–20 hours to exert its inhibitory effect, AH produces an immediate diminution of NK cell activity.[39,40] Moreover, treating AH with anti-TGF-β antibody does not remove its NK-inhibitory activity. Gel filtration chromatography of rabbit AH has revealed that a single 10–12 kDa protein fraction is responsible for the immediate inhibitory effect on NK cell-mediated cytolytic activity. Amino acid sequence analysis of this fraction has shown that the molecule shares >90% amino acid homology with macrophage migration inhibitory factor (MIF). Further *in vitro* studies have demonstrated that recombinant MIF produces an immediate inhibition of NK cell-mediated cytolysis similar to that produced by AH. Thus, the intraocular milieu possesses at least two NK-inhibitory molecules, MIF and TGF-β. The former exerts its effect immediately, while the latter mediates a delayed, protracted inhibition of NK cytolysis in the eye.

Although the intraocular milieu provides uveal melanomas sanctuary from NK cell-mediated attack, once metastatic uveal melanoma cells leave the eye, they must evade NK cells within the bloodstream and within the parenchyma of the liver—two sites of intense NK activity. If NK cell-mediated immune surveillance plays a significant role in controlling uveal melanoma metastases, one might predict that successful metastases need to be endowed with properties that inhibit NK cell activity outside of the immunologically privileged confines of the eye. Two possibilities come to mind. First, the expression of MHC Class I molecules is known to protect tumor cells from NK cell-mediated lysis by sending an 'off' signal to NK cells.[41] Thus, upregulating MHC Class I molecules would be an effective strategy for metastases to escape destruction in the bloodstream and liver. A second strategy for evading NK surveillance, is for the melanoma cells to create their own immune privileged milieu by secreting NK inhibitory factors such as TGF-β and MIF. Two studies on human melanoma patients lend support to the hypothesis that MHC Class I antigen expression favors the development of uveal melanoma metastases. Verbik and co-workers demonstrated that only 4% of the tumor cells from a primary uveal melanoma expressed MHC Class I molecules; by contrast, the incidence of Class I expression was nine times higher in melanoma cells isolated from four different liver metastases in the same patient.[42] Further support for this hypothesis comes from studies by Blom and co-workers who examined 30 primary uveal melanomas and found a significant correlation between the expression of MHC Class I molecules and poor prognosis.[43]

Corneal endothelial and lens epithelial cells express little or no MHC Class I antigen, yet these tissues do not suffer from NK cell-mediated assault, because of the protective effect of NK-inhibitory molecules in the AH that bathe the cells lining the anterior chamber. Interestingly, numerous tissues in the eye, including cells from the uveal tract, produce MIF.[43,44] Is it possible that uveal melanomas constitutively produce MIF as a means of shielding themselves from NK cell-mediated lysis once they depart from the eye? Preliminary results from our laboratory indicate that at least some uveal melanoma cell lines produce sufficient quantities of MIF to protect them from NK cell-mediated lysis. Interestingly, the most potent NK inhibitory effect was found with supernatants from a cell line established from a uveal melanoma metastasis.[45] It remains to be seen if these preliminary findings can be confirmed, but if they are, it would help explain the capacity of uveal melanomas to escape NK cell-mediated elimination in the bloodstream and in the liver.

## SUMMARY AND CONCLUSIONS

The notion that the intraocular milieu is exempt from many immune processes is irrefutable. However, the significance of ocular immune privilege in the pathogenesis of uveal melanoma and retinoblastoma remains unclear. The incidence of uveal melanoma is 16 times less than skin melanoma while retinoblastoma has one of the highest incidences of spontaneous resolution of any tumor. Both of these observations would suggest that immune privilege does not promote tumorigenesis and tumor progression of ocular tumors in humans. However, prospective studies in a variety of animal models indicate that the immune privilege of the eye provides tumors sanctuary from robust systemic immune responses. However, the magnitude and persistence of ocular immune privilege varies. Some highly immunogenic tumors circumvent immune privilege and undergo immunologic rejection in spite of the multiple processes and factors that contribute to ocular immune privilege. Determining which factors circumvent immune privilege could have enormous therapeutic application for intraocular tumor patients, especially those suffering from uveal melanoma and whose survival rates have not improved in the past thirty years.

## ACKNOWLEDGMENTS

This work supported in part by NIH grant CA30276 and an unrestricted grant from Research to Prevent Blindness, Inc.

## REFERENCES

1. Niederkorn JY. Anterior chamber-associated immune deviation. *Chem Immunol.* 1999;73:59–71.
2. Greene HSN LP. The heterologous transplantation of human cancers. *Cancer Res.* 1944;4:352–363.
3. Kaplan HJ, Streilein JW. Immune response to immunization via the anterior chamber of the eye. I. F. lymphocyte-induced immune deviation. *J Immunol.* 1977;118:809–814.
4. Kaplan HJ, Streilein JW, Stevens TR. Transplantation immunology of the anterior chamber of the eye. II. Immune response to allogeneic cells. *J Immunol.* 1975;115: 805–810.
5. Streilein JW, Niederkorn JY. Induction of anterior chamber-associated immune deviation requires an intact, functional spleen. *J Exp Med.* 1981;153:1058–1067.
6. Niederkorn J, Streilein JW, Shadduck JA. Deviant immune responses to allogeneic tumors injected intracamerally and subcutaneously in mice. *Invest Ophthalmol Vis Sci.* 1981;20:355–363.
7. Whittum JA, Niederkorn JY, McCulley JP, Streilein JW. Role of suppressor T cells in herpes simplex virus-induced immune deviation. *J Virol.* 1984;51:556–558.
8. Mizuno K, Clark AF, Streilein JW. Anterior chamber-associated immune deviation induced by soluble antigens. *Invest Ophthalmol Vis Sci.* 1989;30:1112–1119.
9. Mizuno K, Altman NF, Clark AF, Streilein JW. Histopathologic analysis of experimental autoimmune uveitis attenuated by intracameral injection of S-antigen. *Curr Eye Res.* 1989;8:113–121.
10. Streilein JW, Niederkorn JY, Shadduck JA. Systemic immune unresponsiveness induced in adult mice by anterior chamber presentation of minor histocompatibility antigens. *J Exp Med.* 1980;152:1121–1125.
11. Okamoto S, Hara Y, Streilein JW. Induction of anterior chamber-associated immune deviation with lymphoreticular allogeneic cells. *Transplantation.* 1995;59:377–381.

12. Niederkorn JY, Mayhew E, He Y. Alloantigens introduced into the anterior chamber of the eye induce systemic suppression of delayed hypersensitivity to third-party alloantigens through 'linked recognition'. *Transplantation.* 1995;60:348–354.
13. Waldrep JC, Kaplan HJ. Anterior chamber-associated immune deviation induced by TNP-splenocytes (TNP-ACAID). II. Suppressor T-cell networks. *Invest Ophthalmol Vis Sci.* 1983;24:1339–1345.
14. Niederkorn JY. Suppressed cellular immunity in mice harboring intraocular melanomas. *Invest. Ophthalmol Vis Sci.* 1984;25:447–454.
15. Takeuchi M, Alard P, Streilein JW. TGF-beta promotes immune deviation by altering accessory signals of antigen-presenting cells. *J Immunol.* 1998;160:1589–1597.
16. D'Orazio TJ, Niederkorn JY. A novel role for TGF-beta and IL-10 in the induction of immune privilege. *J Immunol.* 1998;160:2089–2098.
17. Geiser AG, Letterio JJ, Kulkarni AB, Karlsson S, Roberts AB, Sporn MB. Transforming growth factor beta 1 (TGF-beta 1) controls expression of major histocompatibility genes in the postnatal mouse: aberrant histocompatibility antigen expression in the pathogenesis of the TGF-beta 1 null mouse phenotype. *Proc Natl Acad Sci USA.* 1993;90:9944–9948.
18. Orcel P, Bielakoff J, De Vernejoul MC. Effects of transforming growth factor-beta on long-term human cord blood monocyte cultures. *J Cell Physiol.* 1990;142:293–298.
19. Inge TH, McCoy KM, Susskind BM, Barrett SK, Zhao G, Bear HD. Immunomodulatory effects of transforming growth factor-beta on T lymphocytes. Induction of CD8 expression in the CTLL-2 cell line and in normal thymocytes. *J Immunol.* 1992;148: 3847–3856.
20. Wilbanks GA, Mammolenti M, Streilein JW. Studies on the induction of anterior chamber-associated immune deviation (ACAID). III. Induction of ACAID depends upon intraocular transforming growth factor-beta. *Eur J Immunol.* 1992;22:165–173.
21. Rook AH, Kehrl JH, Wakefield LM, Roberts AB, Sporn MB, Burlington DB, Lane HC, Fauci AS. Effects of transforming growth factor beta on the functions of natural killer cells: depressed cytolytic activity and blunting of interferon responsiveness. *J Immunol.* 1986;136:3916–3920.
22. Taylor AW, Alard P, Yee DG, Streilein JW. Aqueous humor induces transforming growth factor-beta (TGF-beta)-producing regulatory T-cells. *Curr Eye Res.* 1997;16:900–908.
23. Taylor AW, Streilein JW, Cousins SW. Alpha-melanocyte-stimulating hormone suppresses antigen-stimulated T cell production of gamma-interferon. *Neuroimmunomodulation.* 1994;1:188–194.
24. Nishida T, Taylor AW. Specific aqueous humor factors induce activation of regulatory T cells. *Invest. Ophthalmol Vis Sci.* 1999;40:2268–2274.
25. Griffith TS, Brunner T, Fletcher SM, Green DR, Ferguson TA. Fas ligand-induced apoptosis as a mechanism of immune privilege. *Science.* 1995;270:1189–1192.
26. Schurmans LR, den Boer AT, Diehl L, Van der Voort EI, Kast WM, Melief CJ, Taes KE Jager MJ. Successful immunotherapy of an intraocular tumor in mice. *Cancer Res.* 1999;59:5250–5254.
27. Niederkorn JY, Streilein JW. Intracamerally induced concomitant immunity: mice harboring progressively growing intraocular tumors are immune to spontaneous metastases and secondary tumor challenge. *J Immunol.* 1983;131:2587–2594.
28. Niederkorn JY, Streilein JW. Alloantigens placed into the anterior chamber of the eye induce specific suppression of delayed-type hypersensitivity but normal cytotoxic T lymphocyte and helper T lymphocyte responses. *J Immunol.* 1983;131:2670–2674.
29. Niederkorn JY, Meunier PC. Spontaneous immune rejection of intraocular tumors in mice. *Invest Ophthalmol Vis Sci.* 1985;26:877–884.

30. Knisely TL, Luckenbach MW, Fischer BJ, Niederkorn JY. Destructive and nondestructive patterns of immune rejection of syngeneic intraocular tumors. *J Immunol.* 1987;138: 4515–4523.
31. Knisely TL, Niederkorn JY. Emergence of a dominant cytotoxic T lymphocyte antitumor effector from tumor-infiltrating cells in the anterior chamber of the eye. *Cancer Immunol Immunother.* 1990;30:323–330.
32. Ma D, Alizadeh H, Comerford SA, Gething MJ, Sambrook JF, Anand R, Niederkorn JY. Rejection of intraocular tumors from transgenic mice by tumor- infiltrating lymphocytes. *Curr Eye Res.* 1994;13:361–369.
33. Burnet FM. The concept of immunological surveillance. *Prog Exp Tumor Res.* 1970;13: 1–27.
34. Ortaldo JR, Longo DL. Human natural lymphocyte effector cells: definition, analysis of activity, and clinical effectiveness. *J Natl Cancer Inst.* 1988;80:999–1010.
35. Ma D, Luyten GP, Luider TM, Niederkorn JY. Relationship between natural killer cell susceptibility and metastasis of human uveal melanoma cells in a murine model. *Invest Ophthalmol Vis Sci.* 1995;36:435–441.
36. Ma D, Niederkorn JY. Transforming growth factor-beta down-regulates major histocompatibility complex class I antigen expression and increases the susceptibility of uveal melanoma cells to natural killer cell-mediated cytolysis. *Immunology.* 1995;86: 263–269.
37. Apte RS, Mayhew E, Niederkorn JY. Local inhibition of natural killer cell activity promotes the progressive growth of intraocular tumors. *Invest Ophthalmol Vis Sci.* 1997;38:1277–1282.
38. Cousins SW, McCabe MM, Danielpour D, Streilein JW. Identification of transforming growth factor-beta as an immunosuppressive factor in aqueous humor. *Invest Ophthalmol Vis Sci.* 1991;32:2201–2211.
39. Apte RS, Niederkorn JY. Isolation and characterization of a unique natural killer cell inhibitory factor present in the anterior chamber of the eye. *J Immunol.* 1996;156: 2667–2673.
40. Apte RS, Sinha D, Mayhew E, Wistow GJ, Niederkorn JY. Cutting edge: role of macrophage migration inhibitory factor in inhibiting NK cell activity and preserving immune privilege. *J Immunol.* 1998;160:5693–5696.
41. Ljunggren HG, Ohlen C, Hoglund P, Franksson L, Karre K. The RMA-S lymphoma mutant; consequences of a peptide loading defect on immunological recognition and graft rejection. *Int J Cancer Suppl.* 1991;6:38–44.
42. Verbik DJ, Murray TG, Tran JM, Ksander BR. Melanomas that develop within the eye inhibit lymphocyte proliferation. *Int J Cancer.* 1997;73:470–478.
43. Blom DJ, Luyten GP, Mooy C, Kerkvliet S, Zwinderman AH, Jager MJ. Human leukocyte antigen class I expression. Marker of poor prognosis in uveal melanoma. *Invest Ophthalmol Vis Sci.* 1997;38:1865–1872.
44. Matsuda A, Tagawa Y, Matsuda H, Nishihira J. Identification and immunohistochemical localization of macrophage migration inhibitory factor in human cornea. *FEBS Lett.* 1996;385:225–228.
45. Repp AC, Mayhew ES, Apte S, Niederkorn JY. Human uveal melanoma cells produce macrophage migration-inhibitory factor to prevent lysis by NK cells. *J Immunol.* 2000; 165:710–715.

MARTINE J. JAGER, JESSICA A.W. METZELAAR-BLOK, H. MONIQUE H. HURKS

# 17. Immunogenetics in Uveal Melanoma

## INTRODUCTION

Genetic determinants can influence the biological behavior of tumors in various ways. For example, genes may confer the susceptibility to develop a specific tumor, they may play a role during the outgrowth of the tumor, or they may influence the immunological defense of the body against cancer, for instance in the prevention of metastases. Finally, genes may influence the sensitivity to different forms of treatment.

Uveal melanoma develops only in a few patients, grows slowly, and even large intraocular tumors do not always cause metastases. Furthermore, metastases may stay dormant for many years, suggesting relatively effective defense mechanisms. In uveal melanoma, no gene has been identified as the specific causal factor, and it may be that we are dealing here with a malignancy that occurs randomly, perhaps due to external factors. However, several genes have been identified that could have a relationship with the susceptibility to develop this tumor. As described by Singh et al.[1] (Chapter 4, this book), some genetic determinant is likely to exist.

## PIGMENT AND MC1-R GENE VARIANTS IN UVEAL MELANOMA

The estimated incidence of uveal melanoma is six cases per million per year in Caucasians.[2] Uveal melanoma occurs eight times less frequently in Africans,[3] and only sporadically in Asians. A choroidal nevus is a predisposing lesion, and when the number of melanocytes in the choroid is increased as occurs in congenital ocular melanocytosis and Nevus of Ota, an increased risk of uveal melanoma is seen.[4] In the FAMMM or Dysplastic Nevus Syndrome, increased numbers of cutaneous nevi, cutaneous melanoma, as well as uveal melanoma are seen[5–7] (see Chapters 4–6, this book). These data suggest that pigmentation (skin color) or the number of melanocytes are related to the development of uveal melanoma.

A lot is known about these factors with regard to cutaneous melanoma: in cutaneous melanoma, several phenotypic risk factors have been identified, including the number of melanocytic nevi, presence of atypical nevi, a pale skin, blue eyes, and a tendency to freckle or to burn rather than to tan.[8–13] The presence of red hair

Table 17.1. MC1R gene variants in uveal melanoma patients and in healthy controls.

| Number of MC1R gene variants | Uveal melanoma patients ($n = 162$) | Healthy controls ($n = 255$) |
|---|---|---|
| 0 | 54 (33.3%) | 78 (30.6%) |
| 1 | 72 (44.4%) | 126 (49.4%) |
| 2 | 36 (22.2%) | 51 (20%) |

and oversensitivity to light are associated with the occurrence of certain variants of the gene that codes for the MC1-receptor, the receptor for alfa-melanocyte stimulating hormone (α-MSH). This receptor is expressed on melanocytes and keratinocytes, and binding of α-MSH to its receptor stimulates melanin synthesis. Skin type I and II are characterized by point mutations in this receptor,[14] and the presence of these mutation-containing variants is associated with an increased risk to develop cutaneous melanoma.[15]

Similar associations might be expected in uveal melanoma. Metzelaar-Blok et al.[16] set out to test the distribution of MC1-R gene variants in uveal melanoma. She compared the gene distribution of the MC1-R gene variants in 162 uveal melanoma patients with 255 controls, but found no significant differences between these two groups (Table 17.1). A clear increase in the number of point mutations was seen among uveal melanoma patients with skin type I and II, but this occurred in the controls as well (Table 17.1). These findings are in contrast with studies on cutaneous melanoma, where most patients have skin type II and red/fair hair, and lead to the conclusion that MC1-R variants do not play a role in the susceptibility to develop uveal melanoma.

## EYE COLOR

The two populations were also analyzed with regard to eye color. The uveal melanoma population more frequently had blue eyes, and in comparison with the controls, the observed difference in distribution approached significance ($p = 0.060$). This is in accordance with the findings of Regan et al.,[17] who reported that ocular melanoma is more prevalent among patients with light irises than with dark irises. It may be that lightly colored irises absorb less UV light than dark eyes, and that UV exposure may be a risk factor in developing uveal melanoma. Bito[18] recently discussed the role of the iris in protecting other intraocular tissues from light damage. The iris absorbs most of the light impinging on it, and the more light that reaches the eye, the more iris surface is exposed to it. Sunburn early in life[19] is associated to the later development of uveal melanoma, and several papers discuss other types of exposure to ultraviolet light as a risk factor for uveal melanoma: Holly et al.[20] observed that exposure to UV or black lights, welding burns and snow blindness were associated with an increased risk to develop uveal melanoma. Again, brown irises were found to be protective. Seddon et al.[21] found an association between the development of uveal melanoma and the use of sunlamps, and for caucasians living in the South of the United States. These results indicate, that UV probably plays a role in the induction of uveal melanoma, and that light irises allow more of the light to reach the fundus. Since MC1-R genes were not the essential factor for iris color, it will be interesting to look for other genes that determine iris color, since they may be related to the genetic sensitivity to develop uveal melanoma.

## HLA GENES

As described by Hurks in this book (Chapter 18), HLA expression is important in uveal melanoma, and variations have been observed in the expression levels of HLA Class I antigens. These differences in expression of HLA antigens play a role in antigen recognition, since both cytotoxic T cells and NK cells use HLA Class I molecules to recognize their target. Apart from the importance of quantitative levels of HLA antigens, qualitative differences may also be important. Tumor antigens are presented in the groove of HLA molecules, but tumor-antigen derived peptides vary in their binding affinity to different HLA molecules. Common melanoma antigens are peptides derived from the enzyme tyrosinase, and from the proteins gp100, MAGE-1, MART, or MC1-R, the above mentioned receptor for α-MSH. Tyrosinase, gp100 and MC1-R are differentiation antigens derived from the melanocyte lineage, and MAGE-1 is a germ-cell protein, that is expressed in the testis during embryological development, and re-expressed in some malignancies. Peptides from these proteins have a specific affinity to bind to only some and not all HLA Class I molecules, while other peptides will have binding specificity for another HLA Class I type. One of the peptides derived from gp100 is, for instance, preferentially presented on HLA-A2 molecules.[22]

Since immune responses will only develop against an antigen that is presented in the proper fashion (i.e., on an HLA Class I or II antigen), the genetically-determined presence or absence of an HLA type will define what will happen: only in the presence of the appropriate HLA type will one see the development of an immune response against a certain peptide.

How these polymorphisms exactly influence the development of tumors is as yet unknown, but significant correlations between the presence of certain HLA genes and the occurrence of, for instance, skin melanoma have been described. The presence of HLA-B40 for instance has been found to be related to both the development as well as the clinical progression of cutaneous melanoma.[23]

## HLA-DISEASE ASSOCIATIONS

With regard to uveal melanoma, several investigators studied the association between the occurrence of a certain HLA allele and the development of uveal melanoma (Table 17.2).

Ignatov et al.[24] were the first to report on differences in the distribution of HLA Class I genes between uveal melanoma patients and healthy individuals, finding an increase in the incidence of HLA-A3 and A29, and a decrease in A25 and Bw16. Bertrams et al.[25] compared 81 patients with 1000 controls, and only found an increase in Aw32. Since Dieckhues et al.[26] reported on only five patients, his data are not as relevant. Völker-Dieben et al.[27] used a group of patients with uveal melanoma who had been HLA typed in order to know the HLA type of the cornea.

Table 17.2. HLA frequencies in uveal melanoma, as observed in different studies.

| | Patients | Controls | Decreased | Increased |
|---|---|---|---|---|
| Ignatov et al. 1977[24] | 47 | | A25, Bw16 | A3, A29 |
| Bertrams et al. 1978[25] | 81 | 1000 | – | A32 |
| Dieckhues et al. 1979[26] | 5 | 5046 | – | A1, B27 |
| Völker-Dieben et al. 1983[27] | 69 | 1018 | – | B49 |
| Martinetti et al. 1988[28] | 16 | 388 | – | A32, B14, DR7 |

Their corneas were subsequently donated for corneal transplantation. The HLA distribution in these patients was compared to 1018 controls and Bw49 showed an increased incidence in the patient group. When separating the group according to cell type (pure spindle versus not pure spindle), more differences were observed, with increases in the frequencies of Aw30, Bw49, Bw51, and Bw63 in the pure spindle group. Martinetti et al.[28] looked at only 16 patients, but found an increase in A32, B14 and DR7. Unlike Völker-Dieben, Martinetti found that A32 and B27 were specifically increased in the pure spindle group, and DR3 and DR7 increased in the non-spindle cases. It is interesting that A32 was found in this study as well as in that of Bertrams.

In conclusion, different studies report on a variety of associations between HLA antigens and uveal melanoma, but increases in A32 and DR7 were both observed in two studies. We are working on a further study, in which DNA based typing will be used for the first time in regard to this disease.

## HLA ANTIGENS AND PROGNOSIS

In 1992, Jager et al.[29] investigated the potential contribution of the HLA type to the clinical prognosis of uveal melanoma, using patients from the group that had already been described by Völker-Dieben[27]. We could not retrieve all patients or their HLA type, but managed to obtain histopathological data on 44 eyes containing a uveal melanoma, whose corneas had been used for corneal transplantation between 1976 and 1980. In 42 cases, ten year follow-up or clinical information up to the time of death was available. In one case, the cause of death was unknown, and in one case, no follow-up was available. The data showed that one HLA allele was found to have a significantly different frequency between patients who developed metastases and those that did not. That allele was HLA-B40; five out of eight (62%) HLA-B40-positive patients with uveal melanoma died of metastases, and only five out of 33 HLA-B40 negative patients (15%). It is interesting that one study that looked at cutaneous melanoma found an increased incidence of HLA-B40 in that condition.[30] However, other studies did not find this; they observed either a decrease in HLA-A7,[31] or an increase in B27 in cutaneous melanoma,[32] or an increase in A9 in uveal melanoma patients.[33]

The problem with this finding is that it is difficult to explain. Polymorphisms can influence immune responses by modifications in the antigen-binding site, but also differential expression of individual alleles may be involved. Another option is, that

HLA-B40 is a potent inhibitor of NK-cell function. In a previous study, we observed that patients with a primary uveal melanoma with a high expression of HLA Class I antigens will more often die of metastatic disease.[34] It may be that HLA-B40 is hardly ever down-regulated, and thereby inhibits NK-cell function during metastasis development. Or it may be that it is not HLA-B40 itself that plays a role, but a gene that is in linkage disequilibrium with HLA-B40, and that confers an increased HLA Class I expression or a lower immune responsiveness. This is of course pure speculation, but several candidate genes are in the neighborhood (MIC-A and -B, TNF, Hsp-70, HLA Class II genes).

With regard to HLA Class II molecules, at least two studies found an association between an increased incidence of HLA-DR7, a HLA-Class II antigen, and the development of uveal melanoma (Table 17.1). If these immune response genes conferred a lack of responsiveness against tumor antigens (and thus allowing tumor growth), it may well be that not HLA Class I but HLA Class II-associated immune responses play a role. Ericsson et al.[35] found an association between Class II expression and a bad prognosis, and this may be another indication that HLA Class II antigens are important in uveal melanoma. Since HLA Class II- mediated immune responses often involve CD4+ lymphocytes, it is of interest that we recently showed the importance of CD4 cells in the spontaneous rejection of an intraocular tumor in mice.[36] When Ad5E1-transformed tumor cells are placed in the anterior chamber of a syngeneic C57Bl/6 mouse, intraocular tumor growth occurs, while no growth is seen when these cells are injected subcutaneously.[37] However, after three to four weeks, spontaneous resolution of these tumors is seen. By depletion studies, Schurmans et al.[36] demonstrated, that the responsible T lymphocytes were CD8 negative and CD4 positive, and that the killing mechanism involved HLA Class II and not HLA Class I. Since uveal melanomas often express some HLA Class II,[35] it is possible that anti-HLA Class II directed responses may also occur in the human situation, or that they may be induced in the course of immunotherapeutic approaches. Further studies are necessary to determine whether specific HLA Class II genes are not only associated with the occurrence of a uveal melanoma, but whether they may be related to survival.

## CONCLUSION

While genetic factors such as skin color are involved in the susceptibility to develop uveal melanoma, no specific genes have been identified. It is likely that immune response genes play a role in the defense against the development of uveal melanoma metastases, but up to now it seems that the level of expression of HLA Class I and II antigens on the cells of the primary uveal melanoma is more important than qualitative differences.

## ACKNOWLEDGEMENT

This work was supported by the Dutch Cancer Society, Stichting Haags Oogheelkundig Fonds, Stichting Blinden-Penning and The Nelly Reef Fund.

## REFERENCES


1. Singh AD, Shields CL, De Potter P, Shields JA, Trock B, Cater J, Pastore D. Familial uveal melanoma. Clinical observations on 56 patients. *Arch Ophthalmol* 1996;114:392–399.
2. Egan KM, Seddon JM, Glynn RJ, Gragoudas ES, Albert DM. Epidemiologic aspects of uveal melanoma. *Surv Ophthalmol.* 1988;32:239–251.
3. Scotto J, Fraumeni JF Jr, Lee JAH. Melanomas of the eye and the noncutaneous sites: epidemiologic aspects. *J Natl Cancer Inst.* 1976;56:489–491.
4. Singh AD, De Potter P, Fijal B, Shields CL, Shields JA, Elston RC. Lifetime prevalence of uveal melanoma in Caucasian patients with Oculo(dermal) Melanocytosis. *Ophthalmology.* 1998;105:195–198.
5. Vink J, Crijns MW, Bergman W, Oosterhuis JA, Went LN. Ocular melanoma in families with dysplastic nevus syndrome (DNS). *J Am Acad Dermatol* 1990;23:858–862.
6. Van Hees CL, De Boer A, Jager MJ, Bleeker JC, Kakebeeke HM, Crijns MB, Vandenbroucke JP, Bergman W. Are atypical nevi a risk factor for uveal melanoma? A case control study. *J Invest Dermatol.* 1994;103:202–205.
7. Hammer H, Olah J, Toth-Molnar E. Dysplastic nevi are a risk factor for uveal melanoma. *Eur J Ophthalmol.* 1996;6:472–474.
8. Elwood JM, Gallagher RP, Hill GB, Spinelli JJ, Pearson JC, Threlfall W. Pigmentation and skin reaction to sun as risk factors for cutaneous melanoma: Western Canada Melanoma Study. *Br Med J.* (*Clin Res Ed*) 1984;288:99–102.
9. Rhodes AR, Weinstock MA, Fitzpatrick TB, Mihm MC Jr, Sober AJ. Risk factors for cutaneous melanoma. A practical method of recognizing predisposed individuals. *JAMA* 1987;258:3146–3154.
10. Evans RD, Kopf AW, Lew RA, Rigel DS, Bart RS, Friedman RJ, Rivers JK. Risk factors for the development of malignant melanoma-I; Review of case-control studies. *J. Dermatol Surg Oncol.* 1988;14:393–408.
11. Beitner H, Norell SE, Ringborg U, Wennersten G, Mattson B. Malignant melanoma: aetiological importance of individual pigmentation and sun exposure. *Br J Dermatol* 1990;122:43–51.
12. Lock-Andersen J, Wulf HC, Hnudstorp ND. Interdependence of eye and hair color, skin type and skin pigmentation in a Caucasian population. *Acta Derm Venereol.* 1998; 78:214–9.
13. Lock-Andersen J, Drzewiecki KT, Wulf HC. Eye and hair color, skin type and constitutie skin pigmentation as risk factors for basal cell carcinoma and cutaneous malignant melanoma. A Danish case-control study. *Acta Derm Venereol.* 1999;79:74–80.
14. Valverde P, Healy E, Jackson I, Rees JL, Thody AJ. Variants of the melanocyte-stimulating hormone receptor gene are associated with red hair and fair skin in humans. *Nat Genet.* 1995;11:328–330.
15. Kennedy C, Ter Huurne J, Berkhout M, Gruis N, Bastiaens M, Bergman W, Willemze R, Bouwes Bavinck JN. Melanocortin 1 receptor (MC1R) gene variants are associated with an increased risk for cutaneous melanoma which is largely independent of skin type and hair color. *J Invest Dermattol.* 2001;117:294–300.
16. Metzelaar-Blok JAW, Ter Huurne JAC, Hurks HMH, Keunen JEE, Jager MJ, Gruis NA. Characterization of melanocortin-1 receptor gene variants in uveal melanoma patients. *Invest Ophthalmol Vis Sci.* 2001;42:1951–1954.
17. Regan S, Judge HE, Gragoudas ES, Egan KM. Iris color as a prognostic factor in ocular melanoma. *Arch Ophthalmol.* 1999;117:811–814.
18. Bito LZ. A new approach to the medical management of glaucoma, from the bench to the clinic, and beyond. The Proctor Lecture. *Invest Ophthalmol Vis Sci.* 2001;42; 1126–1133.

19. Tucker MA, Shields JA, Hartge P, Augsburger J, Hoover RN, Fraumeni JF Jr. Sunlight exposure as risk factor for intraocular malignant melanoma. *N Engl J Med.* 1985;313: 789–792.
20. Holly EA, Aston DA, Char DH, Kristiansen JJ, Ahn DK. Uveal melanoma in relation to ultraviolet light exposure and host factors. *Cancer Res.* 1990;50:5773–5777.
21. Seddon JM, Gragoudas ES, Glynn RJ, Egan KM, Albert DM, Blitzer PH. Host factors, UV radiation, and risk of uveal melanoma. A case-control study. *Arch Ophthalmol.* 1990;108:1274–1280.
22. Robbins PF, El-Gamil M, Kawakami Y, Rosenberg SA. Recognition of tyrosinase by tumor-infiltrating lymphovutes from a patient responding to immunotherapy. *Cancer Res.* 1994;54:3124–3126.
23. Pollack MS, Livingstone PO. HLA and DR antigen frequencies in melanoma patients: possible relation to disease prognosis. *Tissue Antigens.* 1985;26:262–265.
24. Ignatov RK, Terentyeura LL, Shulgina NS. A study of antigen distribution of HLA system in melanoma of the uvea (Russian). *Onkol Z.* 1977;14:289.
25. Bertrams J, Spitznas M, Rommelfanger M. Missing evidence for HLA antigen association with Eales'disease, chorioretinitis, central serous retinopathy and malignant choroidal melanoma. *Invest Ophthalmol.* 1978;17:918–920.
26. Dieckhues B, Jünemann G, Küchle HJ, Püttmann T. HLA Antigene bei Augenerkrankungen. *Klin Mbl Augenh.* 1979;175:681–85.
27. Völker-Dieben HJ, D'Amaro J, De Lange P, De Wolff-Rouendaal D. HLA and ABO antigens in patients with malignant choroidal melanoma. *Clin Exp Immunol.* 1983;53: 581–588.
28. Martinetti M, Tafi A, De Paoli F, Dugoujon JM, Cuccia Belvedere M. Immunogenetic heterogeneity of uveal melanoma. *Cancer Detect Prev.* 1988;12:145–148.
29. Jager MJ, Völker-Dieben HJ, De Wolff-Rouendaal D, Kakebeeke-Kemme H, D'Amaro J. Possible relation between HLA and ABO type and prognosis of uveal melanoma. *Doc Ophthalmol.* 1992;82:43–47.
30. Pellegris G, Illeni MT, Vaglini M, Rovini D, Cascinelli N, Masserine C. HLA antigens in malignant melanoma patients. *Tumori.* 1980;66:51–58.
31. Lamm LU, Kissmeyer-Nielsen F, Kjerbye KE, Mogensen B, Petersen NC. HL-A and ABO antigens and malignant melanoma. *Cancer.* 1974;33:1458–1461.
32. Bergholtz B, Brennhovd I, Klepp O, Kaakinen A, Thorsby E. HLA antigens in malignant melanoma. *Cancer.* 1977;39:2342–2344.
33. Cavalier B, Daveau M, Gilbert D, Fontaine M, Cesarini JP, Delpech B. Augmentation de l'antigene HLA-A9 dans les melanomes malins, principalemant dans la formes metastatiques ou les recidives. A propos de 105 melanomes dont 34 formes graves. *C R Acad Sci* 1980;291:241–243.
34. Blom DJR, Luyten GPM, Mooy CM, Kerkvliet S, Zwinderman AH, Jager MJ. Human leucocyte antigen Class I expression: marker of poor prognosis in uveal melanoma. *Invest Ophthalmol Vis Sci.* 1997;38:1865–1872
35. Ericcson C, Seregard S, Bartolazzi A, Levitskaya E, Ferrone S, Kiessling R, Larsson O. Association of HLA Class I and Class II antigen expression and mortality in uveal melanoma. *Invest Ophthalmol Vis Sci.* 2001;42:2153–2156.
36. Schurmans LRHM, Diehl L, Den Boer AT, Sutmuller RPM, Boonman ZF, Medema JP, Van der Voort EIH, Laman J, Melief CJM, Jager MJ, Toes REM. Rejection of intraocular tumors by CD4+ T cells without induction of phthisis. *J Immunol.* 2001;167:5832–5837.
37. Schurmans LRHM, Den Boer Ath, Diehl L, Van der Voort EIH, Kast WM, Melief CJM, Toes REM, Jager MJ. Succesful immunotherapy of an intraocular tumor in mice. *Cancer Res.* 1999;59:5250–5254.

H. MONIQUE H. HURKS AND MARTINE J. JAGER

# 18. HLA Expression in Uveal Melanoma

## HUMAN LEUKOCYTE ANTIGENS

Human leukocyte antigens (HLA) play a central role in immune recognition, both with regard to T cells as well as NK cells. Different functions have been attributed to HLA Class I and II antigens, and while HLA Class I molecules are expressed on almost all cells of the body, expression of HLA Class II antigens is much more restricted (see below). Both classes of antigens may be important in uveal melanoma.

HLA Class I molecules are comprised of the classical (class Ia) HLA-A, -B, and -C antigens and the non-classical (Class Ib) HLA-E, -F, and -G antigens. Both classical and non-classical HLA Class I antigens are cell surface, transmembrane glycoproteins that assemble as heterodimers of a polymorphic heavy chain and a non-polymorphic β2-microglobulin (β2m) light chain.[1,2]

The α1 and α2 domains of the heavy chain form a groove in which endogenously derived peptides, such as melanoma-associated antigens, can be presented to CD8+ (cytotoxic) T cells. The peptide-binding specificity is different for each particular HLA allele. Interaction of the HLA Class I-peptide complex with the T cell receptor (TCR) triggers activation of the T cell, finally leading to cell proliferation, cytokine production and lysis of target cells. In addition to CD8+ T cells, HLA Class I expression is important for the function of natural killer (NK) cells. Human NK cells have two distinct types of surface receptors that interact with HLA Class I molecules and each type of receptor has both inhibitory and activating forms.

The killer cell Ig-like receptors (KIR) bind directly to the conserved sections of individual Class I molecules, whereas the CD94/NKG2 receptor recognizes classical HLA Class I molecules indirectly, using HLA-E as an adapter molecule.[3] In general, low expression of HLA Class I renders a cell more susceptible to NK cell-mediated lysis.

HLA Class II molecules, encoded by the HLA-D locus, are predominantly expressed on antigen-presenting cells such as dendritic cells, B cells, Langerhans cells, macrophages and on activated T lymphocytes. However, inflammatory cytokines, such as interferon-γ (IFNγ) can induce the expression of HLA Class II in other cell types too.[4]

HLA Class II molecules can be subdivided into HLA-DR, HLA-DQ and HLA-DP. In contrast to HLA Class I, HLA Class II polymorphism is mainly located in the β domain of the heavy chain.[5] HLA Class II molecules generally present peptides derived from endocytosed exogenous antigens to CD4+ (helper) T cells, which in turn provide help to cytotoxic T cells and stimulate antibody production by B cells.

## HLA EXPRESSION AND TUMOR IMMUNOSURVEILLANCE

HLA expression plays a crucial role in tumor immunosurveillance. Both CD4+ and CD8+ T cells can only be activated when they recognize tumor-specific antigens, e.g., MAGE, MART-1, or gp100, in association with the appropriate HLA molecules. Therefore, alteration of the HLA phenotype of the tumor may have serious consequences for the host's defense against tumor growth and the development of metastatic disease. Likewise, downregulation of HLA expression may have a negative impact on the efficacy of T cell-based immunotherapy.

The level and pattern of HLA Class I expression has been studied in many different tumor types, including cutaneous and uveal melanoma, and HLA phenotype alterations have been demonstrated in all types of malignancies.[6–9] These altered phenotypes can be classified into five categories: (1) total HLA loss, (2) HLA haplotype loss, (3) HLA locus loss, (4) HLA allelic loss and (5) a compound phenotype representing a combination of phenotypes 1–4.[10,11] Distinct mechanisms underlie the different phenotypes, as reviewed by Garrido et al. (1997)[12] and Algarra et al. (2000).[11] In short, a complete loss of surface HLA Class I expression has been attributed to a lack of β2m-microglobulin synthesis,[6,13] abnormalities in the expression of TAP molecules (peptide transporters necessary in the antigen processing pathway)[6,14] or structural defects within the MHC genes.[7] Loss of a haplotype is predominantly the result of chromosomal loss or abnormalities,[11,15] whereas HLA locus loss can be caused by a genetic as well as by a transcriptional defect.[11,16] The underlying mechanism of allele-specific downregulations is difficult to define. In addition to genetic defects, allele-specific alterations might reflect tumor adaptation to immune pressure.[12,17,18]

Total HLA Class I downregulation is a frequent event, occurring in 16 to 50% of primary tumors.[10,12] Selective, allelic HLA downregulation seems to occur less frequently, in 4–35% of malignancies.[10] However, this is likely to be an underestimate, because of the limited availability of monoclonal antibodies suitable for the immunohistochemical detection of polymorphic HLA determinants. Significant reduction or total loss of HLA is the most effective way for tumor cells to escape CTL elimination, but it simultaneously renders a cell more susceptible to NK cell lysis. Therefore, selective, partial HLA downregulation can be an effective compromise of tumor cells to escape both cytotoxic T cells and NK cells. It needs to be mentioned that tumors are often very heterogeneous: several HLA phenotypes can be present within one tumor. This may explain, in part, the limited response rates of immunotherapies. Moreover, it implies that a combination of therapies, directed at phenotypically different tumor cells, will induce a more effective antitumor immune response and hence reduce the capacity of tumor cells to develop new escape variants.

## HLA CLASS I EXPRESSION ON UVEAL MELANOMA

### MONOMORPHIC HLA CLASS I EXPRESSION

The expression of HLA Class I antigens on uveal melanoma has been extensively investigated using immunohistochemistry on paraffin and cryostat tissue sections and using FACS analysis on human uveal melanoma cell lines. All phenotypes of HLA Class I downregulation as described by Garrido[12] have been observed, except the total HLA loss phenotype.[9,19,20] In the study of De Waard-Siebinga et al. (1996),[19] using the monoclonal antibodies W6/32 (recognizing monomorphic HLA-A,B,C) and BBM1 (directed to the β2-microglobulin of the Class I heavy chain), all 23 primary uveal melanomas showed a high level of HLA Class I expression, i.e. at least 50% of the cells within a tumor stained positively. No associations were found with prognostic markers such as tumor diameter, prominence or scleral invasion. On the other hand, a positive correlation was found between the expression of monomorphic HLA Class I determinants and the presence of tumor infiltrating CD3+ and CD4+ T cells and CD11b+ monocytes/macrophages. The correlation with CD8+ T cells did not reach significance.[21] In contrast to the study of De Waard-Siebinga et al. (1996),[19] Ericsson et al. (2001)[22] found a downregulation of β2m expression (i.e., less than 30% of tumor cells were stained positive) in 35 of 65 primary uveal melanoma lesions analyzed, using the monoclonal antibody L368. This downregulation was significantly correlated with patient survival (see next paragraph).

### HLA EXPRESSION AS A PROGNOSTIC MARKER

In the study of Blom et al. (1997), locus-specific HLA Class I expression was determined.[9] The monoclonal antibodies HCa2 and HC10 were used to stain respectively HLA-A and HLA-B on paraffin sections of 30 primary uveal melanomas. Expression levels of HLA-A and -B were significantly correlated. Large variations in expression were observed between different uveal melanomas. Complete loss of HLA-A was observed in 10 tumors (33%), whereas HLA-B expression was absent in 12 tumors (40%). A high expression of HLA-B was related to the presence of prognostically unfavorable non-spindle cells. No significant correlations were observed between HLA-A or -B expression and other prognostic parameters such as largest tumor diameter, Mib-1 score or mitotic rate. In contrast to the study on monomorphic HLA antigens of De Waard-Siebinga et al. (1996),[19] the locus-specific HLA expression was of significant prognostic value: a low expression of HLA-A and HLA-B molecules was significantly correlated with a better patient survival (Fig. 18.1). Multiple regression analysis showed that the contribution of HLA-A expression to survival exceeded that of tumor diameter and Mib-1 score.[9] This observation that expression of HLA-A and HLA-B is a marker of poor prognosis is recently confirmed by two other studies.[22,23] Ericsson et al. (2001)[22] show that high expression of HLA-B, as well as high expression of β2m and HLA Class II antigens is significantly associated with poor clinical outcome. In another recent study, reduced expression of TAP molecules was demonstrated in uveal melanoma.[24] Although in the majority of tumors, this TAP downregulation was very

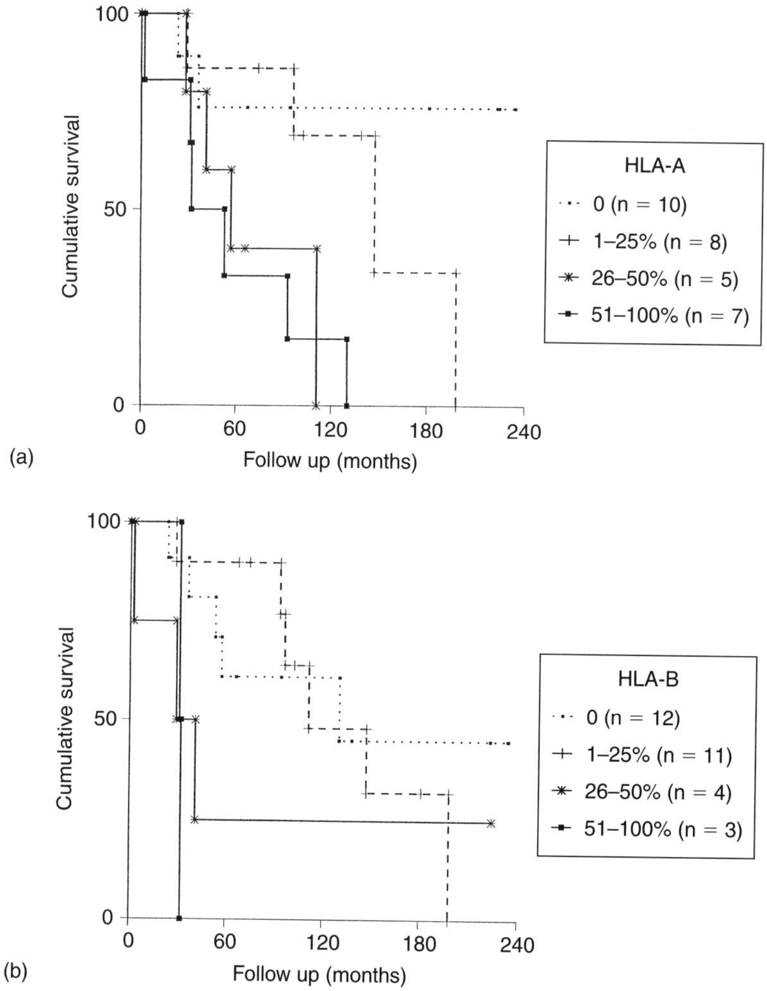


Fig. 18.1. Kaplan–Meyer survival curves for 30 patients, depicting the probability of death due to uveal melanoma versus expression of HLA-A (a) and HLA-B (b). The level of expression was scored semiquantitatively as a percentage of positive cells. Figures are derived from Blom et al. (1997).[9] (Reproduced with permission of Investigative Ophthalmology of Visual Science.)

moderate, it was associated with progression to metastatic disease. Whether the reduced expression of TAP was correlated with reduced expression of HLA Class I was not investigated, but this prognostic finding seems to be in contrast with the correlation between HLA Class I downregulation and a favorable prognosis as observed by others.[9,22,23] In a study involving 41 uveal melanomas, Krishnakumar et al.[46] showed a correlation between a high expression of HLA Class I and II, β2m and antigen-processing molecules, and extrascleral extension as well as the formation of liver metastases.

## THE ROLE OF NK CELLS IN UVEAL MELANOMA

The finding that a low expression of HLA in primary lesions is associated with a favorable clinical course was unexpected and unique for uveal melanoma. Generally, a decreased expression of HLA may facilitate tumor escape from cytotoxic T cells and in other cancers low HLA Class I expression has been associated with tumor progression and/or reduced survival.[25–30] In these malignancies, tumor-antigen-specific CTLs play a major role in controlling tumor growth. In uveal melanoma, the bad prognosis associated with a high HLA Class I expression, supports a protective role for NK cells in the development of metastatic disease, as NK cells can attack target cells more efficiently in the absence of HLA Class I molecules. This hypothesis is strengthened by the study of Ma et al. (1995),[31] who found that the development of hepatic metastases in mice injected with uveal melanoma cells was inversely correlated with the degree of NK cell-mediated lysis. In addition, patients with advanced metastatic disease often show abnormal NK cell function and/or number.[32] Finally, since uveal melanoma metastases spread hematogenously, especially NK cell lysis may be an important first line of defense. In most other types of cancer, spreading occurs mainly lymphatically, suggesting a more crucial role for cytotoxic T cells.

## ALLELE-SPECIFIC DOWNREGULATION

In the former paragraphs, the correlation between a low HLA Class I expression and a better patient survival is described. Low HLA Class I-expressing uveal melanoma cells that leave the eye and enter the bloodstream will be lysed by NK cells. This suggests that the metastatic cells that succeed to settle down in the liver display high HLA Class I expression. Indeed, we observed high expression levels of HLA-A and -B in four different metastases derived from one HLA Class I positive primary uveal melanoma.[33] The question then arises why cytotoxic T cells do not adequately react to these HLA Class I expressing tumor cells. One of the possible answers is the occurrence of HLA allele-specific downregulation. By this mechanism, melanoma cells can avoid recognition by a specific population of CTLs, while expression of the remaining HLA Class I alleles prevents lysis by NK cells.

Using a broad panel of allele-specific monoclonal antibodies suitable for FACS analysis, the polymorphic HLA Class I surface expression of six uveal melanoma cell lines (five derived from a primary tumor and one cell line obtained from a skin metastasis) was determined.[20] In order to upregulate HLA expression, cells were also cultured with IFN$\alpha$ or IFN$\gamma$. In general, the expression of the HLA-A alleles was high and could be further upregulated by both IFN$\alpha$ and IFN$\gamma$. The expression of the HLA-B alleles was low or even negative and variable effects were observed after IFN treatment. In three cell lines, the expression of one B allele could not be restored by IFN$\alpha$ and IFN$\gamma$, whereas the other B allele showed an enhanced expression level upon IFN stimulation. Finally, the metastatic cell line OMM-1 showed a structural lack of expression of both B alleles, indicating an HLA-B locus-specific loss. In this *in vitro* study, the frequency of structural allelic HLA loss was high (50%). If the frequency is just as high *in vivo*, it may complicate the development of immunotherapy in uveal melanoma. T cell-based vaccination protocols are restricted by a specific HLA allele (at the moment predominantly HLA-A2). Loss of this specific allele renders the tumor elusive for the population of CTLs restricted by this allele. Therefore, the expression of this specific allele together with a functional antigen processing machinery in malignant lesions should be an important selection criterion to include patients in T cell-based immunotherapy trials.[10]

Thus, it is important to establish the frequency of selective HLA downregulation in uveal melanoma primary tumors and metastases. However, analysis of the expression of HLA Class I allospecificities in tissue sections is hampered by the limited availability of allele-specific monoclonal antibodies. In a small study of seven uveal melanoma patients, no specific loss of HLA-A2 or HLA-A3 expression was found.[19] In a more recent study, involving 20 HLA-A2 genotyped patients, two primary uveal melanomas (10%) displayed a lack of HLA-A2 expression. In cutaneous melanoma, loss of HLA-A2 expression has been found in 25% of primary lesions and in 31% of metastatic lesions.[8,34]

## DO UVEAL MELANOMA CELLS EXPRESS HLA-G ?

HLA-G is a non-classical HLA Class I molecule, preferentially expressed in fetal placental tissues. In contrast to the classical HLA-A, -B, and -C Class I molecules, HLA-G is characterized by a tissue-restricted distribution and a limited polymorphism.[35] An important function of HLA-G in immunosurveillance is the inhibition of NK cell-mediated cytolysis. This inhibition can be achieved either by direct interaction of HLA-G with inhibitory receptors (KIR) expressed by NK cells or indirectly by activating the CD94/NKG2A receptor using HLA-E as an adapter molecule.[36,37] In addition to its NK cell inhibitory capacities, HLA-G has also been shown to inhibit T cell functions, at the level of proliferation as well as cytolysis.[38] Because of these immunosuppressive properties HLA-G expression may be involved in tumor immunosurveillance, especially since tumors frequently display altered HLA Class I phenotypes.

As NK cells seem to be important players in the immunological defense against uveal melanoma, it was investigated whether uveal melanoma cells express HLA-G to escape immunosurveillance.[39] Eleven human uveal melanoma cell lines were analyzed for the expression of HLA-G by FACS analysis, immunocytochemistry, Western blotting and RT-PCR followed by Southern blotting. Two HLA-G specific monoclonal antibodies were used, 87G and MEM-G/1. In addition, HLA-G expression was determined on frozen tissue sections of 17 primary uveal melanomas. With all HLA-G detection methods, no evidence for HLA-G expression by uveal melanoma cells was found. Furthermore, IFNγ could not induce HLA-G expression in the uveal melanoma cell lines. Notably, all cell lines expressed HLA-E and this expression could be significantly enhanced by IFNγ. The conclusion of this study was that in uveal melanoma, HLA-G does not play a role, neither directly nor indirectly via HLA-E, in tumor escape from cellular immunity.[39]

The lack of HLA-G transcription in uveal melanoma may again reflect a difference in HLA expression characteristics between uveal melanoma and other tumors.

Several studies have demonstrated HLA-G transcription in different types of tumors, including cutaneous melanoma.[40–42] However, also lack of HLA-G transcription by tumor cells has been reported.[43,44] HLA-G protein expression is only rarely found.[40,41,43,44]

## SUMMARY

Downregulation of HLA expression is a common feature in many different types of cancer and may have serious consequences for the immune recognition of tumor cells by cytotoxic T cells and NK cells. In uveal melanoma, a low expression of HLA Class I in primary tumors was correlated with a better patient survival, suggesting a protective role for NK cells in the development of metastatic disease.[45] Low HLA Class I-expressing uveal melanoma cells that leave the eye and enter the bloodstream will be lysed by NK cells. High HLA Class I expressing tumor cells escape NK cell lysis and may succeed to settle down in the liver. HLA allele-specific downregulation may be a mechanism for these cells to avoid killing by cytotoxic T cells. Uveal melanoma cells do not express HLA-G as an additional mechanism to escape immunosurveillance. Alterations of HLA Class I phenotype may complicate the development of immunotherapy in uveal melanoma. Different HLA phenotypes may require different therapeutic approaches. Therefore, it is important to screen uveal melanomas for deficiencies in HLA expression before the patients enter a specific immunotherapy trial.

## ACKNOWLEDGEMENTS

This study was supported by Stichting Haags Oogheelkundig Fonds, Stichting Blinden-Penning and the Nederlandse Vereniging ter Voorkoming var Blindheid.

## REFERENCES

1. Bjorkman PJ, Parham P. Structure, function, and diversity of Class I major histocompatibility complex molecules. *Annu Rev Biochem.* 1990;59:253–288.
2. Shawar SM, Vyas JM, Rodgers JR, Rich RR. Antigen presentation by major histocompatibility complex Class I-B molecules. *Annu Rev Immunol.* 1994;12:839–880.
3. Gardiner CM. Natural killer cells. *Curr Biol.* 1999;9:R716.
4. Andalib AR, Lawry J, Ali SA, Murray AK, Sisley K, Silcocks P, Herlyn M, Rees RC. Cytokine modulation of antigen expression in human melanoma cell lines derived from primary and metastatic tumour tissues. *Melanoma Res.* 1997;7:32–42.
5. Shackelford DA, Kaufman JF, Korman AJ, Strominger JL. HLA-DR antigens: structure, separation of subpopulations, gene cloning and function. *Immunol Rev.* 1982;66: 133–187.
6. Wang Z, Margulies L, Hicklin DJ, Ferrone S. Molecular and functional phenotypes of melanoma cells with abnormalities in HLA Class I antigen expression. *Tissue Antigens.* 1996;47:382–390.
7. Garrido F, Cabrera T, Lopez-Nevot MA, Ruiz-Cabello F. HLA Class I antigens in human tumors. *Adv Cancer Res.* 1995;67:155–195.
8. Natali PG, Nicotra MR, Bigotti A, Venturo I, Marcenaro L, Giacomini P, Russo C. Selective changes in expression of HLA Class I polymorphic determinants in human solid tumors. *Proc Natl Acad Sci USA.* 1989;86:6719–6723.

9. Blom DJ, Luyten GP, Mooy C, Kerkvliet S, Zwinderman AH, Jager MJ. Human leukocyte antigen Class I expression. Marker of poor prognosis in uveal melanoma. *Invest Ophthalmol Vis Sci.* 1997;38:1865–1872.
10. Hicklin DJ, Marincola FM, Ferrone S. HLA Class I antigen downregulation in human cancers: T-cell immunotherapy revives an old story. *Mol Med Today.* 1999;5:178–186.
11. Algarra I, Cabrera T, Garrido F. The HLA crossroad in tumor immunology. *Hum Immunol.* 2000;61:65–73.
12. Garrido F, Ruiz-Cabello F, Cabrera T, Perez-Villar JJ, Lopez-Botet M, Duggan-Keen M, Stern PL. Implications for immunosurveillance of altered HLA Class I phenotypes in human tumours. [Review] [67 refs]. *Immunol Today.* 1997;18:89–95.
13. D'Urso CM, Wang ZG, Cao Y, Tatake R, Zeff RA, Ferrone S. Lack of HLA Class I antigen expression by cultured melanoma cells FO-1 due to a defect in β2m gene expression. *J Clin Invest.* 1991;87:284–292.
14. Cromme FV, Airey J, Heemels MT, Ploegh HL, Keating PJ, Stern PL, Meijer CJ, Walboomers JM. Loss of transporter protein, encoded by the TAP-1 gene, is highly correlated with loss of HLA expression in cervical carcinomas. *J Exp Med.* 1994;179: 335–340.
15. Jimenez P, Canton J, Collado A, Cabrera T, Serrano A, Real LM, Garcia A, Ruiz-Cabello F, Garrido F. Chromosome loss is the most frequent mechanism contributing to HLA haplotype loss in human tumors. *Int J Cancer.* 1999;83:91–97.
16. Ferrone S, Marincola FM. Loss of HLA Class I antigens by melanoma cells: molecular mechanisms, functional significance and clinical relevance. [Review] [57 refs]. *Immunol Today.* 1995;16:487–494.
17. Real LM, Jimenez P, Canton J, Kirkin A, Garcia A, Abril E, Zeuthen J, Ruiz-Cabello F, Garrido F. In vivo and in vitro generation of a new altered HLA phenotype in melanoma-tumour-cell variants expressing a single HLA-class-I allele. *Int J Cancer.* 1998;75: 317–323.
18. Sette A, Chesnut R, Fikes J. HLA expression in cancer: implications for T cell-based immunotherapy. *Immunogenetics.* 2001;53:255–263.
19. De Waard-Siebinga I, Houbiers JGA, Hilders CG, De Wolff-Rouendaal D, Jager MJ. differential expression of HLA-A and -B on uveal melanoma as determined by immunohistology. *Ocular Immunol inflam.* 1996; 4:1–14.
20. Hurks HM, Metzelaar-Blok JA, Mulder A, Claas FH, Jager MJ. High frequency of allele-specific down-regulation of HLA Class I expression in uveal melanoma cell lines. *Int J Cancer.* 2000;85:697–702.
21. De Waard-Siebinga I, Hilders CG, Hansen BE, Van Delft JL, Jager MJ. HLA expression and tumor-infiltrating immune cells in uveal melanoma. *Graefes Arch Clin Exp Ophthalmol.* 1996;234:34–42.
22. Ericsson C, Seregard S, Bartolazzi A, Levitskaya E, Ferrone S, Kiessling R, Larsson O. Association of HLA Class I and Class II antigen expression and mortality in uveal melanoma. *Invest Ophthalmol Vis Sci.* 2001;42:2153–2156.
23. Dithmar SA, Crowder J, Jager MJ, Vigniswaran N, Grossniklaus HE. HLA-I-Antigen expression korreliert mit dem histologischen Zelltyp uvealer Melanome. *Ophthalmologe.* 2002;99:625–628.
24. Cresswell AC, Sisley K, Laws D, Parsons MA, Rennie IG, Murray AK. Reduced expression of TAP-1 and TAP-2 in posterior uveal melanoma is associated with progression to metastatic disease. *Melanoma Res.* 2001;11:275–281.
25. Van Duinen SG, Ruiter DJ, Broecker EB, Van der Velde EA, Sorg C, Welvaart K, Ferrone S. Level of HLA antigens in locoregional metastases and clinical course of the disease in patients with melanoma. *Cancer Res.* 1988;48:1019–1025.

26. Vitale M, Rezzani R, Rodella L, Zauli G, Grigolato P, Cadei M, Hicklin DJ, Ferrone S. HLA Class I antigen and transporter associated with antigen processing (TAP1 and TAP2) down-regulation in high-grade primary breast carcinoma lesions. *Cancer Res.* 1998;58:737–742.
27. Hicklin DJ, Wang Z, Arienti F, Rivoltini L, Parmiani G, Ferrone S. β2-Microglobulin mutations, HLA Class I antigen loss, and tumor progression in melanoma. *J Clin Invest.* 1998;101:2720–2729.
28. Concha A, Esteban F, Cabrera T, Ruiz-Cabello F, Garrido F. Tumor aggressiveness and MHC Class I and II antigens in laryngeal and breast cancer. *Semin Cancer Biol.* 1991; 2:47–54.
29. Kageshita T, Hirai S, Ono T, Hicklin DJ, Ferrone S. Down-regulation of HLA Class I antigen-processing molecules in malignant melanoma: association with disease progression. *Am J Pathol.* 1999;154:745–754.
30. Levin I, Klein T, Kuperman O, Segal S, Shapira J, Gal R, Hart Y, Klein B. The expression of HLA Class I antigen in prostate cancer in relation to tumor differentiation and patient survival. *Cancer Detect Prev.* 1994;18:443–445.
31. Ma D, Luyten GP, Luider TM, Niederkorn JY. Relationship between natural killer cell susceptibility and metastasis of human uveal melanoma cells in a murine model. *Invest Ophthalmol Vis Sci.* 1995;36:435–441.
32. Whiteside TL, Herberman RB. Role of human natural killer cells in health and disease. *Clin Diagn Lab Immunol.* 1994;1:125–133.
33. Blom DJ, Schurmans LR, Waard-Siebinga I, Wolff-Rouendaal D, Keunen JE, Jager MJ. HLA expression in a primary uveal melanoma, its cell line, and four of its metastases. *Br J Ophthalmol.* 1997;81:989–993.
34. Kageshita T, Wang Z, Calorini L, Yoshii A, Kimura T, Ono T, Gattoni-Celli S, Ferrone S. Selective loss of human leukocyte Class I allospecificities and staining of melanoma cells by monoclonal antibodies recognizing monomorphic determinants of Class I human leukocyte antigens. *Cancer Res.* 1993;53:3349–3354.
35. Kirszenbaum M, Djoulah S, Hors J, Le GI, de Oliveira EB, Prost S, Dausset J, Carosella ED. HLA-G gene polymorphism segregation within CEPH reference families. *Hum Immunol.* 1997;53:140–147.
36. Lee N, Llano M, Carretero M, Ishitani A, Navarro F, Lopez-Botet M, Geraghty DE. HLA-E is a major ligand for the natural killer inhibitory receptor CD94/NKG2A. *Proc Natl Acad Sci USA.* 1998;95:5199–5204.
37. Pazmany L, Mandelboim O, Vales-Gomez M, Davis DM, Becker TC, Reyburn HT, Seebach JD, Hill JA, Strominger JL. Human leucocyte antigen-G and its recognition by natural killer cells. *J Reprod Immunol.* 1999;43:127–137.
38. Carosella ED, Dausset J, Rouas-Freiss N. Immunotolerant functions of HLA-G. *Cell Mol Life Sci.* 1999;55:327–333.
39. Hurks HM, Valter MV, Wilson L, Hilgert I, Van den Elsen PJ, Jager MJ. Uveal melanoma: no expression f HLA-G. *Invest Ophthalmol Vis Sci.* 2001;42:3081–3084.
40. Paul P, Cabestre FA, Le Gal FA, Khalil-Daher I, Le Danff C, Schmid M, Mercier S, Avril MF, Dausset J, Guillet JG, Carosella ED. Heterogeneity of HLA-G gene transcription and protein expression in malignant melanoma biopsies. *Cancer Res.* 1999;59: 1954–1960.
41. Real LM, Cabrera T, Collado A, Jimenez P, Garcia A, Ruiz-Cabello F, Garrido F. Expression of HLA G in human tumors is not a frequent event. *Int J Cancer.* 1999;81: 512–518.
42. Cabestre FA, Lefebvre S, Moreau P, Rouas-Friess N, Dausset J, Carosella ED, Paul P. HLA-G expression: immune privilege for tumour cells? *Semin Cancer Biol.* 1999; 9:27–36.

43. Pangault C, Amiot L, Caulet-Maugendre S, Brasseur F, Burtin F, Guilloux V, Drenou B, Fauchet R, Onno M. HLA-G protein expression is not induced during malignant transformation. *Tissue Antigens.* 1999;53:335–346.
44. Davies B, Hiby S, Gardner L, Loke YW, King A. HLA-G expression by tumors. *Am J Reprod Immunol.* 2001;45:103–107.
45. Jager MJ, Hurks HMH, Levitskaya J, Kiessling R. HLA expression in uveal melanoma: there is no rule without some exception. *Hum Immunol.* 2002;63:444–451.
46. Krishnakumar S, Abhyankar D, Lakshim-Sundaram A, Pushparaj V, Palanivelu Shanmugan M, Biswas J. Major histocompatibility antigens and antigen-processing molecules in uveal melanoma. *Clin Cancer Res.* 2003;9:4159–4164.

GERASIMOS ANASTASSIOU

# 19. Cell Adhesion Molecules: A Brief Review of Their Structure and Function. Their Role in Uveal Melanoma

## INTRODUCTION

Cell adhesion is critical for the genesis and maintenance of both three-dimensional structure and normal function in tissues. The biochemical entities mediating cell adhesion are multiprotein complexes comprising three broad classes of macromolecules: the adhesion receptors, the extracellular matrix molecules, and the adhesion plaque proteins.[1] Cell adhesion receptors are typically transmembrane glycoproteins that mediate binding to extracellular matrix (ECM) molecules or to counter-receptors on other cells; these molecules determine the specificity of cell–cell or cell–ECM interactions. An exciting concept that has emerged from recent cell biological research is that cell adhesion complexes are not simply static architectural entities. Rather, they are dynamic units that are capable of capturing and integrating signals from the extracellular environment. Moreover, the functions of cell adhesion complexes are precisely regulated by biochemical events within the cell. Thus, cell adhesion receptors are at a nexus of two-way signalling between the cell and its' external environment. This chapter will focus on the main families of the cell adhesion molecules (CAM) and their implication in tumor biology and immunology. Furthermore, it will review published data concerning these molecules and uveal melanoma.

## CELL ADHESION MOLECULES: CLASSIFICATION

To date, five main families of cell adhesion molecules are known each with a large number of members: the integrins, the members of the immunoglobulin gene superfamily, the selectins, the CD44-family, and the cadherins.

*Integrins* form a family of membrane-spanning cell-surface proteins that promote cell–cell and cell–matrix adhesion. The integrins are composed of two different subunits, the alpha and beta chains. Both alpha and beta subunits are type-I transmembrane glycoproteins with a single hydrophobic transmembrane segment and a short cytoplasmic part. The extracellular domains of the subunits form the alpha/beta-heterodimers.[2,3] Integrins co-localise with various components of the cytoskeleton in focal contacts and adhesion plaques and, consequently, the cytoplasmic domains of the integrins are thought to interact with cytoskeletal proteins, in particular, talin, α-actinin and actin. These properties endow integrins with the ability to serve as a link between the cytoskeleton and the ECM. A binding site for several (but not all) integrins on the ECM proteins has been identified as being the tripeptide Arg-Gly-Asp (RGD).[4,5] Fourteen different alpha and eight beta chains have been detected to date. The alpha and beta chains form a multitude of receptors in their various combinations: some of them have affinity to components of the ECM (i.e., collagen, laminin, fibronectin and vitronectin), and others to cell bound ligands on leukocytes and endothelial cells (Table 19.1).[6]

Table 19.1. The integrin receptors and their ligands.

| Integrin αβ heterodimer | β subunit | Other names | α subunit | Other names | Ligands of the integrin heterodimer |
|---|---|---|---|---|---|
| *VLA family* | | | | | |
| VLA-1 | β1 | VLAβ, CD29, gpIIa | α1 | CD49a | Laminin, (collagen I, IV) |
| VLA-2 | | | α2 | CD49b | Collagen I–VI, (laminin) |
| VLA-3 | | | α3 | CD49c | Fibronectin, laminin, collagen I, kalinin |
| VLA-4 | | | α4 | CD49d | VCAM-1, fibronectin |
| VLA-5 | | | α5 | CD49e | Fibronectin |
| VLA-6 | | | α6 | CD49f | Laminin, merosin |
| β1α7 | | | α7 | | Laminin |
| β1α8 | | | α8 | | |
| β1αv | | | αv | CD51 | Fibronectin |
| *LEUCAM family* | | | | | |
| LFA-1 | β2 | CD18 | αL | CD11a | ICAM-1, -2, -3 |
| Mac-1 | | | αM | CD11b | ICAM-1, fibrinogen, C3bi |
| P150,95 | | | αX | CD11c | C3bi |
| *CYTOADHESIN family* | | | | | |
| CD41a, gpIIbIIIa | β3 | GpIIIa, CD61 | αIIb | GpIIb, CD41 | Fibrinogen, fibronectin, Vitronectin, von Willebrand factor |
| Vitronectin receptor | | | αv | CD51 | Vitronectin, Fibrinogen, von Willebrand factor, laminin, thrombospondin, fibronectin |
| β4α6 | β4 | | α6 | CD49f | Laminin |
| β5α v | β5 | βx, βs | αv | CD51 | Vitronectin, fibronectin |
| β6α v | β6 | | αv | CD51 | Fibronectin |
| β7α4, LPAM-1 | β7 | βp | α4 | CD49d | Fibronectin, VCAM-1, ligand on Peyers Patch HEV |
| β8αv | β8 | | αv | CD51 | |

Integrins and especially the members of the Leucam family are required for a broad range of leukocyte functions, including T-helper and B-lymphocyte responses, natural killing, antibody-dependent cytotoxicity mediated by monocytes and granulocytes, and adherence of leukocytes to endothelial cells, fibroblasts and epithelial cells.[7,8] Thus, integrin receptors have a central role in the functions of the immune system throughout life.[9] Integrin expression has been also studied extensively in human tumors. A multitude of studies have provided evidence that changes in integrin expression on tumor cells is a crucial step towards tumor progression and dissemination.[10–12] Thus, integrins display putative therapeutically useful targets.[13] Various integrin-based therapy regimens are currently under clinical and experimental investigation.[14–17]

*The immunoglobulin gene superfamily* contains some of the most known CAM. This superfamily comprises more than 70 members, including the MHC antigens, the T cell receptor, the immunoglobulins, CD2, CD3, CD4, CD8, and the CAM (i.e., ICAM-1, -2, -3, VCAM-1, NCAM, and PECAM). All the members of the Ig superfamily share the Ig domain, composed of 90–110 amino acids arranged in a sandwich of two sheets of anti-parallel β-strands, which is usually stabilised by a disulphide bond at its centre. An interesting structural feature of the CAM of the Ig superfamily is that, in contrast to Ig's and MHC antigens, which have paired Ig domains, the domains of the CAM are unpaired.[18,19] Table 19.2 summarises the expression sites and the ligands of the CAM members of the Ig superfamily.

The CAM of the Ig superfamily are involved in almost any known pathway (e.g., antigen recognition, T cell activation, natural killing, cytotoxicity of monocytes, leukocyte–endothelial cell interaction, and many others) of the immune system.[9] Their role is of fundamental importance although there remains a large amount to be clarified. Since some of the CAM are also expressed on the surface of tumor cells it became obvious that these molecules are also involved in tumor immunology. The loss of CAM on the tumor surface may help these cell to overcome the immune surveillance. On the other hand, the expression of CAM on the tumor surface may enable the disseminated tumor cells to leave the lymphatic circulation or blood stream and, thus, enable them to establish distant colonies. Since the expression of most of the CAM of the Ig superfamily is inducible by inflammatory cytokines[20] and reversible within some hours, it is theoretically possible for a tumor cell under certain environmental circumstances to change the CAM phenotype in order to successfully metastasise.

*Selectins* represent the smallest and most recently identified family of CAM. Only three members exist: L-, E-, and P-selectin. All three of them were originally found by different approaches but, due to additional information gained by cloning and sequencing, it rapidly became clear that these molecules are strikingly similar.[21] The selectins have an extracellular, a transmembrane and a cytoplasmic domain. At the amino terminus is a 120 amino acid domain homologous to C-type lectins which shares greater than 60% homology within the three selectins. Adjacent to the lectin domain is a sequence of nucleotides resembling epidermal growth factor (EGF). Following the EGF domain, there are variable number of short consensus repeats of approximately 60 amino acids. Two subgroups were identified according to the tissue distribution of the selectins: the leukocyte

Table 19.2. Members of the immunoglobulin gene superfamily.

| Molecule | Size (Ig-domains) | Expression | Ligands |
|---|---|---|---|
| ICAM-1 | | | |
| Intercellular adhesion molecule-1 | 90–115 kD (5) | Endothelial cells, leukocytes, tumor cells, epithelial cells, a.o. | LFA-1 (CD11a/CD18), Mac-1 (CD11c/CD18) |
| ICAM-2 | | | |
| Intercellular adhesion molecule-2 | 46–65 kD (2) | Endothelial cells, monocytes, dendritic cells, lymphocytes | LFA-1 (CD11a/CD18) |
| ICAM-3 | | | |
| Intercellular adhesion molecule-3 | 116–140 kD (5) | Lymphocytes, monocytes, neutrophils, subset of dendritic cells | LFA-1 (CD11a/CD18), Mac-1 (CD11c/CD18) |
| VCAM-1 | | | |
| Vascular cell adhesion molecule-1 | 90–110 kD (7) | Endothelial cells, tumor cells, dendritic cells, macrophages | VLA-4 (CD49d/CD29), $\alpha 4\beta 7$ |
| PECAM-1 | | | |
| Platelet endothelial cell adhesion molecule-1 | 130–140 kD (6) | Platelets, T-cells, endothelial cells, monocytes, granulocytes. | PECAM-1, others |
| NCAM | | | |
| Neural cell adhesion molecule | 175–220 kD (5) | Neurons, subset of T-cells, NK-cells, tumor cells. | NCAM, others |

selectin (L-selectin, expressed on lymphocytes and neutrophils) and the endothelial selectins (E-, and P-selectin, expressed on endothelial cells; P-selectin also expressed on platelets and megakaryocytes). Beside homophylic binding among selectins (i.e., L-selectin with E-, or P-selectin) numerous other ligands (i.e., sialyl Lewis X, GlyCAM-1, lymph node vascular addressin, CD24) have been identified over the last decade.[22]

The major function of the selectins is to regulate the interactions that occur between leukocytes and vascular endothelial cells, the initial and controlling step in the movement of leukocytes into both lymphoid and non-lymphoid organs.[23] In this way, the selectins enable neutrophils and monocytes to enter sites of inflammation.[24] Apart from their crucial role in the inflammatory cascade, selectins may also be involved in the metastatic process. Experimental data supports the role of endothelial selectins as homing receptors for disseminated CD24 positive tumor cells which could thereby extravasate into tissues.[25,26]

*The CD44 proteins* form an other family of cell surface adhesion molecules. The multiple protein isoforms are encoded by a single gene by alternative splicing. The human CD44 gene is composed of two groups of exons. One group, comprising exons 1–5 and 16–20, encodes the standard isoform (CD44s). The remaining 10 variable exons 6–15 (v1–10) can be alternatively spliced and theoretically no less than 1000 variants could be generated.[27] Molecules containing the variable exons are called CD44v. The CD44 standard isoform contains 363 amino acids and has a molecular mass of 37 kD. The protein consists of three domains: the cytoplasmic (72 amino acids), the transmembrane (21 amino acids), and the extracellular one (270 amino acids). The variable region is the point in the extracellular domain at which up to 381 amino acids are inserted at a site between exons 5 and 16 of the RNA transcript. Due to a number of post-translational modifications, the CD44 protein may vary significantly, and in some cases the molecular mass may exceed 200 kD. The major ligand of CD44 is hyaluronic acid, an ubiquitously found component of the ECM. Further components of the ECM such as collagen, fibronectin, and laminin may also serve as ligands for CD44 proteins.[28] The cytokine osteopontin was also reported to bind in a specific, dose-dependant manner to CD44.[29]

Whereas CD44s is expressed on the majority of human tissue types, the expression of CD44v is much more restricted. CD44v isoforms are found in haematopoetic cells and in reactive lymph node cells. Only a few cell types do not express any CD44 isoforms, including hepatocytes and pancreatic acinar cells.[28] The CD44 proteins are involved in many immunological pathways. CD44 expression is significantly elevated in activated T-cells and mediates the extravasation of the T-cells into sites of inflammation.[30] In addition, the presence of CD44v seems to be very important for the migration of dendritic cells from peripheral organs to lymph nodes.[31] In neoplasia, a number of unusual CD44 transcripts relative to those in corresponding normal tissue have been reported. The main implication of CD44 was suspected in the process of metastasis since many parallels between metastasis and lymphocyte migration exist. This was confirmed by experimental data which clearly demonstrated the putative role of CD44 in metastasis.[32,33] However, there appears to be considerable cell-type and tumor-type specificity for the functions of this family of CAM since both pro-invasive and tumor-suppressing properties have been described.[34]

*The cadherin protein family* has been steadily growing, reaching the number of about 50 different cadherins in both vertebrates and invertebrates. Moreover, this number of cadherin genes was doubled by the recent description of 52 human proto-cadherin genes.[35] Despite these developments, the 'classical' cadherins (E-, N-, and P-cadherin) have been extensively studied and serve as prototype molecules for the whole cadherin superfamily. E-cadherin is a transmembrane glycoprotein with an extracellular part comprising five ectodomain (EC) modules of about 110 amino acid residues with conserved calcium binding sequence motifs. The complete ectodomain is indeed stabilised by multiple calcium ions.[36] The ectodomains of the cadherin molecules at the intercellular junctions of epithelial cells are responsible for cell contact. However, structural linkage with the cytoskeleton is needed for full functionality. This is mediated by specific protein complexes bound to the cytoplasmic part of the cadherins: i.e. catenin proteins at adherens junctions and plakoglobin, plakophilin and desmoplakin proteins at desmosomal plaques.[37]

Cadherins are expressed in a cell-, tissue- and development specific manner. Historically, cadherins' function has been perceived to be to link cells and to stabilise these links through interaction with the cytoskeleton. The consequences of such adhesions can have dramatic effects on tissue stability and morphogenetic processes such as cell rearrangement, cell migration, tissue formation and the establishment and maintenance of neural networks.[38] Defective cadherin function can render non-invasive cells invasive,[39] and induced expression of various cadherins in invasive cells can suppress their invasiveness in a cell-contact-dependent manner.[40] Cadherin function is not limited to the physical interactions among groups of cohering cells; cadherins can also participate in signalling events between and within cells that affect differentiation, proliferation and migration.[41]

## CELL ADHESION MOLECULES AND UVEAL MELANOMA

### THE IMMUNOGLOBULIN GENE SUPERFAMILY

The earliest report on CAM in uveal melanoma was published by Van der Pol et al.,[42] who detected immunoreactivity with an *ICAM-1* monoclonal antibody in a series of 25 uveal melanomas. Since this initial description, three additional groups also investigated the immunohistochemical expression of ICAM-1 in uveal melanoma. Natali et al.[43] found a preferential expression of ICAM-1 in lesions with the mixed and epithelioid cell type in their series of 12 uveal melanomas, while Carrel et al.[44] failed to detect any immunoreactivity in ten uveal melanomas using another ICAM-1 antibody. Our group reported on a larger series of 90 clinically monitored uveal melanomas,[45] finding a strong ICAM-1 positivity in the majority of the tumors. In 73 out of 90 tumors (81%), more than 75% of the tumor cells stained ICAM-1 positive. Interestingly, those tumors with less than 75% ICAM-1 positivity metastasised significantly more often than those with greater than 75% positivity for this marker (odds ratio: 7.5, $p = 0.001$). Even in multivariate analysis with other prognostically significant parameters (e.g., tumor location, scleral infiltration), this observation remained statistically significant and therefore, we postulated that ICAM-1 might be a novel prognostic marker in uveal melanoma. In experiments with cell lines, Creyghton et al.[46] demonstrated that ICAM-1 was upregulated by IFN-gamma and TNF-alpha, but not by IFN-alpha.

The expression of *NCAM* in uveal melanoma has been the subject of two immunohistochemical reports. Mooy et al.[47] studied 32 primary lesions as well as 29 metastatic lesions of uveal melanoma, using two antibodies. One antibody recognised all major isoforms of NCAM, and the other recognised the HNK-1 epitope in some of the isoforms only. They found that NCAM was significantly more often expressed in aggressive, rapidly metastasising primary tumors and in metastases ($p = 0.02$ and 0.04, respectively). HNK-1 was significantly more often expressed in larger tumors ($p = 0.04$). In liver metastases, HNK-1 immunoreactivity was significantly less frequently expressed than NCAM ($p = 0.005$). Based on these observations, the authors suggested that the NCAM isoforms which lack the HNK-1 epitope may play a role in the organ specific metastatic behaviour of uveal melanomas. We have also studied the NCAM expression in 87 clinically monitored

Table 19.3. Summary of the studies on uveal melanomas and members of the immunoglobulin gene superfamily.

| Study | Material | Molecules examined | Main outcome |
|---|---|---|---|
| Van der Pol et al.[42] | Cryosections $N=25$ | ICAM-1 | • Strong ICAM-1 positivity |
| Natali et al.[43] | Cryosections $N=12$ | ICAM-1 | • Strong ICAM-1 positivity<br>• Association with cell type |
| Carrel et al.[44] | Cryosections $N=10$ | ICAM-1 | • All lesions ICAM-1 negative |
| Creyghton et al.[46] | Cell lines $N=4$ | ICAM-1 | • Strong ICAM-1 positivity<br>• Upregulation by IFN-$\gamma$ and TNF-$\alpha$ |
| Mooy et al.[47] | Cryosections $N=61$ | NCAM, HNK-1 | • Strong NCAM positivity in aggressive tumours and in metastases<br>• HNK-1 less frequent than NCAM in liver metastases |
| Anastassiou et al.[45] | Paraffin sections $N=90$ | ICAM-1, NCAM, VCAM-1 | • Lack of ICAM-1 correlates with the development of metastasis<br>• NCAM only on spindle cells<br>• VCAM-1 only weakly positive |

uveal melanomas using a single antibody recognising the three major NCAM isoforms.[45] In our studies, NCAM was negative in 73 out of 87 tumors (84%). We only observed NCAM positivity on spindle but not on epithelioid tumor cells. We could not determine a relationship between NCAM expression and metastasis development, as is the case with ICAM-1, in uveal melanoma.

In our clinicopathological study, we also investigated the expression of *VCAM-1* in 88 uveal melanomas.[45] Only 24 out of the 88 tumors (27%) showed some clusters of VCAM-1 positive tumor cells. We found no association between VCAM-1 expression with any of the clinicopathological parameters included in our analyses. No further reports on VCAM-1 or other of the remaining CAM of the immunoglobulin gene superfamily in uveal melanoma exist in the literature to date.

## THE INTEGRINS

Two early reports examined the expression of integrins by immunohistochemistry in 36[48] and 12[49] uveal melanomas, respectively. Ten Berge et al.[48] found that alpha 2 and alpha 4 expression were rare in uveal melanoma, but most lesions expressed alpha 3, alpha 5 and alpha 6. They also failed to detect the alpha v beta 3 integrin receptor in any of the primary uveal melanomas, while the alpha v beta 5 integrin receptor was found in all tumors. The authors did not find any association between integrin expression and any histopathological parameters in their study and, therefore, concluded that determination of the integrin expression profile is not suitable for categorising uveal melanomas as less malignant and highly malignant lesions. Rohrbach et al.[49] found that alpha 6 was expressed only by a small portion of tumor cells in three out of 12 examined uveal melanomas. The authors speculated that the non-epithelial uveal melanomas, which produce only minimal basement membrane material, would have no need for laminin receptors. Interestingly, in a recent report Elshaw et al.[50] found that both laminin receptors (i.e., alpha 1 and alpha 6) as well the VCAM-1 receptor (i.e., alpha 4) were absent on melanocytes but expressed on uveal melanoma cells.

Since the description of the alpha v beta 3 integrin receptor in uveal melanoma by Ten Berge and co-workers, this receptor has become the subject of intense investigation due to evidence that this integrin is involved in both tumor angiogenesis and metastasis of cutaneous melanoma. Natali et al.[51] could verify the observation by Ten Berge et al.[48] that alpha v beta 3 is not expressed on uveal melanoma cells. On the other hand, three groups detected alpha v beta 3 in uveal melanoma cell lines.[46,50,52] Marshall et al.[52] also described an absence of expression of beta 6 and beta 8 in the uveal melanoma cells examined, while beta 1 and beta 5 were detectable. In addition, Creyghton et al.[46] showed that the expression of alpha 1–3 was up-regulated when tumor cells were co-cultured with IFN-alpha, IFN-gamma and TNF-alpha. Similar, Baker et al. found a differential expression of VLA-1, -2, -6 in tumor cells growing in cell culture.[53]

In the recent past, two interesting reports were published by the Canadian group, Larouche et al.,[54] who performed transfection experiments with uveal melanoma cells. Thereby, they provided evidence that the transcriptional activity directed by the alpha 4 promoter sequences was inversely correlated to the potential of uveal melanoma to yield metastases. Additional experiments in electrophoretic mobility shift assays (EMSA) demonstrated that the binding of the nuclear proteins likely to account for transcription of the alpha 4 gene to alpha 4.1 (namely Bp1, Bp2, Bp4, and Bp5) was dramatically reduced in uveal melanoma, but not in normal uveal melanocytes. The authors concluded that the alpha 4 integrin may play a role in the ability of tumor cells to evade the primary tumor and form metastases. Beliveau et al.,[55] investigating alpha 5 integrin, fibronectin and MMPs in four uveal melanoma cell lines, found that the most tumorigenic cell line lacked the expression of alpha 5 integrin and, in addition, secreted a distinctive MMP with a molecular weight of 117 kDa. In a later report of the same group the alpha 5 integrin receptor displayed a differential role towards tumorigenicity in two uveal melanoma cell lines.[56]

We also conducted an immunohistochemical study with 90 clinically monitored uveal melanomas.[57] Since only very few monoclonal antibodies suitable for paraffin-embedded tissue exist, the number of integrin receptors we could screen was limited. We also assessed the microvascular architecture of the tumor and looked for possible associations between these and integrins. We found an association between the expression of VLA-2 in tumors and the presence of vascular networks ($p = 0.05$). Tumors with less than 25% VLA-3 positive cells infiltrated the sclera more frequently than those with more than 25% VLA-3 cell positivity ($p = 0.05$). Tumors expressing less than 50% alpha(v) positive cells were of the mixed or epithelioid cell type ($p = 0.05$) and, with less statistical precision, were

Table 19.4. Summary of the studies on integrin expression in uveal melanomas.

| Study | Material | Molecules examined | Main outcome |
|---|---|---|---|
| Ten Berge et al.[48] | Cryosections $N = 36$ | $\alpha$1–6, $\alpha$v, $\alpha v\beta 3$, $\alpha v\beta 5$, $\beta 1$, $\beta 4$ | • No pattern of expression<br>• No association with histopathological parameters<br>• $\alpha v\beta 3$ not detected |
| Rohrbach et al.[49] | Cryosections $N = 12$ | $\alpha 6\beta 1$ | • Only weak positive |
| Creyghton et al.[46] | Cell lines $N = 4$ | $\alpha$1 – 6, $\alpha$v, $\alpha v\beta 3$, $\alpha v\beta 5$, $\beta 1$, $\beta 2$, $\beta 4$ | • Variable expression<br>• $\alpha v\beta 3$ positivity in one cell line<br>• Upregulation of $\alpha$1–3 by IFN-$\alpha$, IFN-$\gamma$ and TNF-$\alpha$ |
| Natali et al.[51] | Cryosections $N = 12$ | $\alpha$v, $\alpha v\beta 3$ | • $\alpha v\beta 3$ not detected |
| Marshall et al.[52] | Cell lines $N = 3$ | $\alpha v\beta$1,-3,-5,-6,-8 | • $\alpha v\beta$1,-3,-5, positive<br>• $\alpha$ v$\beta$6,8 negative |
| Larouche et al.[54] | Cell lines $N = 2$ | $\alpha 4$ | • Inverse correlation with the metastatic potential |
| Beliveau et al.[55] | Cell lines $N = 4$ | $\alpha 5$ | • The most tumorigenic cell line was $\alpha 5$ negative |
| Anastassiou et al.[57] | Paraffin sections $N = 90$ | $\alpha$2,-3,-v | • Association between $\alpha 2$ and vascular patterns<br>• No association with the development of metastasis |
| Elshaw et al.[50] | Cell lines $N = 10$ | $\alpha$1–6, $\alpha v\beta 3$, $\beta 1$ | • $\alpha 1\beta 1$, $\alpha 4\beta 1$, and $\alpha 6\beta 1$ were absent on melanocytes but expressed on melanoma cells |
| Baker et al.[53] | Short term culture $N = 10$ | $\alpha 1\beta 1$, $\alpha 2\beta 1$, $\alpha 6\beta 1$ | • Integrins were differentially expressed during cell culture |
| Beliveau et al.[56] | Cell lines $N = 2$ | $\alpha 5\beta 1$ | • $\alpha 5\beta 1$ had differential influence upon tumorigenicity in two distinct cells lines |

associated with the presence of extraocular growth ($p = 0.07$). We could not find any association between integrin expression (alpha 2, alpha 3, and alpha v) and the development of metastases.

## THE CD44 PROTEINS

Very little is known about this family of CAM in uveal melanoma. Creyghton et al.[46] found an abundant expression of the CD44 standard protein in 4 cell lines. Co-culture of the tumor cells with IFN-alpha, IFN-gamma and TNF-alpha did not alter CD44 expression. Danen et al.[58] examined three of the four previously investigated cell lines[46] and an additional 12 tumors by immunohistochemistry for the expression of CD44 standard and variant proteins. All uveal melanomas strongly stained with antibodies to the standard portion of CD44. No expression of the CD44 variant 7 was found, whereas v5, v6 and v10 were expressed in 2/12, 5/12 and 8/12 cases, respectively. Variant 6 was slightly expressed on the examined cell lines, while v5, v7 and v10 were absent. The authors did not find any association between CD44 expression and any of the histopathological prognostic parameters. The latest report on CD44 and uveal melanoma was presented by Song et al.[59] in a series of 40 tumor tissues. They found CD44 positivity in 63% of the tumors, and an association between CD44 expression and scleral infiltration ($p = 0.01$).

## THE CADHERINS AND THE SELECTINS

So far, only one report on uveal melanoma and cadherin expression exists.[60] Our group examined 16 tumor specimens for E- and N-cadherin expression by microarray analysis (RNA level) and immunohistochemistry (protein level). Our data showed that N-cadherin is absent in uveal melanomas. E-cadherin was differentially expressed and showed no association to histopathology. These findings are contrary to the results from cutaneous melanomas, which lack E-cadherin and abundantly express N-cadherin.[61] A recent study demonstrated a potential influence of beta-catenin (a cytoplasmic protein forming a complex with the intracellular domain of E-cadherin), on invasive potential of uveal melanoma cells.[62]

There are no reports on uveal melanoma and selectins in the literature to date.

## CONCLUSIONS

From the above review, it is clear that our knowledge about CAM in uveal melanoma is very limited. In many cases, we do not even have any basic information such as the expression of the molecules (e.g., selectins). On the other hand, many of the published reports can be considered only to be preliminary since most cohorts of tumors examined were small. In addition, many of the reports present immunohistochemical data or expression analysis by FACS using cell lines and do not give any information about the function of the CAM in uveal melanoma. CAM, however, remain an interesting field for further research in uveal melanoma.

## REFERENCES


1. Gumbiner BM. Cell adhesion: the molecular basis of tissue architecture and morphogenesis. *Cell.* 1996;84:345–357.
2. Hynes RO. Integrins: versatility, modulation, and signaling in cell adhesion. *Cell.* 1992;69:11–25.
3. Dedhar S. Integrins and tumor invasion. *Bioessays.* 1990;12:583–590.
4. Ruoslahti E, Pierschbacher MD. New perspectives in cell adhesion: RGD and integrins. *Science.* 1987;238:491–497.
5. Loftus JC, O'TooleTE, Plow EF, Glass A, Frelinger ALd, Ginsberg MH. A beta 3 integrin mutation abolishes ligand binding and alters divalent cation-dependent conformation. *Science.* 1990;249:915–918.
6. Ruoslahti E. Integrins. *J Clin Invest.* 1991;87:1–5.

7. Kishimoto TK, Larson RS, Corbi AL, Dustin ML, Staunton DE, Springer TA. The leukocyte integrins. *Adv Immunol.* 1989;46:149–182.
8. Springer TA, Dustin ML, Kishimoto TK, Marlin SD. The lymphocyte function-associated LFA-1, CD2, and LFA-3 molecules: cell adhesion receptors of the immune system. *Annu Rev Immunol.* 1987;5:223–252.
9. Springer TA. Adhesion receptors of the immune system. *Nature.* 1990;346:425–434.
10. Varner JA, Cheresh DA. Integrins and cancer. *Curr Opin Cell Biol.* 1996;8:724–730.
11. Guan JL, Shalloway D. Regulation of focal adhesion-associated protein tyrosine kinase by both cellular adhesion and oncogenic transformation. *Nature.* 1992;358:690–692.
12. Akiyama SK, Olden K, Yamada KM. Fibronectin and integrins in invasion and metastasis. *Cancer Metastasis Rev.* 1995;14:173–189.
13. Velasco-Velazquez MA, Molina-Guarneros JA, Mendoza-Patino N, Sullivan Lopez J, Mandoki JJ. Integrins and integrin-associated molecules: targets for the development of antimetastatic therapies. *Rev Invest Clin.* 1999;51:183–193.
14. Van Hagen PM, Breeman WA, Bernard HF, Schaar M, Mooij CM, Srinivasan A, Schmidt MA, Krenning EP, De Jong M. Evaluation of a radiolabelled cyclic DTPA-RGD analogue for tumour imaging and radionuclide therapy. *Int J Cancer.* 2000;90: 186–198.
15. Mitjans F, Meyer T, Fittschen C, Goodman S, Jonczyk A, Marshall JF, Reyes G, Piulats J. In vivo therapy of malignant melanoma by means of antagonists of alpha v integrins. *Int J Cancer.* 2000;87:716–723.
16. Gutheil JC, Campbell TN, Pierce PR, Watkins JD, Huse WD, Bodkin DJ, Cheresh DA. Targeted antiangiogenic therapy for cancer using Vitaxin: a humanized monoclonal antibody to the integrin alpha v beta 3. *Clin Cancer Res.* 2000;6:3056–3061.
17. De Fougerolles AR, Sprague AG, Nickerson-Nutter CL, Chi-Rosso G, Rennert PD, Gardner H, Gotwals PJ, Lobb RR, Koteliansky VE. Regulation of inflammation by collagen-binding integrins alpha 1 beta 1 and alpha 2 beta 1 in models of hypersensitivity and arthritis. *J Clin Invest.* 2000;105:721–729.
18. Polte T, Newman W, Gopal TV. Full length vascular cell adhesion molecule 1 (VCAM-1). *Nucl Acids Res.* 1990;18:5901.
19. Simmons D, Makgoba MW, Seed B. ICAM, an adhesion ligand of LFA-1, is homologous to the neural cell adhesion molecule NCAM. *Nature.* 1988;331:624–627.
20. Dustin ML, Springer TA. Role of lymphocyte adhesion receptors in transient interactions and cell locomotion. *Annu Rev Immunol.* 1991;9:27–66.
21. Lasky LA, Singer MS, Yednock TA, Dowbenko D, Fennie C, Rodriguez H, Nguyen T, Stachel S, Rosen SD. Cloning of a lymphocyte homing receptor reveals a lectin domain. *Cell.* 1989;56:1045–1055.
22. Vestweber D. The selectins and their ligands. *Curr Top Microbiol Immunol.* 1993;184:65–75.
23. Vestweber D. Selectins: cell surface lectins which mediate the binding of leukocytes to endothelial cells. *Semin Cell Biol.* 1992;3:211–220.
24. Butcher EC. Leukocyte-endothelial cell recognition: three (or more) steps to specificity and diversity. *Cell.* 1991;67:1033–1036.
25. Fogel M, Friederichs J, Zeller Y, Husar M, Smirnov A, Roitman L, Altevogt P, Sthoeger ZM. CD24 is a marker for human breast carcinoma. *Cancer Lett.* 1999;143: 87–94.
26. Aigner S, Ramos CL, Hafezi-Moghadam A, Lawrence MB, Friederichs J, Altevogt P, Ley K. CD24 mediates rolling of breast carcinoma cells on P-selectin. *Faseb J.* 1998;12: 1241–1251.
27. Tolg C, Hofmann M, Herrlich P, Ponta H. Splicing choice from ten variant exons establishes CD44 variability. *Nucleic Acids Res.* 1993;21:1225–1229.

28. Goodison S, Urquidi V, Tarin D. CD44 cell adhesion molecules. *Mol Pathol.* 1999;52: 189–196.
29. Weber GF, Ashkar S, Cantor H. Interaction between CD44 and osteopontin as a potential basis for metastasis formation. *Proc Assoc Am Physician.* 1997;109:1–9.
30. DeGrendele HC, Estess P, Siegelman MH. Requirement for CD44 in activated T cell extravasation into an inflammatory site. *Science.* 1997;278:672–675.
31. Weiss JM, Renkl AC, Sleeman J, Dittmar H, Termeer CC, Taxis S, Howells N, Schopf E, Ponta H, Herrlich P, Simon JC. CD44 variant isoforms are essential for the function of epidermal Langerhans cells and dendritic cells. *Cell Adhes Commun.* 1998;6:157–160.
32. Reeder JA, Gotley DC, Walsh MD, Fawcett J, Antalis TM. Expression of antisense CD44 variant 6 inhibits colorectal tumor metastasis and tumor growth in a wound environment. *Cancer Res.* 1998;58:3719–3726.
33. Gunthert U, Hofmann M, Rudy W, Reber S, Zoller M, Haussmann I, Matzku S, Wenzel A, Ponta H, Herrlich P. A new variant of glycoprotein CD44 confers metastatic potential to rat carcinoma cells. *Cell.* 1991;65:13–24.
34. Herrlich P, Morrison H, Sleeman J, Orian-Rousseau V, Konig H, Weg-Remers S, Ponta H. CD44 acts both as a growth- and invasiveness-promoting molecule and as a tumor-suppressing cofactor. *Ann NY Acad Sci.* 2000;910:106–118; discussion 118–120.
35. Wu Q, Maniatis T. A striking organization of a large family of human neural cadherin-like cell adhesion genes. *Cell.* 1999;97:779–790.
36. Pertz O, Bozic D, Koch AW, Fauser C, Brancaccio A, Engel J. A new crystal structure, $Ca^{2+}$ dependence and mutational analysis reveal molecular details of E-cadherin homoassociation. *Embo J.* 1999;18:1738–1747.
37. Nollet F, Kools P, Van Roy F. Phylogenetic analysis of the cadherin superfamily allows identification of six major subfamilies besides several solitary members. *J Mol Biol.* 2000;299:551–572.
38. Steinberg MS. Adhesion in development: an historical overview. *Dev Biol.* 1996;180: 377–388.
39. Yap AS. The morphogenetic role of cadherin cell adhesion molecules in human cancer: a thematic review. *Cancer Invest.* 1998;16:252–261.
40. Foty RA, Steinberg MS. Measurement of tumor cell cohesion and suppression of invasion by E- or P-cadherin. *Cancer Res.* 1997;57:5033–5036.
41. Knudsen KA, Frankowski C, Johnson KR, Wheelock MJ. A role for cadherins in cellular signaling and differentiation. *J Cell Biochem Suppl.* 1998;31:168–176.
42. Van der Pol JP, Jager MJ, De Wolff-Rouendaal D, Ringens PJ, Vennegoor C, Ruiter DJ. Heterogeneous expression of melanoma-associated antigens in uveal melanomas. *Curr Eye Res.* 1987;6:757–765.
43. Natali PG, Bigotti A, Nicotra MR, Nardi RM, Delovu A, Segatto O, Ferrone S. Analysis of the antigenic profile of uveal melanoma lesions with anti-cutaneous melanoma-associated antigen and anti-HLA monoclonal antibodies. *Cancer Res.* 1989;49: 1269–1274.
44. Carrel S, Schreyer M, Gross N, Zografos L. Surface antigenic profile of uveal melanoma lesions analysed with a panel of monoclonal antibodies directed against cutaneous melanoma. *Anticancer Res.* 1990;10:81–89.
45. Anastassiou G, Schilling H, Stang A, Djakovic S, Heiligenhaus A, Bornfeld N. Expression of the cell adhesion molecules ICAM-1, VCAM-1 and NCAM in uveal melanoma: a clinicopathological study. *Oncology.* 2000;58:83–88.
46. Creyghton WM, De Waard-Siebinga I, Danen EH, Luyten GP, Van Muijen GN, Jager MJ. Cytokine-mediated modulation of integrin, ICAM-1 and CD44 expression on human uveal melanoma cells in vitro. *Melanoma Res.* 1995;5:235–242.

47. Mooy CM, Luyten GP, De Jong PT, Jensen OA, Luider TM, Van der Ham F, Bosman FT. Neural cell adhesion molecule distribution in primary and metastatic uveal melanoma. *Hum Pathol* 1995;26:1185–1190.
48. Ten Berge PJ, Danen EH, Van Muijen GN, Jager MJ, Ruiter DJ. Integrin expression in uveal melanoma differs from cutaneous melanoma. *Invest Ophthalmol Vis Sci.* 1993;34: 3635–3640.
49. Rohrbach JM, Wild M, Riedinger C, Kreissig I, Thiel HJ. Premetastatic uveal melanoma cells do not express laminin receptors. *Ger J Ophthalmol.* 1994;3:144–147.
50. Elshaw SR, Sisley K, Cross N, Murray AK, MacNeil SM, Wagner M, Nichols CE, Rennie IG. A comparison of ocular melanocyte and uveal melanoma cell invasion and the implication of alpha 1 beta 1, alpha 4 beta 1 and alpha 6 beta 1 integrins. *Br J Ophthalmol.* 2001;85:732–738.
51. Natali PG, Hamby CV, Felding-Habermann B, Liang B, Nicotra MR, Di Filippo F, Giannarelli D, Temponi M, Ferrone S. Clinical significance of alpha (v) beta 3 integrin and intercellular adhesion molecule-1 expression in cutaneous malignant melanoma lesions. *Cancer Res.* 1997;57:1554–1560.
52. Marshall JF, Rutherford DC, Happerfield L, Hanby A, McCartney AC, Newton-Bishop J, Hart IR. Comparative analysis of integrins in vitro and in vivo in uveal and cutaneous melanomas. *Br J Cancer.* 1998;77:522–529.
53. Baker JK, Elshaw SR, Mathewman GE, Nichols CE, Murray AK, Parsons MA, Rennie IG, Sisley K. Expression of integrins, degradative enzymes and their inhibitors in uveal melanoma: differences between in vitro and in vivo expression. *Melanoma Res.* 2001; 11:265–273.
54. Larouche N, Larouche K, Beliveau A, Leclerc S, Salesse C, Pelletier G, Guerin SL. Transcriptional regulation of the alpha 4 integrin subunit gene in the metastatic spread of uveal melanoma. *Anticancer Res.* 1998;18:3539–3547.
55. Beliveau A, Berube M, Rousseau A, Pelletier G, Guerin SL. Expression of integrin alpha 5 beta 1 and MMPs associated with epithelioid morphology and malignancy of uveal melanoma. *Invest Ophthalmol Vis Sci.* 2000;41:2363–2372.
56. Beliveau A, Berube M, Carrier P, Mercier C, Guerin SL. Tumorigenicity of the mixed spindle-epithelioid SP6.5 and epithelioid TP17 uveal melanoma cell lines is differentially related to alpha 5 beta 1 integrin expression. *Invest Ophthalmol Vis Sci.* 2001;42: 3058–3065.
57. Anastassiou G, Schilling H, Djakovic S, Bornfeld N. Expression of VLA-2, VLA-3, and alpha (v) integrin receptors in uveal melanoma: association with microvascular architecture of the tumour and prognostic value. *Br J Ophthalmol.* 2000;84:899–902.
58. Danen EH, Ten Berge PJ, Van Muijen GN, Jager MJ, Ruiter DJ. Expression of CD44 and the pattern of CD44 alternative splicing in uveal melanoma. *Melanoma Res.* 1996; 6:31–35.
59. Song J, Luo C, Xia R, Jiang S. Expression of CD44 molecule and its significance in uveal and conjunctival melanomas. *Hua Hsi I Ko Ta Hsueh Hsueh Pao.* 1998;29:38–41.
60. Anastassiou G, Tschentscher F, Zeschnigk M, Bornfeld N. Cadherin expression in uveal melanoma. *Exp Eye Res.* 2002;74:423–425.
61. Hsu MY, Wheelock MJ, Johnson KR, Herlyn M. Shifts in cadherin profiles between human normal melanocytes and melanomas. *J Invest Dermatol Symp Proc.* 1996;1: 188–194.
62. Kim K, Daniels KJ, Hay ED. Tissue-specific expression of beta-catenin in normal mesenchyme and uveal melanomas and its effect on invasiveness. *Exp Cell Res.* 1998; 245:79–90.

IAN A. CREE, FEDERICA DI NICOLANTONIO AND MICHAEL H. NEALE

# 20. Chemotherapy of Uveal Melanoma

## INTRODUCTION

Uveal melanoma differs substantially from cutaneous melanoma, and is even more chemoresistant.[1] Because it is a rare tumor with an incidence of around 6 per million in Caucasian populations, uveal melanoma has not attracted much interest from the pharmaceutical industry, or from many oncologists. The purpose of this chapter is therefore to redress the balance a little. A tumor that kills around 50% of the patients it affects and accounts for 13% of melanoma deaths is surely worthy of greater interest.

Uveal melanoma is a slow-growing tumor with few mitoses and even fewer apoptoses. Labelling of cells in the cell cycle by S-phase markers such as Ki67 show that only around 1% of cells are actually proliferating. Uveal melanoma cells spread hematogenously by necessity, as there are no lymphatics in the choroid or orbit. The commonest site of metastasis is the liver, and patients often present with metastatic disease at a stage too advanced for them to withstand chemotherapy.

To date, chemotherapy for this tumor has been disappointing, with few responses and little benefit to patients, even in comparison with cutaneous melanoma.[2–5] However, new data from several sources suggest that chemotherapy may be possible and that the future of chemotherapy for uveal melanoma is unlikely to be as bleak as past experience might suggest.

## CHEMOTHERAPEUTIC DRUGS

Chemotherapy has evolved from the early days of alkylating agents such as cyclophosphamide and melphalan to encompass more than 40 agents and several classes of drugs with differing mechanisms of action (Table 20.1). Initial ideas centred on the use of alkylating agents to target proliferating cells within tumors. Because all chemotherapeutic drugs are toxic, the idea of using them at intervals to allow the normal proliferating tissue such as bone-marrow to recover became the way in which most chemotherapy was and is still given (Fig. 20.1a). Recognition of resistance was explained by the Goldie–Coldman hypothesis, which suggested that optimum chemotherapy depends upon the interval between doses, the efficacy of the chemotherapy and the mutation rate of the cells. Thus dose intensity becomes the main determinant of response.[6,7] The use of bone marrow stimulation by cytokines such as granulocyte colony stimulating factor (G–CSF) has allowed dose

Table 20.1. Chemotherapeutic drugs and mechanisms of action. This list is far from exhaustive, but does include most of those used at some time to treat melanoma.

| Class | Drug name | Mechanism of action |
|---|---|---|
| Alkylating agents | Cyclophosphamide, Melphalan, Treosulfan | DNA damage by methylation of bases |
| Platinum | Cisplatin, Carboplatin, Oxaliplatin | Formation of platinum adducts on DNA |
| Topoisomerase inhibitors | Doxorubicin, Epirubicin, Mitoxantrone, Etoposide, Topotecan | Inhibition of topoisomerases, enzymes which unravel DNA during transcription of DNA |
| Vinca alkaloids | Vincristine, Vinblastine, Vindesine, Vinorelbine | Inhibition of microtubule assembly required for mitosis |
| Taxanes | Paclitaxel, Docetaxel | Inhibition of microtubule depolymerization |
| Anti-metabolites | 5-fluorouracil, Methotrexate, Cytosine arabinoside, Gemcitabine | Incorporate incorrect bases into DNA and RNA |

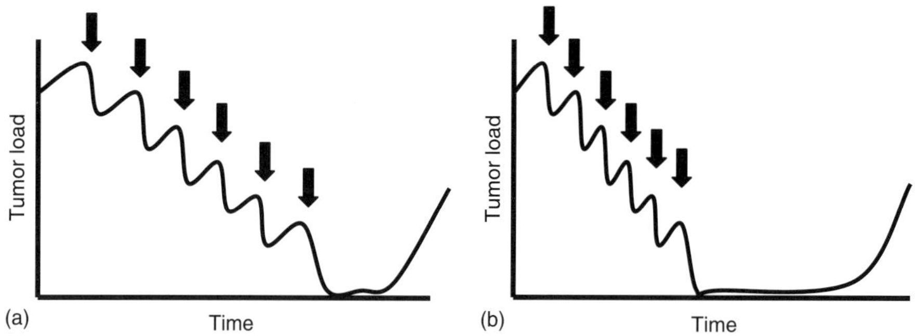


Fig. 20.1. The theoretical effect of chemotherapy on tumor load. (a) Multiple doses are given leading to progressive reduction in tumor burden, though residual cells may still re-grow and lead to recurrence. (b) Dose intensification with shorter intervals allows less time for re-growth of cells between cycles of chemotherapy, and the bone marrow can be induced to proliferate between cycles with cytokines (e.g. G–CSF). However, overall survival may not be improved if residual cells are present at the end of treatment.

intensification, with less time between each cycle of chemotherapy (Fig. 20.1b). In addition, it has been recognized that higher individual doses of drugs can be used if they are given sequentially rather than in combination (Fig. 20.2).

However, in the case of solid tumors with low proliferation rates, these models are clearly a considerable simplification of a very complex process. It is now recognised that chemotherapy has much more complex effects based not just on pharmacokinetic considerations, but also on the response of cancer cells to the agents used.

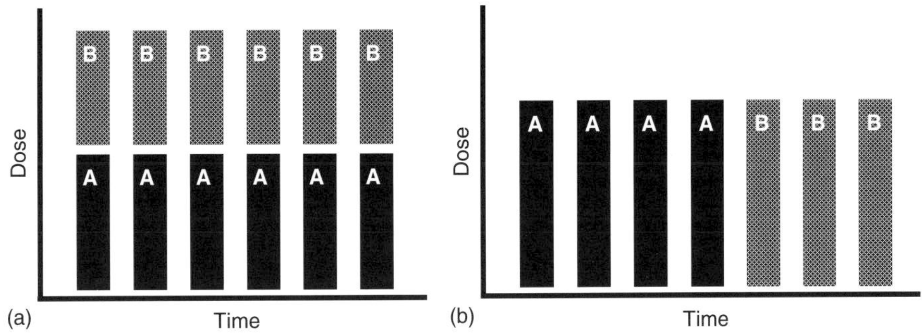


Fig. 20.2. (a) Combination chemotherapy is intended to circumvent resistance. In the example, six cycles of a combination of drugs (A + B) are given. (b) Sequential chemotherapy (A → B) also overcomes resistance by giving more than one agent, but allows higher dosage of individual drugs, and often uses a larger number of cycles.

Studies of the molecular consequences of exposure to chemotherapy have become common during the last decade, keeping pace with the explosion of knowledge about the molecular causes of cancer. This is likely to be particularly useful in the future as more specific agents become available.

## PREVIOUS ATTEMPTS

There are no published randomized trials of chemotherapy in uveal melanoma and few large series or phase II trials have been reported. The largest series was published in 1995 by the MD Anderson in Texas.[8] This showed beyond any doubt that DTIC and DTIC-containing regimens have no place in the treatment of this disease. Despite a small series from Philadelphia suggesting that the aptly named and most aggressive form of DTIC-containing chemotherapy (BOLD—bleomycin, vincristine, lomustine and DTIC) with interferon-α had some activity,[9] a subsequent EORTC study failed to show any benefit (Ocular Oncology Group, Kivelä et al.[30]) and toxicity was an issue in these patients, most of whom have poor hepatic function.

Given the poor results of systemic chemotherapy, various groups turned to the investigation of intra-hepatic arterial chemotherapy.[10] This has potential because of the biology of uveal melanoma: metastasis to the liver is usual, occurring in around 90% of patients with secondary disease, and occurs by haematogenous spread from the eye, where there are no lymphatics. Surgical resection of metastases has been associated with improved survival.[11] Recent results using an alkylating agent (fotemustine) by intrahepatic administration have been particularly encouraging.[12,13]

The undoubted immunogenicity of melanoma[14] (see below) has resulted in several trials of chemoimmunotherapy. BOLD + interferon had some effect in early trials,[9] and some positive effects were also reported by Terheyden et al.[15] using fotemustine systemically with interferon and interleukin-2 (IL-2). This area remains interesting, but there is little evidence that it will provide any major advance over chemotherapy alone. In most patients the added toxicity of interferon or IL-2 is probably not justified.

## ADJUVANT THERAPY

Uveal melanoma has usually spread before diagnosis and it is widely recognized that adjuvant treatment to deal with these clinically silent micrometastases would be advantageous. Animal experiments suggested that adjuvant chemotherapy might be effective,[16] but these have not yet been followed up in the clinic, mainly because there is little evidence of efficacy of chemotherapy in metastatic disease.

In cutaneous melanoma, interferon-α has been shown to produce an improved survival in about 10% of patients with high-risk disease.[17,18] The mechanism of action of interferon is obscure—this cytokine has direct anti-proliferative effects, but also affects the immune system and is anti-angiogenic in tumors dependent upon basic fibroblast growth factor (bFGF), as uveal melanoma seems to be (Boyd et al., unpublished). As a result, interferon-α2b was chosen by the group at St Bartholomew's hospital and Moorfields Eye Hospital for a randomized adjuvant study in patients with high risk uveal melanoma (defined by largest tumor diameter). The study is recruiting slowly (PN Plowman, personal communication), and no results are available. Further evidence in support of this approach has been provided by Dithmar et al.,[19] who showed that interferon was able to reduce the number and growth of hepatic metastases in an animal model.

## CHEMOSENSITIVITY AND NEW REGIMENS

The poor response to systemic cytotoxic agents was confirmed in chemosensitivity assays with primary uveal melanoma cells by Myatt et al.[20] Only a few agents showed any effect at all, and there was considerable variation in the activity of the more effective agents between individual tumors. The best DNA-damaging agent was treosulfan, an alkylating agent that methylates the guanine bases at the $O^7$ position, so that its effects are less susceptible to repair by $O^6$-methylguanylmethyl transferase (MGMT) than other drugs.[21] These findings prompted the author's laboratory to try inhibiting DNA repair in treosulfan-exposed cells by the addition of gemcitabine. This agent is a cytosine analogue which inhibits DNA polymerases at sub-cytotoxic concentrations. Since DNA polymerases are required for most DNA repair pathways, there was a possibility that the damage caused by treosulfan would be prolonged sufficiently for the cells to undergo growth arrest or apoptosis. DNA damage leads to up-regulation of the tumor suppressor gene p53, which is wild-type in nearly all uveal melanomas,[22] and results in growth arrest or apoptosis in most cell types.[23] The strategy seemed to work,[4] though formal proof of the mechanism is still lacking.

In the clinic, treosulfan + gemcitabine has proved useful in uveal melanoma patients (Keilholtz et al., unpublished; Pfohler et al.[31]) and, paradoxically, in other tumor types,[24] though as yet formal trials of this combination have yet to be conducted in patients with metastatic melanoma. Two regimens with similar dose intensity are in regular use: one based on a three-weekly cycle length has proved particularly helpful and data from heavily pre-treated ovarian cancer patients is

Table 20.2. Previous attempted chemotherapy for uveal melanoma.

| Reference | Regimen | Response rate | Median survival |
|---|---|---|---|
| Bedikian et al.[8] | DTIC containing | <1% | 7 months |
| Nathan et al.[9] | BOLD | 20% | NA |
| EORTC (Unpublished) | BOLD | NA | ?12 months |
| Terheyden et al.[15] | Fotemustine + IL2 + IFN-α | 1/3 (33%) | 8, 16 & 49 months |
| Cantore et al.[10] | Intrahepatic cisplatin | 3/8 (38%) | 15 months |
| Leyvraz et al.[12] | Intrahepatic fotemustine | 12/30 (40%) | 14 months |
| Salmon et al.[13] | Intrahepatic fotemustine | N/A ($n = 75$) | 9 months |

available.[24] The series collected by members of the Ocular Oncology Group[30] include a complete response (Uwe Reinhold, unpublished) and several patients with minor responses or prolonged stable disease using this regimen (Table 20.2). These data are encouraging, but require clinical trial confirmation. In the interim, many oncologists are giving DTIC, sometimes in combination, with no published evidence that this is of any real benefit.

## MOLECULAR DEVELOPMENTS

It is clear that cancer is an acquired genetic disease: multiple mutations, biochemical changes in DNA such as hypermethylation, or gene amplification lead to the formation of a clonal proliferation. This clone and sub-clones arising as a result of genetic instability inherent to many cancers may undergo further changes during chemotherapy, changing its phenotype as a response to drug exposure. Uveal melanoma differs substantially from cutaneous melanoma at the molecular level, and recent studies have implicated several pathways.

Molecular markers shed some light on the resistance of uveal melanoma. MDR1 expression is present in cell lines[25] and in primary tumors.[26,27] This drug efflux pump is thought to be an important mediator of resistance to some drugs, notably topoisomerase inhibitors and vinca alkaloids. There are a number of active inhibitors of PgP now in clinical development,[28] and these may prove useful in rendering uveal melanoma susceptible to anthracyclines in particular.[27] The only note of caution here relates to LRP, which is expressed by 57% of tumors[27] and is not affected by PgP inhibitors.

## CURRENT RECOMMENDATIONS

The decision of treat patients with uveal melanoma is currently based mainly on unpublished data. There are no phase II or III trial data and only series of patients are available on which to base recommendations. This situation is unsatisfactory and the first recommendation must be to enter patients into clinical trials whenever this is possible.

That said, there will be patients who request chemotherapy outside clinical trials and it is quite clear that most skin melanoma or DTIC based regimens are inadequate. Those who are willing to accept an experimental regimen are likely, on currently rather insecure evidence, to be best served by the following regimen:

Treosulfan 5 $g/m^2$ IV day1 + gemcitabine 1 $g/m^2$ d1, q 3 week.

Unfortunately treosulfan is not available in North America except on a named patient basis. Treosulfan is obtainable from Medac GmbH, Theaterstr. 2–6, 22880 Wedel Germany and gemcitabine from Eli Lilly (Eli Lilly and Company Lilly Corporate Center, Indianapolis, Indiana 46285 USA). The regimen is well tolerated with little neutropenia if used first-line. The dose of gemcitabine can be reduced to avoid excessive fatigue or neutropenia in later cycles. There is certainly an argument for treating patients until progression or until side effects become unacceptable.[31]

## FUTURE DEVELOPMENTS

Uveal melanoma exhibits tumor latency: it can be many years, even decades before metastases become apparent.[11,29] This tumor is therefore a prime candidate for successful adjuvant treatment, the aim of which is eradicate or differentiate the metastatic cells if possible, and to prolong the period of latency if not. Unfortunately the mechanisms of tumor latency are poorly understood, and to date there is no adjuvant therapy available for patients with large uveal melanomas in whom there is a 50% chance that they will die from metastatic disease, though the results of several studies are awaited.

For metastatic disease, the Treosulfan + Gemcitabine regimen may provide good palliation, and the results of clinical trials are awaited. Cure of metastatic disease is not currently possible, but we now know how important angiogenesis is to uveal melanoma and there is evidence that the tumor cells alter their antigenic status to evade immune surveillance.[14] Individualised multi-modality treatment using all three approaches to attack the tumor may become feasible within the next five years and could provide more success.

## SUMMARY

Uveal melanoma is a slow-growing tumor that shows even greater chemoresistance than cutaneous melanoma. It does not respond to the standard DTIC-based chemotherapy regimens, although intrahepatic arterial infusion of fotemustine has been shown to have some effect in a proportion of cases where this is feasible. Nevertheless, increasing knowledge of the molecular biology of this tumor and the ability to design new drugs or use existing ones more effectively provide some grounds for optimism. Uveal melanoma is susceptible to some alkylating agents and inhibitors of DNA repair such as gemcitabine can enhance their effect. The combination of treosulfan + gemcitabine is now undergoing clinical trials and early data is encouraging with at least one documented complete response in the first 14 patients treated. Uveal melanoma is a rare tumor and clinical trials are therefore both difficult to perform and to fund. Translational research can assist the process of new regimen and drug development. However, the multi-centre developmental approach, which has been so successful in improving treatment of the primary tumor, is essential to the development of chemotherapy for secondary disease.

## ACKNOWLEDGEMENTS

I am grateful to members of the Ocular Oncology Group of the EORTC, Dr Takami Sato, Mr John Hungerford, Dr R Simpson, Dr Shelley Boyd, Drs Carol and Jerry Shields, for useful discussion of many of the issues surrounding chemotherapy of this tumor. Some of the work described in this chapter was funded by a donation from Schering Plough Ltd.


## REFERENCES


1. Cree IA. Cell cycle and melanoma—two tumours from the same cell type. *J Pathol.* 2000;191:112–114.
2. Boaziz C, Mazeron JJ, Morere JF, Breau JL, Israël L. [Malignant melanoma of the uvea]. *Bull Cancer.* 1993;80:577–583.
3. Pyrhönen S. The treatment of metastatic uveal melanoma. *Eur J Cancer.* 1998;34 Suppl 3:S27–S30.
4. Neale MH, Myatt N, Cree IA, Kurbacher CM, Foss AJE, Hungerford JL, Plowman PN. Combination chemotherapy for choroidal melanoma: ex vivo sensitivity to treosulfan with gemcitabine or cytosine arabinoside. *Br J Cancer.* 1999;79:1487–1493.
5. Woll E, Bedikian A, Legha SS. Uveal melanoma: natural history and treatment options for metastatic disease. *Melanoma Res.* 1999;9:575–581.
6. Coppin C, Coldman AJ, Goldie JH. Modelling the effect of chemotherapy intensity. *Prog Clin Biol Res.* 1990;354B:103–116.
7. Kaufman D, Chabner BA. Clinical strategies for cancer treatment. In: Chabner BA, Longo DL, Philadelphia, Lipincott-Raven, eds *Cancer Chemotherapy and Biotherapy,* 2nd edn, 1996:pp. 1–16.
8. Bedikian AY, Legha SS, Mavligit G, Carrasco CH, Khorana S, Plager C, Papadopoulos N, Benjamin RS. Treatment of uveal melanoma metastatic to the liver: a review of the M.D. Anderson Cancer Center experience and prognostic factors. *Cancer.* 1995;76: 1665–1670.
9. Nathan FE, Berd D, Sato T, Shield JA, Shields CL, De Potter P, Mastrangelo MJ. BOLD + interferon in the treatment of metastatic uveal melanoma: first report of active systemic therapy. *J Exp Clin Cancer Res.* 1997;16:201–208.
10. Cantore M, Fiorentini G, Aitini E, Davitti B, Cavazzini G, Rabbi C, Lusenti A, Bertani M, Morandi C, Benedini V, et al. Intra-arterial hepatic carboplatin-based chemotherapy for ocular melanoma metastatic to the liver. Report of a phase II study. *Tumori.* 1994;80:37–39.
11. Aoyama T, Mastrangelo MJ, Berd D, Nathan FE, Shields CL, Shields JA, Rosato EL, Rosato FE, Sato T. Protracted survival after resection of metastatic uveal melanoma. *Cancer.* 2000;89:1561–1568.
12. Leyvraz S, Spataro V, Bauer J, Pampallona S, Salmon R, Dorval T, Meuli R, Gillet M, Lejeune F, Zografos L. Treatment of ocular melanoma metastatic to the liver by hepatic arterial chemotherapy. *J Clin Oncol.* 1997;15:2589–2595.
13. Salmon RJ, Levy C, Plancher C, Dorval T, Desjardins L, Leyvraz S, Pouillart P, Schlienger P, Servois V, Asselain B. Treatment of liver metastases from uveal melanoma by combined surgery-chemotherapy. *Eur J Surg Oncol.* 1998;24:127–130.
14. Zierhut M, Streilein JW, Schreiber H, Jager MJ, Ruiter D, Ksander BR. Immunology of ocular tumours. *Immunol Today.* 1999;20:482–485.

15. Terheyden P, Kämpgen E, Rünger TM, Bröcker EB, Becker JC. [Immunochemotherapy of metastatic uveal melanoma with interferon alfa-2b, interleukin-2 and fotemustine. Case reports and review of the literature]. *Hautarzt*. 1998;49:770–773.
16. Sanborn GE, Niederkorn JY, Gamel JW. Efficacy of dacarbazine (DTIC) in preventing metastases arising from intraocular melanomas in mice. *Graefes Arch Clin Exp Ophthalmol*. 1992;230:192–196.
17. Kirkwood JM, Strawderman MH, Ernstoff MS, Smith TJ, Borden EC, Blum RH. Interferon alfa-2b adjuvant therapy of high-risk resected cutaneous melanoma: the Eastern Cooperative Oncology Group Trial EST 1684. *J Clin Oncol*. 1996;14:7–17.
18. Kirkwood JM. Adjuvant interferon in the treatment of melanoma. *Br J Cancer*. 2000;82:1755–1756.
19. Dithmar S, Rusciano D, Lynn MJ, Lawson DH, Armstrong CA, Grossniklaus HE. Neoadjuvant interferon alfa-2b treatment in a murine model for metastatic ocular melanoma: a preliminary study. *Arch Ophthalmol*. 2000;118:1085–1089.
20. Myatt N, Cree IA, Kurbacher CM, Foss AJE, Hungerford JL, Plowman PN. The ex vivo chemosensitivity profile of choroidal melanoma. *Anti-Cancer Drugs*. 1997;8:756–762.
21. Hartley JA, O'Hare CC, Baumgart J. DNA alkylation and interstrand cross-linking by treosulfan. *Br J Cancer*. 1999;79:264–266.
22. Chana JS, Wilson GD, Cree IA, Alexander RA, Myatt N, Neale M, Foss AJ, Hungerford JL. c-myc, p53 and bcl-2 expression and clinical outcome in uveal melanoma. *Br J Ophthalmol*. 1999;83:110–114.
23. Lane DP. Cancer. p53, guardian of the genome. *Nature*. 1992;358:15–16.
24. Grecu OM, Kurbacher CM, Peter Mallmann P, Howard W, Bruckner HW, Cree IA. Treosulfan and gemcitabine in heavily pretreated patients with breast and ovarian cancer: Laboratory study and clinical pilot trial of the ISCO Clinical Study Group. ASCO 2001, Abstract 2500.
25. Van der Pol JP, Blom DJ, Flens MJ, Luyten GP, De Waard-Siebinga I, Koornneef L, Scheper RJ, Jager MJ. Multidrug resistance-related proteins in primary choroidal melanomas and *in vitro* cell lines. *Invest Ophthalmol Vis Sci*. 1997;38:2523–2530.
26. Dunne BM, McNamara M, Clynes M, Shering SG, Larkin AM, Moran E, Barnes C, Kennedy SM. MDR1 expression is associated with adverse survival in melanoma of the uveal tract. *Hum Pathol*. 1998;29:594–598.
27. Satherley K, De Souza L, Neale MH, Alexander RA, Myatt N, Foss AJE, Hungerford JL, Hickson ID, Cree IA. Relationship between expression of topoisomerase II isoforms and chemosensitivity in choroidal melanoma. *J Pathol*. 2000;192:174–181.
28. Mistry P, Stewart AJ, Dangerfield W, Okiji S, Liddle C, Bootle D, Plumb JA, Templeton D, Charlton P. *In vitro* and *in vivo* reversal of P-glycoprotein-mediated multidrug resistance by a novel potent modulator, XR9576. *Cancer Res*. 2001;61:749–758.
29. Sato T, Babazono A, Shields JA, Shields CL, De Potter P, Mastrangelo MJ. Time to systemic metastases in patients with posterior uveal melanoma. *Cancer Invest*. 1997;15:98–105.
30. Kivelä T, Suciu S, Hansson J, Kruit WH, Kuoristo MS, Kloke O, Gore M, Hahka-Kemppinen M, Parvinen LM, Kumpulainen E, Humblet Y, Pyrkonen S. Bleomycin, vincristine, lomustine and decarbazine (BOLD) in combination with recombinant interferon alpha-2b for metatstatic uveal melanoma. *Eur J Cancer*. 2003;39:1115–1120.
31. Pfohler C, Cree IA, Ugurel S, Kuwert C, Haass N, Neuber K, Hengge U, Corrie PG, Zutt M, Tilgen W, Reinhold U. Treosulfan and gemcitabine in metastatic uveal melanoma patients: results of a multicenter feasibility study. *Anticancer Drugs*. 2003;17:337–340.

# INDEX